C. Thomas Gualtieri

Neuropsychiatry and Behavioral Pharmacology

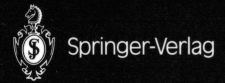
Springer-Verlag

Neuropsychiatry
and
Behavioral Pharmacology

C. Thomas Gualtieri

Neuropsychiatry and Behavioral Pharmacology

Springer-Verlag
New York Berlin Heidelberg London
Paris Tokyo Hong Kong Barcelona

C. Thomas Gualtieri
Medical Director
at North Carolina Neuropsychiatry
Chapel Hill, NC 27516
and
at Rebound, Inc.
Hendersonville, TN 37077, USA

Gualtieri, C. Thomas
    Neuropsychiatry and behavioral pharmacology / C. Thomas Gualtieri.
        p.   cm.
    Includes bibliographical references.
    ISBN 0-387-97314-1 (alk. paper)
    1. Neuropsychiatry. 2. Psychopharmacology. 3. Brain—Wounds and
injuries—Complications and sequelae. 4. Brain—Diseases—
Complications and sequelae. I. Title.
    [DNLM: 1. Behavior—drug effects. 2. Brain Injuries—
complications. 3. Brain Injuries—psychology. 4. Organic Mental
Disorders—psychology. 5. Psychotropic Drugs—therapeutic use.   WL
354 G912n]
    RC343.Q35   1990
    616.8—dc20
    DNLM/DLC   90-9805

Printed on acid-free paper.

Text prepared on Xerox Ventura Publisher using author-supplied WordPerfect disks.
Printed and bound by Edwards Brothers, Inc., Ann Arbor, MI.
Printed in the United States of America.

9 8 7 6 5 4 3 2 1

ISBN 0-387-97314-1 Springer-Verlag New York Berlin Heidelberg
ISBN 3-540-97314-1 Springer-Verlag Berlin Heidelberg New York

To Anthony Powell, his brothers and sisters, 1990.

Contents

Introduction

Neuropsychiatry is applied neuroscience. The brain, not behavior, is its point of departure. In this, it is distanced from the concerns of traditional psychiatry, which is built around the primacy of behavior. The neuropsychiatrist is concerned with brain, and behavior is derivative.

Neuropsychiatry has been defined, in the past, with a narrow view of its proper domain: disorders that are clearly related to a lesion, like stroke; or to a degenerative disease, like Alzheimer's or Parkinson's; or to a systemic condition that affects brain, like Lupus, for example. Our interest, and the concern of this book, is with a different class of neuropsychiatric conditions, and they are hardly ever dealt with in the literature. They are the behavioral syndromes that arise as a result of congenital or acquired brain injuries.

So, this is what we are about: the neuropsychiatric effect of traumatic brain injury, the behavioral syndromes associated with mental retardation, and a few of the development disabilities of childhood. The subject of our concern is, therefore, unique. It is different from the usual concern of neuropsychiatrists, behavioral neurologists, and neuropsychologists. There is also a different approach to the subject.

The concern is not with lesions but with prototypes, prototypes of mechanisms that govern brain, and disorders of brain. It is with the clinical meaning of specific neurophysiological processes, like kindling, reciprocal inhibition and activation, long-term potentiation, and time-dependent sensitization; of specific neuropharmacologic processes; of the laws that govern the expression of human traits, collectively known by the name of behavioral genetics; and of the interaction between these elements and the personal ecology of the neuropsychiatric patient. The paradigms and mechanisms around these elements are only imperfectly understood. But they are, quite clearly, the presage of how we shall, someday, come to understandthe brain and its disorders.

Since neuropsychiatry is an applied science, it borrows models and paradigms from all of the preclinical neurosciences. Since it is a clinical science, it employs these models in the service of diagnosis and treatment. The art is in deciding which model is most appropriate to a give clinical circumstance; there is always a wide range of theoretical and empirical structures to choose among. This book is about a few clinical conditions where cogent models are at hand, and seem to be germane to diagnosis and treatment.

The book is oriented towards developmental neuropsychiatry: that is, the congenital and the acquired disorders of relatively young people. It is concerned with relatively static conditions; the neurodegenerative disorders, that are usually the mainstay of neuropsychiatry, are not dealt with here.

Although the patients we shall discuss have static disorders, some degree of functional recovery may always be expected. Treatment is designed not to slow the course of degeneration, but to enhance natural, compensatory healing processes. The clinical problems we shall address are the severe behavior disorders of children, of retarded people, of people with epilepsy and of victims of traumatic brain injury. They are clinical problems for which effective treatment may be expected to bring years of useful and productive living.

Treatment is the focus. There is clearly a need for a manual of practical therapeutics in this field. There is no current book oriented to the requirements of professionals in developmental neuropsychiatry, that presents practical advice within a theoretical framework. Treatment is also a window. It is a way to test the validity of theoretical models in the real world. It is, after all, a very good way to discover whether a neuroscientific paradigm has practical value. It is also a good place to generate ideas. In our opinion, one should never consider a field of clinical endeavor to be entirely derivative of basic science. There is an integrity to the applied sciences that is co-equal with the "purity" of the basic sciences.

The treatment with which we are most directly concerned is psychopharmacology, but we prefer the term *behavioral pharmacology*. That is because the therapeutic approach to our unconventional patients is only rarely syndromic, in the sense of the Kraepelinian DSM-3. Approaches to treatment that are symptommatic, functional or hypothetical, as we shall describe, deserve to occupy an equal rank with approaches that are purely syndromic, in terms of psychiatric orthodoxy. Treatments are oriented to changes in specific target behaviors, to improvement in specific cognitive or regulatory functions, or to testing specific hypotheses concerning the etiopathogenesis of a disorder. It is the special method one uses to deal with psychiatric problems in patients who cannot be classified by psychiatrists. It is entirely empirical, and it places more reliance on treatment response over time than on front-end diagnostic exercises.

This book is about a diverse group of patients—patients with whom we are very familiar, clinical problems that have been the focus of our research and teaching. The organization of the book is not comprehensive, however, since it is built around a few conditions with which we have had a great deal of experience. The interests of our research group have always been around the psychopharmacology of unusual populations. Events have conspired to lend a certain unity to our work, a framework that is captured in the title of the book, if not in its subsequent construction.

But the problems are new and interesting, and since they have not been, as a rule, the subject of a great deal of research by other clinical scientists, it is possible that our opinion will appear novel. Not as signal insights or as fundamental truths, perhaps, but, at least, as new perspectives.

CHAPTER 1

The Neuropsychiatric Sequelae of Traumatic Brain Injury

The number of people with disabilities from serious brain injury is growing fast; they are one of the largest populations of neuropsychiatric patients in the United States. There are two reasons for this extraordinary phenomenon.

The first reason is that patients who have sustained severe head injuries, for example in motor vehicle accidents, are now more likely to survive, compared even to ten years ago. Med-Evac technology and intensive neurosurgical care are better. The statistic, often cited, is that 10 years ago 90% of closed head injury (CHI) victims died. Today, 90% survive. Each year there are about 500,000 new brain injury victims in the United States; each year, 75,000 or 100,000 victims of traumatic brain injury (TBI) are left with significant disability (Kraus, 1987).

As we have learned more about the neurobehavioral consequences of severe head injury, we have also learned to appreciate the milder but similar consequences of mild head injury. People who have survived severe head injuries are around to tell what it is like, and they tell us what the victims of mild head injuries have been saying all along. This is a difference in degree, obviously, but not a difference in kind. A few years ago, victims of "postconcussion syndrome" were thought to be hypochondriacs, or "compensation neurotics." Now we appreciate that their problems are real. The second reason why the number of TBI patients is increasing is that we have learned what the neuropsychiatric consequences of "mild" brain injury really are.

The problems of mild head injury victims have been documented in epidemiologic studies (Colohan et al., 1986; Rimel et al., 1981; Rutherford et al., 1979; Gronwall and Wrightson, 1974; Alves et al., 1986; Barth et al., 1983). Research with laboratory animals has confirmed that comparatively mild injuries can have lasting neuropathic sequelae, that neural tissue can be seriously damaged, or even destroyed, by comparatively mild trauma to the head (e.g., Jane et al., 1982).

Until recently, the only professionals with any interest in TBI were the clinical neuropsychologists, and until recently they were a small, unimportant group of specialists within psychology. Their clinical work was largely confined to the Veterans Hospitals, where they worked with the victims of battlefield injuries. There would be a spate of new head injury research after every war; for example, the work of Kurt Goldstein after World War I, and that of Alexander Luria and William Lishman after World War II.

Although the research of Goldstein, Luria, and Lishman is the foundation of much of what we do today, it is important to remember that the nature of the current problem is very different from what they were contending with. Wartime injuries tend to be penetrating injuries, from high-speed missiles that penetrate a circumscribed area of brain, particularly the frontal lobes. Such injuries cause focal cortical damage. In contrast, the CHI that are most common today, from motor vehicle accidents, falls, and sporting contests, are "acceleration-deceleration" injuries, not penetrating injuries. The pathophysiology and the neurobehavioral sequelae of CHI are very different from those caused by penetrating injuries.

In a CHI, damage is done not only to the cortical surface of brain, but also to subcortical and axial (brainstem) structures. The diffuse degeneration of cerebral white matter is axonal damage that is caused by mechanical forces shearing the fiber at the moment of impact ("diffuse axonal injury," "diffuse white matter shearing injury," "diffuse damage of the immediate impact type"). It has been described in human beings with posttraumatic dementia; similar clinical and structural changes have been produced experimentally in subhuman primates using nonimpact-controlled angular acceleration of the head, in the absence of increased intracranial pressure or hypoxemia (Blumbergs et al., 1989).

Hence, there are two kinds of damage: the specific cortical lesions, which may be focal, and which therefore resemble the circumscribed lesions of penetrating injury victims; and axial or brainstem lesions, which are diffuse and have more diffuse behavioral sequelae.

The victim of a circumscribed cortical lesion may be hemiplegic, or aphasic, or prosopagnosic, or cortically blind; the victim of a CHI may have these problems plus deficits in arousal, attention, self-regulation, memory, and initiation. The latter derive from diffuse injury to subcortical structures. This new class of patients, therefore, is more complex; their problems are not given to the simple, cortical-syndromic classifications that are appropriate for patients with focal cortical lesions.

The identification of cortical lesions has been the foundation of neuropsychology, and the neuropsychological test batteries developed during the 1950s by Luria, Halsted, and Reitan are more appropriate to an older class of patients. Such batteries of tests are still useful, but they are not always sufficient to appraise and measure the disabilities of CHI victims. The complexity of the CHI victim usually requires the evaluation techniques of various disciplines.

The challenge of CHI—its complexity as well as the magnitude of the afflicted population—has attracted the attention of physiatrists, neurologists, psychiatrists, and of therapists in speech and physical and occupational therapy. The rehabilitation centers that have sprung up tend to use an interdisciplinary team model; "case managers" are employed to coordinate the different therapies and the patient's reintegration into his family and the wider community. The model is largely borrowed from developmental disabilities, and there is more in head injury treatment today that is taken from the field of mental retardation than there is from Goldstein and Luria. Head injury rehabilitation is a practical, outcome-oriented field that is not tied to theoretical constructs as neuropsychology has been, or to diagnostic categories, as psychiatry still is, or to the simple brain maps that neurologists still tend to prefer.

One enduring problem for the head injury victim is that he usually receives neuropsychiatric consultation from psychiatrists and neurologists who have no training or experience in the field of head injury, and who tend to interpret the patient's difficulties in terms of conventional psychiatric diagnoses and treatments, or in terms of the conventional neurological examination. As a result, the neuropsychiatric diagnosis and treatment of head injury victims is not always what it ought to be. Far too often, the victim of a mild head injury is treated as if he (or she) were only imagining that something is wrong. If the computer-assisted tomography (CAT) scan is normal, or the EEG, and if there are no focal neurological findings on examination, the patient is told that nothing is wrong with his brain, and the problem must be therefore be "functional," or psychiatric, or that it is "posttraumatic stress." And when such patients go to a psychiatrist, they may be treated with psychotherapy that is irrelevant to the nature of their real deficit or, worse, with drugs that can aggravate it.

On the other hand, we know a great deal more about head injury than such practice would have you believe. The information is scattered, but it is available to anyone who wishes to make a special study. That is why experience with head injury patients is so important. It is not one's professional credentials that speak to expertise in the area of diagnosis and treatment—it is the special study one has made of traumatic brain injury. The most important instrument for the diagnosis of neurobehavioral sequelae of TBI is a physician or a psychologist with experience in TBI. The most effective therapeutic agent is a professional who understands the nature of the problem.

The Neurobehavioral Sequelae of Traumatic Brain Injury

The neurobehavioral sequelae of TBI are effects on complex arrays of behavior, cognition, and emotional expression. They include psychiatric disorders such as depression, psychosis, disinhibition, abulia, dysregulation, hypochondriasis, insomnia, bulimia, and pathological drinking. They also include the traditional neurological sequelae—epilepsy, low arousal, hypersomnolence, posttraumatic headache, and migraine. They include, too, many of the higher cognitive functions that are usually the precinct of the neuropsychologist, like deficits in memory, attention, and executive function.

The neurobehavioral sequelae of TBI necessarily include the interpersonal difficulties that compound the plight of the head injury victim and his family: the interpersonal and professional problems that occur at work; the practical problems in finding appropriate rehabilitation services and in trying to convince carriers to pay for services that are necessary; and, finally, the stresses that arise as patients and families try to negotiate the adversarial climate that all too often arises after brain injury.

TBI usually have well-defined and obvious effects on the motor system, effects on muscle strength, tone, and coordination; well-defined and obvious effects on the understanding and production of speech and language; and well-defined neuropsychological effects that stem from focal lesions to cortex or to subcortical structures, such as hippocampus, striatum, and thalamus, whose functions are understood. There are autonomic and appetitive effects from injury to hypothalamus that are understandable in terms of the established physiology of that organ. There is the global deterioration in cognitive ability that is the consequence of diffuse cortical injury, and the global depression of arousal that is the consequence of diffuse brain injury, especially to the brain stem.

The term "neurobehavioral sequelae," however, also refers to higher order difficulties in behavior and emotional expression that are less obvious and less well defined. Such difficulties are not always interpretable in terms of a specific lesion or a clearly defined brain map. They may not be apparent on neuropsychological tests, and their origins may not be apparent on conventional neurodiagnostic measures like the EEG, the CAT scan, or nuclear magnetic resonance imaging (NMRI). They may resemble the so-called functional psychiatric disorders, although they rarely present as typical psychiatric disorders, and it is a mistake to treat them as if they were. They may arise in the absence of a definable anatomic lesion; they are sometimes the result of subtle biochemical changes in the physiology of neurotransmitters and neuromodulators. They may begin as relatively minor disabilities, on a neuropathic basis, but they may be aggravated and become quite dangerous by virtue of interpersonal stress and professional indifference.

Although there are many TBI patients whose only complaints are "neurobehavioral," most TBI patients present with a mixed clinical picture, with behavioral and emotional changes superimposed upon the more easily defined motoric, linguistic, autonomic, or cognitive deficits. It is really quite impossible to draw meaningful distinctions between the neurological, psychiatric, neuropsychological, and rehabilitative aspects of head injury recovery. The proper understanding of the TBI patient requires an understanding of how different areas of deficit interact and compound each other.

The Postconcussion Syndrome

The postconcussion syndrome (PCS) is a condition observed in patients who have had comparatively mild head injuries, with only transient periods of confusion or unconsciousness, and no anatomic evidence of damage to brain. The classic symptoms of PCS are headache, dizziness, alcohol intolerance, irritability, and difficulty concentrating (Friedmann, 1892). Because the initial trauma is less dramatic, the connection between neurobehavioral sequelae and their traumatic origin is often lost. The patient's difficulties may be attributed to "compensation neurosis" or to other psychological factors. In such circumstances, the inexperienced physician may inadvertently place himself or herself in an adversarial position toward the patient: trying to convince the patient that nothing is wrong, when the patient himself knows better.

(It is interesting to remark that our current notion of "compensation neurosis" was the creation of a nineteenth-century Prussian physician who noted an increase in work-related complaints of injury after railway workers won the right to compensation [Rigler, 1879]. On the other hand, why would the workers complain if there *were* no opportunity for compensation? Nineteenth-century Prussia may not be the most appropriate model for labor relations and occupational medicine.)

The most common symptoms of PCS are chronic and low grade, and they include fatigue or anergia, insomnia, depression, attention and memory deficits, headache, unusual sensations, paraesthesias or neuralgias, and a vague sense that something is wrong. That sense is not so vague, however, that it can be dispelled by a physician who "assures" the patient that nothing is wrong and everything is going to be all right.

The patient may have symptoms of anxiety that can overlap with or be mistaken for posttraumatic stress disorder (PTSD). He may have flashbacks to the accident, preoccupation with it, phobic avoidance, and terrifying dreams. These are typical elements of PTSD; so are attentional lapses and dissociative reactions. It may not always be a simple matter, therefore, to distinguish between the functional reaction to an accident (PTSD) and the emotional and attentional symptoms that are part of the pathophysiology of the PCS.

To make matters even more complicated, the patient may develop what physicians call somatic preoccupations, or even frank hypochondriasis. These may be aggravated by the simultaneous occurrence of whiplash or of lower back injury, the persistence of posttraumatic headache, and, finally, the presence of vague sensations, migratory dysesthesias, and paraesthesias. It is an irony of PCS, where so many patients are mistaken for hypochondriacs, that somatic preoccupation and hypochondriasis may actually be manifestations of brain injury.

The symptoms of PCS are those that we usually associate with psychological or interpersonal disturbance: mild depression, lack of motivation, anxiety, insomnia, sexual dysfunction, loss of ambition, headache, dizziness, weakness, easy fatigue, absentmindedness, a quick temper, easy frustration, impatience, and difficulty getting along with people. There may be unusual sensory phenomena, like anosmia (loss of smell), dysgeusia (bad taste), hypacusis (sensitivity to certain noises), photosensitivity (sensitivity to bright light), or paresthesias (tingling sensations). The cognitive effects include inattention, lack of concentration, inability to read, memory lapses, and disorganization. These are the sequelae of traumatic injury to axial and to brainstem structures.

In the first year after brain injury, the patient may be given to "spells." These are sudden events, sensations, or focal weakness or changes in mental state that last for only a few moments, and that resemble, for all the world, mild focal seizures. PCS patients should be permitted at least a few such spells, especially if the EEG is normal. They tend to remit, as time goes by. If the patient really does have posttraumatic epilepsy, the diagnostic picture will be clear enough in time.

The PCS patient may present with anguish. Although the injury was comparatively mild, the subsequent experience is insufferable. Insomnia, headache, inability to concentrate, restlessness, irritability, sexual dysfunction, dizziness, and vague and unusual sensations like hypacusis or photosensitivity are aggravated by the insensitivity and ignorance of physicians. The inevitable consequence is confusion and dismay about the problem, its nature, and its origins, and this of course only compounds the desperation, insomnia, and somatic preoccupations of the patient. The patient may become mistrustful or hostile or even paranoid, especially if the insurance company is less than forthcoming or if the forensic proceedings around the accident are bitterly adversarial.

PCS patients may also have elements of frontal lobe or temporal lobe syndromes, but they tend to be less disabling than those seen in the more severely injured patients described further on.

There are two essential treatments for the PCS: one is psychological, and one is pharmacological. The most important element of psychological treatment is counseling about the normal course of recovery. Patients need to be educated about the problems they are having, and how they stem, naturally and physiologically, from the injury they have sustained. They have to know what to expect, and the meaning of what they are experiencing. They need guidance in how to cope with their physical and their psychological symptoms, with their neuropsychological deficits, and with their altered temperament, level of energy, and sexuality. They need counseling about their jobs, family relations, and legal proceedings. They need an advocate, a guiding hand, a source of reassurance. Their somatic complaints require respectful attention. Referral to other specialists and recourse to neurodiagnostics should be intelligent and prudent, not a crude, shotgun approach. Patients deserve to be kept out of the hands of quacks. They also need to be protected from physicians whose point of view is so thoroughly modern that they believe no problem exists unless it is demonstrated on a scan of some sort.

When a patient is told that he has a brain injury, there is the inevitable conclusion that the situation is irremediable. The patient should be told, and told with conviction, that nothing can be further from the truth. That the brain is more capable of healing than any other organ system. That healing is a natural process, that it is fostered by a personal attitude of hope, and by the support of one's family. That it can be retarded by impatience, frustration, rage, or self-pity. That a deficit in one area is no less than the opportunity to develop new strengths in another.

Pharmacological treatments are best let alone, because drugs have an uncertain effect in head injury patients, and their side effects may actually retard the course of recovery. But there are occasions when prudent pharmacotherapy can accomplish a great deal.

For problems with sleep, one prefers the serotonergic drugs, like L-tryptophan or trazodone. Amitryptiline is not a good choice because it is so anticholinergic (Mattila et al., 1978); fluoxetine may be a good choice, but it is a new drug, and not proven in this patient group (Cassidy, 1989). If the severe insomnia of PCS can be controlled, much of the daytime anguish and irritability may disappear as well.

For problems with low energy, mild depression, abulia, inattention, and poor memory, one prefers the dopamine agonists such as methylphenidate. For emotional incontinence and irritability to the point of rage, one may elect a trial of carbamazepine or of valproate. Alternatively, one may try one of the serotonergic antidepressants. For problems of anxiety, restlessness, akathisia, somatic preoccupation and mild depression, the drug of choice is buspirone.

Personality Changes

Family members may report that the TBI patient is a "different person." The most dramatic changes are those that characterize the frontal and the temporal lobe patients, whom we shall describe further on. It is important to remember, however, that there is no single personality type that characterizes the brain injury patient. The changes that may occur in temperament, motivation, cognitive style, level of energy, and response to stress or to frustration are not consistent or even predictable.

One can imagine the ordeal of having to adjust to a spouse, a parent, or a child who has experienced a dramatic personality change. This is the bitterest pill the family of a head injury victim has to take. Not only is he handicapped; he (the victim) is *another person* who is handicapped.

On the other hand, the more common consequence of mild TBI, especially of closed head injuries, is the exaggeration of preexisting personality traits. This is probably why some clinicians, and many family members, are reluctant to attribute psychological difficulties following TBI to the injury. A person who was impulsive and given to poor judgment before an injury will be even more so after CHI. Someone who was temperamental, or emotionally unstable, or given to temper will be even less stable after a CHI. People who were overly reflective or philosophical may turn to obsessions or cosmic ruminations, people who are sticky to begin with will get turgid, people who are eccentric or willful or stubborn will only be more so. So, when one alludes to such changes as the effects of TBI, someone may counter with the argument that the patient was "always like that." Well, he probably was. Now he still is, only more so.

Head injury may aggravate negative personality characteristics, or it may change a minor personal weakness into a major area of difficulty. Only on the rarest occasions will a head injury actually diminish a preexisting negative trait—rarely, but it may happen. One of our patients was impulsive, rowdy, and a philanderer before his injury. After a trauma affecting the convexity of the frontal lobes, he became a docile homebody who had no initiative to go out, and preferred nothing more than to stay home and take care of the baby. Actually, he had an abulic syndrome, and a rocking stereotypy, but his wife liked it just fine.

Brain injury may also exaggerate the negative traits one associates with the different life stages. This creates real problems in diagnosis, because we all know that personality changes can occur simply by virtue of passage through a life stage like adolescence or middle age. It is not easy to decide that an adolescent who loses interest in school, who hangs out with bad kids, and who is argumentative at home is suffering the sequelae of a head injury. Middle-aged people with chronic fatigue or sexual disinterest or somatic preoccupations or hypochondriasis are not unfamiliar types, but these problems can be the result of head injury. School kids may begin to look like hyperactive or learning-disabled school kids. In old people, the effects of TBI may simply look like the onset of dementia. (In old people, TBI can also unmask an underlying but undetected dementia, or it may accelerate the development of dementia).

There is an explanation for this phenomenon, because CHI tend to damage frontal lobe and axial structures that are responsible for regulating behavior and emotional response. Everyone has some negative personality trait to hold in check. When one loses the brain structures that delimit the extremes of behavior, when one loses the energy to hold them in check, the result is not new pathology, but an old attribute that is newly pathological. It is similar to what Hughlings Jackson referred to as a "release" phenomenon, when negative attributes are released, so to speak, from cortical control. Jackson used the term to refer to specific neurological functions, but it is also a valid principle for the development of neurobehavioral problems after TBI.

The exaggeration of negative attributes is an aspect of TBI that may have larger consequences. We know, for example, that systems that are allowed to fluctuate between exaggerated extremes may destabilize, and we know that quantitative changes may evolve into qualitative changes. A canoe that is constantly rocking may finally capsize. An electron that is continually activated will ultimately jump to a new orbit. A brain system that is kindled long enough will ultimately seize. So, the psychological consequences of dysregulation may ultimately go beyond the bounds of mere exaggeration of negative traits. If the dysregulation is allowed to continue unchecked, the consequences may grow more serious.

Consider the head injury patient who becomes negativistic, irritable and prone to temper outbursts and assaultive behavior. He loses his job and his family as a consequence. As his life is degraded even further by loneliness and alienation, he may become depressed and suicidal. A head injury patient who is impulsive, with poor judgment and no concept of safety is a good candidate for a second head injury—the more so if he has derangements in time perception or space perception, and even more so if he drinks or consumes illicit drugs. A head injury patient who loses his personal ambitions and values may drop out of school, or out of the competitive job market, in spite of efforts to remediate or to structure his career. As he sinks lower down the socioeconomic ladder, he will be prone to all the problems that come from poverty and personal neglect.

Thus, it is important to address the early psychological sequelae of CHI, to restore the modulatory functions of axial brain structures pharmacologically, or to compensate for excesses of behavior by giving the patient a controlled and structured environment. If one does not take such precautions, the outcome will likely be further destabilization and evolution to psychopathology.

This is not the inevitable consequence of TBI by any means, and a much larger number of TBI cases, especially mild cases, have a much more sanguine outcome. The disabilities that follow mild TBI may last for weeks or months or even years, but there is always the likelihood of improvement, or even complete resolution of symptoms. Improvement may be spontaneous, or it may require a course of treatment. With the proper treatment, most patients do very well.

Posttraumatic Headache

Headache is the most common problem following mild head injury; it is central to the diagnosis of PCS, and it is also a common problem in patients who have had severe TBI. It is one of the most persistent symptoms following head injury, and it is one of the most difficult symptoms to treat. It may be a nonspecific diagnosis, just plain headache, or it may be a specific headache syndrome, like migraine, basilar migraine, or cluster headache. Posttraumatic headaches may be constant, intermittent, or paroxysmal. They may be spontaneous, or they may be precipitated by stress, exertion, or fatigue. They usually diminish in severity as time goes by, but they may not. What usually happens is that patients learn to live with headache; they accept the small degree of relief that may come with drugs like ibuprofen, and they carry on.

The typical posttraumatic headache is described as a dull ache, or less frequently as a throbbing sensation. It may be focal or diffuse, unilateral or bilateral. It is not typically paroxysmal, although it is not uncommon to meet a patient who complains of a constant, dull headache upon which are superimposed intermittent, paroxysmal attacks. The cephalgias may be described as stabbing, bursting, hammering, or there may simply be a sense of fullness, dizziness, or fuzziness in the head (Appenzeller, 1987). There may be elements suggestive of migraine, such as nausea and vomiting, or the need to rest quietly in a dark room, but it is said that "true" migraine is uncommon following TBI (Appenzeller, 1987). (Posttraumatic migraine may be more commonly encountered in children than it is in adults [Heyck, 1975]).

We do not really understand the mechanism of posttraumatic headaches. They may be related to scars or small neuromas in the scalp, or to meningeal adhesions, scars, or cysts, or to neurochemical events in the innervation of the cerebral vasculature. They may be related to whiplash cervical injuries, headaches of musculoskeletal or tension type with neck pain and vertigo. But it is the rare patient with posttraumatic headache for whom an etiopathogenetic diagnosis may be made.

Posttraumatic headaches do not necessarily arise immediately after the injury. In fact, generalized headache usually makes its onset with some delay after the injury (Appenzeller, 1987).

Basilar migraine (basilar artery migraine, BAM) is a commonly misdiagnosed disorder, an intense vascular headache anteceded by aura, or prodromata to indicate dysfunction in the brain stem, cerebellum and occipital cortex (Bickerstaff, 1962), the area supplied by the basilar artery and its branches. The accompanying symptoms may include visual impairment (transient amaurosis, reduction in vision, diplopia), vertigo, ataxia, paraesthesias, weakness, and dysarthria (Sturzenegger and Meienberg, 1985). There may be transient loss of consciousness, and EEG abnormalities are not uncommon. The latter may be persistent, even between headaches; therefore, BAM may be misdiagnosed as epilepsy (Jacome, 1987). The fact that both BAM and complex partial epilepsy may respond to the anticonvulsant carbamazepine (CBZ) may complicate the diagnosis, although it is customary to treat BAM with a beta blocker rather than CBZ.

BAM commonly occurs in adolescent girls (Sturzenegger & Meienberg, 1985), and it may arise after uncomplicated whiplash injuries (Jacome, 1986).

Treatment of posttraumatic headache is the treatment of headache. It is appropriate to consider the same range of treatments that are effective (or marginally effective, if you will) for patients whose headache is not traumatic in origin. Sedating drugs, depressants, and opiates should be avoided. Drugs with negative cognitive effects, like amitryptiline, and drugs that may cause depression, like the beta blockers, should be used very carefully, or not at all. If the headache is not relieved by ibuprofen or similar nonsteroidal antiinflammatory drugs (NSAIDs), or by acetaminophen, one may consider a calcium channel blocker like verapamil. Cranial electrostimulation is a nonpharmacological approach that is occasionally helpful (see Chapter 5, this volume).

Although the pharmacological and the behavioral treatment of posttraumatic headache are less than ideal, it is reasonable to be assuring to the patient. Although posttraumatic headache may be persistent, it usually subsides with the passage of time, and the patient may be thus reassured. Often, one will observe alleviation of posttraumatic headache when other neurobehavioral sequelae of CHI, like anxiety, fatigue, depression, and social isolation are successfully handled.

The Frontal Lobe Syndromes

The frontal and the temporal lobes are vulnerable to TBI by virtue of their anterior position and exposure to the cribiform plate, a bony structure against which brain tissue may be shorn during a traumatic episode.

The frontal lobes are a vast expanse of brain tissue that subsume a broad range of functions: motor control (the motor strip and the premotor strip), expressive language (Broca's area), regulation (the orbitofrontal surface) and executive behavior (the convexity). So it is presumptuous to talk about a unitary "frontal lobe syndrome." Nevertheless, one does. To be more precise, neuropsychiatrists refer to two frontal lobe syndromes, one arising from lesions to the convexity, and the other arising from lesions to the orbital surface of the frontal lobe. The model for the first is lobotomy; the second, sociopathy.

The extensive convex surfaces of the frontal lobes were, at one time, a mystery to neurologists and to psychologists; they were felt to be gratuitous organs that could be dispensed with (at the whim of the Veterans Administration, no less). It was this belief that led to the psychosurgical procedure known as "prefrontal lobotomy," and this bizarre medical experiment was finally terminated when it was discovered that not only did the frontal convexity indeed have a role to play in the genesis of behavior, but that the role was central. This expanse of brain tissue seems to subsume the highest order of personality—initiative, will, drive, volition. Patients with lesions in this area tend to have little spontaneous behavior or initiative; they do not initiate interaction, although they are perfectly pleasant if someone else does. If you watch them sitting in the waiting room, you may be struck by their quiet, passive demeanor.

The companion symptoms are really quite extraordinary: the patients may deny their disability (anosagnosia); they may be compliant to a fault, or, alternatively, as stubborn as mules. They are not flexible as people, or as thinkers, and they prefer to deal with simple, agreeable issues. They have difficulty when the rules are changed, when there is the requirement for readjustment to a new set of demands. They tend to get stuck in a rut; a personal rut, or a cognitive rut. In extreme cases this may be so dramatic that they perseverate or engage in stereotyped behavior. They tend to be socially inappropriate, but in an innocent kind of way, like a bumpkin. They are not very good in complex or ambiguous situations, they prefer structure and predictability in their environment, they are not good planners, and they have real difficulty with complex tasks. They are easily distracted, they can be absentminded, they can stare off for long periods without a thought in their head.

One of our patients had bifrontal lesions of the convexity. He took the earnings from his settlement and built a small grocery at a country crossroads. There was no business. He stayed there. The milk in his cooler was out of date, the cans of food were old and dusty, and the few customers who lived nearby—hardly anyone lived nearby—stopped coming. He didn't leave the place until his money ran out and he had used up all his credit. Then he moved back to town. The store was a total write-off.

Another patient had bilateral lesions in the frontal pole when he got tossed around in a cement mixer. He was prone to "spells"; he would sit and stare into space, immobile, attentive to nothing in his environment and responsive to no stimulus save physical touch. He was not in nonconvulsive status; he had severe attentional lapses, which responded favorably to dopamine agonist treatment.

Some frontal patients are said to be "abulic," from the Greek words "without appetite." Such patients are not especially motivated to do anything, simply for lack of will, and they spend their days quietly, doing as little as they possibly can. It is not that they are uninterested, or disinterested; it is the capacity for interest at all that is missing. They may also have parkinsonian signs: masklike faces, cogwheeling, positive glabellar tap. That, and the reliability of their response to the antiparkinsonian drug amantadine (Gualtieri et al., 1989) reaffirms one's belief in the axis of corpus striatum-frontal convexity.

One of our patients, with bilateral lesions of the convexity, was really quite polite and responsive during the examination, and during the interview would respond appropriately, although passively and without much expressiveness. When she was sitting in the waiting room, though, she would just sit, immobile, and stare into space. She would never read or fidget or talk to the receptionist. She lived by herself. At home, she would just sit, sometimes watching TV, sometimes not. She hardly had the initiative to feed herself. She made instant coffee, but that was about all. As time went on, she just seemed to waste away.

The second frontal lobe syndrome is the result of injury to the inferior-medial (orbitofrontal) surface of the frontal lobe. The primary symptoms are disinhibition and dysregulation. The psychiatric model is the sociopathic personality.

The disinhibited patient may be an innocent, not unlike a hyperactive kid, with witzelsucht, the compulsion to joke, excitability, short attention span, impulsiveness, restlessness, and emotional lability. He may be sexually disinhibited, with either promiscuous behavior or lewd talking or both. Impulsive behavior and extremes of temperament may take a destructive turn, with substance abuse, reckless driving, or scrapes with the law. As a rule, such patients are not so violent as patients with temporal lobe injuries, but they are extremely susceptible to the effects of alcohol and other downers (like the benzodiazepines); they may be prone to what is called pathological intoxication, and under such circumstances they can be assaultive. The orbitofrontal patient has lost his capacity for self-control, or more commonly, is capable of losing it very easily in unstructured settings or when he is stressed or under the influence of an intoxicant.

The author had the privilege, during his youth, to serve as a general physician in a couple of rough, rural Southern communities. There was a Saturday-night denizen of the Emergency Room; the young man whose idea of a good time was a few beers at a roadhouse and then a good fight. It was not until many years later that the behavioral neurology of rednecks became apparent. Combine the impulsive, aggressive behavior of the frontal lobe patient with an elevated pain threshold (also the consequence of an orbitofrontal lesion), the disinhibiting influence of even a small amount of alcohol, and the inability to learn enduring lessons from unpleasant experience, and you have the familiars of a country ER.

On the other hand, under structured circumstances, the orbitofrontal patient does quite well. When scrutiny is intense, or when the situation is structured or novel, he may be polite and compliant—"Chesterfieldian" in his manners and consideration for others. Let the structure lapse, though, and Lord Chesterfield will retire, and the devil will rise again.

The orbitofrontal surface is the rostral projection of the ascending reticular activating system, a latticework of neurons that arise in the brain stem and project monoaminergic neurotransmitters to the diencephalon, limbic cortex, and frontal lobe. The function of this network is regulation: at the brainstem level, regulation of arousal; in the diencephalon, of appetitive behaviors; and in the limbic and frontal cortex, of higher level behavior and emotional expression. The frontal patient with a lesion in this region has a limited capacity to regulate and control behavior in response to feedback from the environment; he has difficulty conforming to societal norms or to social cues, he cannot control overreactions to novel or to stressful circumstances, and is likelier to respond to stress by acting out some untoward motor program than by internalizing his reactions and getting anxious or worried or insecure. In fact, he has a limited capacity for experiencing such emotions at all. Psychosurgical procedures are still done to ablate this pathway, in fact, in patients with severe, disabling anxiety who do not respond to conventional treatments. Surgical procedures in this area may also be brought to bear to control certain intense pain syndromes.

Psychiatrists occasionally talk about "pure" sociopaths, people who are capable of the most egregious transgressions but who are wholly incapable of experiencing remorse for their actions, even when confronted. Some of these characters are identical to frontal lobe patients with lesions of the orbital surface. It is a kind of disconnection syndrome. Impulsive behavior is released from inhibitory cortical regulation, and the capacity to integrate behavior in line with established social norms has been removed. There is no capacity to self-reflect, to view oneself in an alternative framework, for example, as others do. There is limited capacity for self-correction, most notably when the consequences of misbehavior are painful. There is a tendency to repeat the transgression whenever the opportunity presents itself. And there is agnosia for the deficit.

These two frontal lobe syndromes, the disinhibited orbitofrontal and the abulic convexity lesion, comprise the largest group of CHI patients with defined cortical syndromes. Both syndromes are characterized by poor judgment, inability to plan, unrealistic ambitions, and limited insight into the nature of their deficits.

Dopamine agonist drugs are sometimes helpful in patients with the orbitofrontal syndrome, especially the psychostimulants; amantadine may also be helpful. The therapeutic model is not the parkinsonian patient, it is the hyperactive child (see Chapter 14, this volume).

The Temporal Lobe Syndromes

The temporal lobe syndromes are even more variable than the frontal lobe syndromes. Different regions of the temporal lobes are responsible for receptive language, high-level integration of sensory input, memory, and emotional expression. The temporal lobe syndromes, then, as they occur following TBI, may refer to disorders of receptive language (that are dealt with extensively in the aphasia literature); disorders of sensation or of sensory integration, some of the amnestic syndromes, and a wide range of "emotional" or "functional" psychiatric disorders.

The most severe impairments of memory are associated with bilateral temporal lobe injury to the anterior horn of the hippocampus. What is called a "dense" anterograde amnesia, the failure to encode new memories, is the result of bilateral temporal lobectomy, including the hippocampus. The most dramatic cases were surgical patients, like the famous case from Connecticut, H.M. Usually, the amnesia associated with severe TBI is "patchy" rather than dense, that is, some memories are successfully encoded while others are not. In TBI, temporal lobe amnesia is usually complicated by a component of inattention, which is frontal or axial, as the case may be, rather than temporal. When dopamine agonist therapy is directed against a memory deficit, it should, optimally, effect the consolidation of long-term memory as well as affecting attentional processes that allow the encoding process to begin (Evans, Gualtieri & Patterson, 1987).

When the early neurosurgeons performed their operations for severe temporal lobe epileptics, they sometimes went as far back as the anterior hippocampus; had they gone further, they would have reproduced the experiment of Kluver and Bucy (1937). Monkeys with bilateral temporal lobectomies involving the amygdala appear to be incapable of mounting an emotional response to any circumstance, and their day is passed in bland endeavors, especially stereotyped activity like mouthing and self-stimulation. Kluver-Bucy symptoms (KBS) are occasionally seen in severe TBI patients during the coma-recovery period. Partial KBS, a grossly incapacitating condition with symptoms that resemble autism, may persist in some patients (see Chapter 10, this volume).

Rather than emotional indifference, or "psychic blandness," the temporal lobe patient is usually given to excess of emotional expression: uncontrollable rage attacks, for example, sudden unprovoked episodes of crying or laughing (emotional incontinence), or sudden changes in mood (emotional lability). The psychiatrists sometimes use the term intermittent explosive disorder, and the neurologists are given to "episodic dyscontrol." After aphasia, it is probably the most common behavioral manifestation of temporal lobe injury, and it is certainly the most dramatic, with significant forensic as well as interpersonal aspects. The animal model for "episodic dyscontrol" is a lesion in the septum or the amygdala, two deep temporal nuclei that are usually included as part of the "limbic" brain.

The specific treatment for episodic dyscontrol is carbamazepine, and alternatives are valproic acid, lithium, beta blockers, and, for emotional incontinence, amitryptiline or fluoxetine. It is not a difficult disorder to treat.

Frontal lobe patients with lesions of the orbital surface may also be given to episodes of violent rage, and the distinction between frontal and temporal lobe patients may not always be made on the basis of the topography of the behavior. Rather, the correlates of the behavior, and the results of neurodiagnostic and neuropsychological testing, are required to localize the source. On the other hand, CHI are usually associated with damage to several areas of brain.

Major affective disorders frequently arise in patients with temporal lobe injury, although there is disagreement whether they are more likely to occur in right (Flor-Henry, 1979) or left (Robinson et al., 1983a) temporal lobe lesions. In fact, it is likely that the anterior region of both hemispheres plays a role in the expression of affective symptoms (Ross and Rush, 1981). The affective disorders that occur after TBI may be either unipolar or bipolar, and they are virtually indistinguishable from the "functional" affective disorders psychiatrists contend with all the time. In fact, affective disorders arising from temporal lobe lesions are probably the only neurobehavioral consequence of TBI that is indistinguishable from the conventional psychiatric condition.

The treatment of affective disorders following TBI is usually the same that one would prescribe for a conventional psychiatric disorder, and the antidepressants and lithium are usually effective. One may be more inclined to consider a dopamine agonist to treat an anergic depression; however, one must remember that virtually all the tricyclics may have negative effects on motor performance (Gualtieri, 1988) and that some of the anticholinergic antidepressants may impair memory performance (Mattila et al., 1978). Bupropion would be an ideal antidepressant for TBI patients if it were not for its proclivity to lower the seizure threshold; that side effect, however, may well be overstated, because most of the antidepressants have the same effect. Trazodone and fluoxetine are, as a consequence, enjoying some currency among psychiatrists who treat TBI patients.

Lithium, also, is a drug that may impair motor performance, and it is said to slow the speed of mental processing (Judd et al., 1977; Kusumo and Vaugn, 1977).

Carbamazpine and valproate may be better choices for the TBI patient who is bipolar.

Flor-Henry (1979) is also identified with the attribution of schizophreniform psychosis to left temporal lobe injury. This observation, however, has been superseded by subsequent descriptions of the psychosis of temporal lobe epilepsy; although the association between a left temporal focus and schizophrenia may well be correct, at least statistically, a unilateral temporal lesion will likely kindle a mirror focus long before psychotic symptoms develop. The psychosis of temporal lobe epilepsy, furthermore, is not identical to typical schizophrenia; for one, negative symptoms are less likely to occur—a relative sparing of the "ego"; for another, the patient will usually show additional features suggestive of the "interictal personality" of temporal lobe epilepsy. The delusions and hallucinations, for example, are more commonly religious in nature, and the patient may be given to typical rage outbursts and violent behavior. The treatment of the psychosis of temporal lobe epilepsy is primarily with an anticonvulsant like carbamazepine or valproic acid, and only secondarily with low doses of a high-potency neuroleptic, like fluphenazine or pimozide, that will not lower the seizure threshold. It is not uncommon for temporal lobe psychotics also to develop depressive symptoms, which, in turn, require specific antidepressant therapy.

Hyposexuality is a typical temporal lobe symptom. We have seen several TBI patients with mixed temporal and frontal lobe syndromes, with disinhibition and sexually explicit language combined with hyposexuality and absolute disinterest in acting on the consequences of their leering insinuations. An ironic combination, to be sure.

Once, we were called to consult on behalf of a middle-aged man who had sustained severe temporal and frontal lobe damage in a motor vehicle crash. He had been a Nashville policeman who was in hot pursuit of a criminal when his squad car was struck broadside by a city garbage truck. As you might imagine, the city of Nashville was committed to this fellow's rehabilitation, and no expense was spared to find the best services money could buy.

He had a preoccupation with sex, and talked about nothing else. He wandered off, at every opportunity, toward downtown where he intended to find a woman of the night on Music City Row. Finally, desperate to suppress this preoccupation and willing to go any length to win his cooperation with rehab, the staff resolved to satisfy his desires. They even found one of his old girlfriends, who was willing to sacrifice her virtue to his recovery.

Their assignation was interrupted, though; he was polite and friendly, but he was as disinterested in the act as he had been preoccupied with the pursuit. However, this epiphany had no lasting effect. His rambling and preoccupations responded, rather, to a slight increase in the blood level of CBZ.

The interictal personality of temporal lobe epilepsy has been described, at length by other authors and we have alluded to the syndrome in another chapter (see Chapter 6, this volume). We shall also discuss the development of posttraumatic (temporal lobe) psychosis further on in this chapter. It is appropriate to emphasize, at this juncture, however, that epilepsy is not the primary mediating event in the development of personality traits or of symptoms that have been traditionally described in association with temporal lobe epilepsy.

The Thalamic Syndrome

This disorder is usually seen in stroke patients or in tumor patients, but relatively circumscribed injury to thalamus can also occur after TBI. After a variable length of time has elapsed following an insult to thalamus, and as sensation begins to recover, some patients develop pain and hyperpathia on the side contralateral to the lesion (Levin et al., 1983) In TBI patients, the problem may be bilateral, by virtue of more extensive damage to thalamic structures. The pain is spontaneous, or else provoked by external stimuli that one would ordinarily not consider to be noxious. It is usually constant, but it may be paroxysmal. The quality is often described as an unfamiliar disagreeable sensation, like paraesthesia, formication, gnawing, crushing, burning, or freezing (Levin et al., 1983).

The syndrome was first described by Dejerine and Roussy in 1906, and it is sometimes referred to as Dejerine's syndrome. "Thalamic pain syndrome" is another term for it known, but it is not invariably associated with an identifiable lesion of the thalamus (Leijon et al., 1989).

TBI patients with elements of the thalamic syndrome are almost never able to actually describe their experience of pain and dysesthesia, because there are usually cognitive and linguistic deficits as well. Like the Kluver-Bucy syndrome after TBI, it is most commonly observed during the coma-recovery phase, when the patient is confused and disoriented as well as dysesthetic. This may compound problems of diagnosis.

The commonest clinical presentation is a patient at Rancho 3 or 4 who reacts intensely, and in the most negative way, to any new stimulus; a noise, the physical touch of attendants or of therapists, or the mere approach of another individual. The patient may scream, utter obscenities, or lash out physically. One of our patients would flash the bird at the approach of any new person, although he could tolerate the proximity of a familiar nurse. The noxious stimulus that tended to evoke this extreme reaction was someone, anyone but his favorite nurse, looking him in the eye.

The recommended treatment for this problem, when it occurs in a coma-recovery patient, is simple. Minimize stimulation, rely on familiar faces and familiar stimuli, and introduce new things slowly and gradually. Then, wait for the problem to pass, as it usually does. In the interim, family members and staff need to be counseled about the nature of the problem, and how to handle it.

Very little has been written about the pharmacological treatment of this syndrome (Nuzzo and Warfield, 1985). The rationale for the use of carbamazepine is probably based on the utility of that drug for trigeminal neuralgia; although the locus is different, the mechanism of action may be relevant. Milder cases of dysesthesia have been treated with amitryptiline, although that is a drug to avoid, if one can, in patients who are cognitively impaired. In a recent study, however, amitryptiline was found to be more effective than CBZ for the control of "poststroke pain" (Leijon and Boivie, 1989). If one assumes that it is the serotonergic effect of amitryptiline that mitigates the pain response of a disesthetic patient, one might be tempted to try other serotonergic drugs, or the serotonin cascade treatment that we have described elsewhere in this volume (see Chapter 7).

The fellow who used to flash the bird responded to amantadine, actually (Gualtieri et al., 1989), although he had done poorly on CBZ and amitryptiline (AMI). The dopamine agonist was effective, one presumes, because it seemed to enhance his general level of alertness and cognitive processing.

There is a small class of patients who exhibit a total lack of spontaneous activity at rest and extremely intense symptoms only under stimulation (Bakchine et al., 1989). One such patient, described by Bakchine et al. (1989), was described as "hypersyntonic," referring to an exacerbated, immediate apprehension of the external world, with immediate reaction associated with difficulty in apprehending the relative salience of stimuli. This may also be described as hypervigilance with intense hyperreactivity. One such patient had manic symptoms under stimulation, with bilateral orbitofrontal lesions and right temporoparietal injury (Bakchine et al., 1989). Another patient, with similar symptoms, had a circumscribed right thalamic infarct (Bougousslavsky et al., 1988). Disinhibition, loss of selectivity, irritability, and lack of initiative and perseveration, normally thought to be frontal lobe signs, are not unknown in association with thalamic lesions as a consequence of disruption of frontal lobe projections, especially from the dorsomedian nucleus (Bougousslavsky et al., 1988). Bakchine et al. (1989) described successful treatment with clonidine. We have used the combination of beta blockers with clonidine.

Agitation During Coma Recovery

This is the most dramatic and severe behavioral outcome of TBI, the extremely unstable phase that occurs when a patient has regained consciousness after a period of time in coma. It is usual for such patients to be disoriented and confused, and they usually have some behavioral and emotional instability as well. The level of arousal is low, even though they may seem hypervigilant, intense, and hyperreactive to environmental stimuli. Their attention span is short; they are extremely distractible, and they may have severe anterograde amnesia. Stereotyped motor behaviors are common, including elements of the Kluver–Bucy syndrome (see Chapter 10, this volume). Emotional lability is also the rule, or even its more extreme form, emotional incontinence, with sudden and unprovoked outbursts of laughter or crying. Patients may show dysesthesia, an extreme reaction to any novel stimulus or person, as if the sight or sound of someone new were painful or terrifying. They may be extremely hostile, with coprolalia, racial epithets, and sudden assaultive behavior. If they can walk, they may wander away with no regard for personal safety or the norms of decency. Their behaviors are disorganized, and the commonest element of affective expression is agitation.

The most important thing to remember about this period is that is a phase, a part of the recovery process, a physiological event that must be respected and interfered with as little as possible. It is usually transient, and heroic behavioral or pharmacological interventions are usually contraindicated. The patient has to be protected and kept comfortable, of course, and some degree of maintenance rehabilitation therapy should be kept up, but the best action during this period of instability is to wait it out.

It is remarkable what simple environmental measures will do to alleviate the problems of the agitated coma-recovery patient. Keeping the patient with a single, familiar nurse; adjusting the level of light and ambient noise; redirecting the patient to a safer environment; and putting Velcro tape on the doorknobs to discourage elopement. It is only in the most severe, and prolonged cases of postcoma agitation that pharmacological intervention is necessary. When agitation occurs in the neurosurgical ICU, with a patient pulling tubes and resisting treatments that are life sustaining, it may be necessary to intervene sooner with an effective drug. But in the rehabilitation unit, there has to be at least some tolerance for difficult behaviors and some capacity to adjust the physical environment and level of staffing.

The evaluation of the coma-recovery patient who is agitated or hypoaroused requires first a medical workup to exclude metabolic or infectious disorders and neurological evaluation for seizures, hydrocephalus, or intracranial hemorrhage. The alcoholic patient may require thiamine injection. The psychological evaluation should address environmental measures that can increase agitation, especially overstimulation, or confusion arising from isolation and unfamiliarity.

The conventional psychiatric differential that would include schizophreniform psychosis, organic affective disorder, and intermittent explosive disorder is not usually helpful, and one's choice of medication is usually guided more by trial and error than by psychiatric diagnosis. There is the clinical inclination to treat temporal lobe patients with CBZ, whether they be psychotic or affective or explosive.

On the one hand, diagnosis by location of the injury is of limited value; coma, and the agitation that occurs during coma recovery, are almost invariably associated with brainstem injury. On the other hand, the brain map may be a guide to pharmacotherapy, and because coma and postcoma are states of axial compromise, monoamine agonists may represent "rational pharmacotherapy." The location of cortical injury may also explain why a patient is disturbed by a particular circumstance, however, and how a proper environmental program should be developed. The patient with an occipital lesion may not respond to a program that requires processing visual information. A patient with extensive temporal lobe injuries may have Kluver–Bucy symptoms that are disturbing to staff and to family, who must be counseled to tolerate these problems to a degree, to redirect activities when possible, and to abide, patiently, their passage (see Chapter 10, this volume). It is said that CBZ is effective for KBS-type problems; that may be an overstatement, but it is a reasonable try in an area of endeavor guided by trial and error.

Trial and error but not "trial and hurt." The first principle of pharmacotherapy during the coma-recovery stage is to avoid drugs that may impede the recovery process, or that may impair the patient's limited ability to process information and to respond effectively. The second principle, or, rather, a corollary of the first, is to minimize the prescription of neuroleptic drugs. Although neuroleptic drugs are probably the most commonly prescribed agents for patients with postcoma agitation, the only unequivocal indication for this class of drugs is for central hyperthermia. In fact, central hyperthermia may be distinguished from septic pyrexia by virtue of the patient's response to neuroleptic drugs.

Neuroleptics are probably the most commonly prescribed drugs for agitation during the coma-recovery period, and that is because they have a reliable sedating effect, over the short term. So, the patient who is acutely agitated and is resisting the most essential medical supports, may be treated with a parenteral neuroleptic for a brief period of time. It is necessary, though, to minimize neuroleptic treatment even in extreme cases, because the drugs are not particularly effective over the long term; they tend to lower the seizure threshold, they may actually promote autonomic instability or neuromuscular rigidity, and they may even retard the cortical recovery process (Feeney et al., 1982).

The problem with treatment for agitation during the coma-recovery period is that there are so many pharmacological alternatives to neuroleptics and so many useful drugs to choose among that none has achieved established primacy. So, one may be perfectly justified in prescribing the psychotropic anticonvulsants, carbamazepine (CBZ) or valproic acid (VPA), lithium (Li), verapamil (VML), naltrexone, or a beta blocker; rarely, one might achieve success with an antidepressant or a benzodiazepine. In a given patient, any of these drugs might be expected to work quite well with a minimum of sedation if the doses are judicious and if the patient is monitored carefully. But none of these drugs will work reliably. That is, it is unlikely to get a good result in more than 40% of the patients who are treated.

In our rehabilitation centers, the drug of choice for postcoma agitation is the mixed dopamine agonist amantadine (Chandler et al., 1988; Gualtieri et al., 1989). We have explained the rationale for dopamine agonist therapy in head injury patients in previous papers (e.g., Gualtieri, 1988). In a few words, the idea is to compensate for damage to subcortical or axial neurons that project to striatal, limbic, and frontal cortex; the neurotransmitter dopamine is a central figure, it seems, in the neuropharmacology of CHI (van Woerkum et al., 1977; Vecht et al., 1975). One may expect success with amantadine in more than half the patients one treats with the drug; it is not sedating, and at moderate doses it may actually raise the seizure threshold and promote arousal, attention, and motor performance. The side-effect profile is favorable, especially when it is compared to the usual alternatives, and the major problems are paradoxical excitement, which is a rare event, and seizures, which are extremely rare.

Amantadine is also preferable to the psychostimulants methylphenidate and amphetamine for the coma-recovery patient who is underaroused, somnolent, and unmotivated. Some of these patients may be more abulic and akinetic than somnolent and unmotivated. There is a posttraumatic parkinsonism that responds favorably to this antiparkinsonian drug.

The syndrome of Dejerine, associated with thalamic infarct, is a terrible problem because the patient appears to respond to any novel stimulus—the approach of a new person, a change in venue, ambient noise—with extreme agitation, hostility, and fear, with screaming or even assaultive behavior. It is as if the merest stimulation were painful, and we refer to such patients as dysesthetics. Such patients may be treated with amantadine, or CBZ, or with serotonergic drugs like tryptophan, amitryptiline, nortryptiline, or fluoxetine. Another alternative is clonidine.

A drug that is effective during this period may not be necessary or even harmless over the longer term. It is a different brain one treats after this unstable period has resolved, and it is often a mistake to continue treatment when the patient has entered the phase of postrecovery.

The Prediction of Outcome

Traumatic brain injuries are classified as "mild," "moderate," or "severe" on the basis of the patient's score, during the immediate postinjury period, on the Glasgow Coma Scale (GCS)—that is, on the basis of the depth of coma (Rimel et al., 1982). The GCS measures verbal response, eye-opening, and motor response to promptings by the examiner.

As a general rule, the depth of coma is predictive of outcome; so is the duration of coma, and so is the extent of brain tissue destruction. In fact, these three elements are interrelated. The fact that the outcome of an injury is related to the severity of the injury may seem like a truism, but it is actually a good example of the Rule of Severity, a clinical corollary to Lashley's Law of Mass Action. It is no less than the guide to prediction of outcome relative to any cerebral insult.

The severity of outcome following TBI may be inferred directly from measures of the severity of injury. The same is true in other areas of neuropsychiatry. The severity of outcome following cerebral infection or perinatal hypoxia, for example, is predicted by the extent of infection and the degree to which it has destroyed tissue. This principle, the "continuum of casualty," is one of the foundations of developmental medicine. In epilepsy, outcome is predicted by the extent of the encephalopathy that has given rise to seizures in the first place. The indicators of bad prognosis indicators in epileptic patients—mental retardation, number of seizures, evidence of focality, difficulty in achieving anticonvulsant control—are all, in fact, measures of encephalopathy. A similar range of factors determine the outcome of posttraumatic epilepsy.

In psychiatry, the prognosis of schizophrenia is determined by the degree to which psychosis is superimposed upon encephalopathy. The so-called negative schizophrenic is actually a patient with deficit symptoms. The old Kraeplinian term, dementia praecox, is much more descriptive of the course such patients endure. And when one encounters such patients in centers for developmentally handicapped individuals, as one often does, their treatment and their day-to-day management is not so different from the treatment and management of the retarded. The "positive schizophrenics," on the other hand, are less likely to experience such a deteriorating course; they respond more favorably to medical treatments, and they are less likely to show evidence of encephalopathic change.

Even in childhood autism the outcome is determined, not by the severity of the autistic symptoms, but rather by the child's level of mental handicap. The outcome of childhood hyperactivity is not related to the severity of the symptoms, but rather to the accumulation of additional handicaps (see Chapter 14, this volume).

Outcome following TBI, therefore, is a paradigm for neuropsychiatry. It is the clearest demonstration of the Rule of Severity since Pasamanick formulated the Continuum of Casualty.

The Rule of Severity is complemented by the Rule of Nonspecificity. The outcome of TBI is only to a degree influenced by the location of the specific lesion. The neurobehavioral sequelae of brain injury are also, to a substantial degree, indeterminate. Whether a patient develops catastrophic consequences like aphasia, epilepsy, psychosis, or dementia after brain injury appears to be influenced by elements external to the injury itself. The age of the patient, the patient's premorbid characteristics, sex, laterality, and genetic proclivities, as well as other factors, may be as important as the location and extent of the lesion. Insofar as these elements are understood, one may speak with confidence of a predictable outcome. Because their full impact is seldom if ever understood, one's confidence is rarely firm.

The third rule is the Law of Reserve. What the patient brings to the injury will influence, to some degree, what he is left with afterward. Nothing influences recovery quite so strongly as the patient's premorbid level of intelligence, mental stability, and family support. Recovery from brain injury, like any human affliction, demands an enormous allocation of personal resources. If one commands a wealth of such resources, to that degree may the reserve be spent in the service of recovery. If one is poor to begin with, to that degree will the process of recovery be limited. And if a patient with a preexisting neuropsychiatric condition experiences severe TBI, not only will the recovery be impeded, but there is the additional risk of exponential deterioration in both conditions.

The physical and the neurobehavioral sequelae of TBI are thus influenced by an array of interacting elements. Of these, initial severity is an important factor but by no means the only important factor. The age of the patient, his personal resources, and the existence of premorbid neuropsychiatric conditions weight the outcome to a substantial degree.

The evaluation of TBI, therefore, entails several steps. First, there is the initial severity of the injury, judged on the basis of the extent of actual damage, and the depth and duration of coma. Then there is the evaluation of the overt physical and neurological consequences of the injury. Next is an appraisal of the patient's premorbid level of function, his psychological reserve on the one hand and on the other his individual areas of weakness. Finally, there is the posttreatment environment, and the degree to which that promotes stability and recovery, or instability and deterioration.

The Trajectory of Recovery

What is called the "trajectory of recovery" is defined, in large part, by these four elements. But it is also an independent variable, an element in itself that will influence outcome in unpredictable ways.

Recovery from TBI is not necessarily linear, a gradual, step-by-step recovery process with increments of improvement spaced evenly over time. It is stepwise. There are times when no change occurs at all—"plateaus"—and times when changes occur in several areas of deficit at a rapid pace. There are even times when the steps go down, when the recovery process seems to reverse itself for a while, when functions are lost that seemed at one time to be returning in force.

Theoretically, the largest part of biological recovery from TBI occurs in the first 2 years after a serious injury. The recovery that occurs thereafter is said to be the result of special interventions, or of learned compensatory strategies. Practically, though, it appears that substantial change may occur, even in patients many years post injury (Gualtieri and Nygard, 1988). We have found that intensive rehabilitation may be successful in patients who are more than 5 years from the point of initial injury. The trajectory of recovery may be enhanced at any point, it seems, after TBI.

The trajectory may be turned to decline at any point as well. There is evidence to suggest that new symptoms of PCS may develop at any time during the first year after mild head injury (Alves et al., 1986). Deterioration in memory performance on neuropsychological testing may develop 2 years after TBI (see Chapter 2, this volume). Severe neuropsychiatric disorders like psychosis and epilepsy may arise many years after an injury (Thomsen, 1984; Salazar et al., 1985); and TBI is an important element in the development of dementia in later life (Mortimer et al., 1985b).

The consideration of untoward long-term sequelae in some TBI patients should not blind the reader to the fact that head injury recovery is one of the most gratifying phenomena to treat in the field of neuropsychiatry. The common belief is that brain damage is irreversible, that because neural tissue is incapable of regeneration, damage to neural structures is permanent and permanently disabling. In fact, that is only half true.

Although there is much about recovery from brain injury that we do not understand, we know that the process is active and dynamic and that it can achieve striking results. The neural hardware may be incapable of complete regeneration, but the software is capable of reprogramming itself to a remarkable degree, and the neurochemical matrix that runs the system can always be readjusted. The environment of the head injury patient can be engineered, with not much difficulty, to minimize the impact of handicap and to optimize the capacity of remaining functions. Although we are all know people with obvious and persistent handicaps that have arisen from brain injury, we have also observed the substantial degree to which function can return, in a healthy person, when conditions were optimal. The trajectory of recovery may not always be as steep as one would prefer, and the final altitude may not be as lofty, but the machine is not necessarily grounded. And of all the elements that influence recovery, confidence that this belief is so may well be the most potent.

Evaluation of the TBI Patient

The evaluation of the coma patient is discussed in a monograph by Plum and Posner (1980), and the evaluation of the agitated patient during the coma-recovery stage is described here. The evaluation of motoric, linguistic, and neuropsychological deficits following TBI has been considered extensively in the relevant literature, but there really is no current guide to the evaluation of the ambulatory patient with relatively mild neurobehavioral sequelae of TBI.

The first instrument for evaluation is the confidence and trust of the patient. TBI patients are usually eager to talk to clinicians who understand TBI. Most of them have had difficult experiences with clinicians who jump to conclusions about their problems, even though it is apparent that they have no experience or knowledge of TBI.

The initial history-taking can convey familiarity with TBI, even in advance of the first visit, if questionnaires are sent to the patient that target particular areas that are germane to their problem; these might have to do with symptoms of postconcussion syndrome in general, and symptoms of memory deficit in particular. The patient should try to come to the initial visit with questionnaires completed and behavioral ratings done by at least one independent observer. (It is always good for an independent party to accompany the patient on the occasion of the first evaluation, to supplement the patient's history and to confirm the recommendations that are made; head injury patients can, after all, have memory impairments, and someone has to remember when the next appointment is. Patients may also be anosagnosic; this peculiar deficit does little to advance the clinical history.)

The patient should bring relevant medical information to the initial evaluation, especially operative reports from the injury, a discharge summary, the results of previous neurodiagnostic and neuropsychological tests, and the appropriate medical records, especially with respect to drug treatment.

The initial history should include the basics: previous medical history, social history, family history (especially for psychiatric, neurological, and developmental disorders) and medication history. The patient's premorbid characteristics should be discussed at length: personality traits, school and work history, family relations, attitudes, psychological difficulties, high-risk behaviors, and substance abuse. The history of the trauma should be covered quite completely: when, how, and why the injury occurred, what the extent of injury was, loss of consciousness, duration of coma and of posttraumatic amnesia, seizures during the immediate posttrauma period, and medications. Then, the history of hospitalization and of subsequent treatment experiences.

The patient should have described his current level of deficit of the questionnaires he completed before the evaluation, so that the discussion of current difficulties can be based upon his responses, and there should be plenty of time to expand on areas of difficulty, their development over the course of time following the injury, and their response to treatment interventions. It is essential to understand how a problem area is actually an impediment to normal function. It is not enough to decide someone has a problem with understanding what he reads. The essential question is how this is a handicap to him. Does it mean he cannot do his job, or does it just mean he looks at the pictures when he reads the comics?

The history should be taken before, during, and after the physical examination. Patients tend to relax after the examination is over, and they are more willing then to share intimacies. The neuropsychiatric examination begins with a regular physical and then a complete neurological examination. One looks for dysmorphic features that may speak to a preexisting developmental problem, and to signs of alcoholism or of drug abuse. The neurological examination is directed especially to the motor system: strength and tone, gait, tandem gait, cerebellar testing (finger to nose, heel to shin), the educated Romberg (feet together, eyes closed, arms outstretched, palms up), fine motor coordination (finger to thumb, the Mandrake test) and motor imitation (fist-palm, fist-chop-slap, Mandrake). One looks for subtle asymmetries in tone, strength, and deep tendon reflexes. One observes for tremor, dyskinesia, mannerisms, or stereotypies. One tests for cogwheeling and glabellar tap, and observes for other signs of parkinsonism.

The Mandrake test, properly executed, is probably the most sensitive sign of prefrontal injury. The patient is asked to imitate the examiner, who gestures hypnotically, as Mandrake the Magician used to do. The patient is asked to overcome his inhibition at such a silly task, but to perform smoothly and gracefully. After a while, the examiner will thrust forth his arms with fingers extended on one side, and a closed fist on the other, and alternate left to right, fingers and fist, and the patient is expected to spontaneously follow the examiner's lead, without a prompt. Then, one may change the pattern of fist-fingers, left-right-right-left-right-right, and then change sets again, with increasing frequency and increasing difficulty to the pattern. This is a test of a variety of prefrontal functions, including motor coordination and imitation, cognitive flexibility, perseveration, frustration tolerance and compliance. It is the motor equivalent of the Luria lines.

One checks for frontal release signs, like the grasp reflex, Hoffmann's sign, the palmomental reflex (PMR), the suck, snout, rooting, and corneomandibular ("bulldog") reflexes. The PMR is the most sensitive to mild subcortical injury in the frontal region. It should be quantitated: left and right, mild, moderate, extreme, and one to six in succession, to test for extinction.

The mental state exam is the third component of the neuropsychiatric examination. A good example may be taken from Strub and Black (1985). The entire examination is rarely done, because many of the items are designed for lower level patients. Instead, in a higher level patient, additional neuropsychological tests are added.

An office physician can test verbal fluency, figural fluency, verbal memory (the Buschke Selective Reminding Task or the Rey Auditory Verbal Learning Test), visual memory (the Rey–Osterreith Complex Figure, the Benton Visual Retention Test), perceptual-motor ability and motor planning (Trails), motor speed and accuracy (Finger Tapping, Grooved Pegboard, Purdue Pegboard), constructional ability (drawing, puzzles), anomia, and astereognosis (an anomia box full of funny little things). Such testing can be done in less than an hour by a physician or by a trained technician. There is also a sophisticated computerized neuropsychological battery than can be administered in a physician's office.

More complicated cases should be referred to a skilled neuropsychologist, of course, but one has to be careful about that. Batteries like the Halsted-Reitan and the Luria Nebraska are long and onerous, and they are also incredibly expensive. What is worse, they may not be as sensitive as the simple battery just described.

There is no "standard" neuropsychological examination, and there is great variability in the quality of the product. A skilled, modern neuropsychologist gives the most sensitive tests of higher cognitive function, regardless of their origin in a "battery." There are some patients who will do well on the neuropsychiatric examination described above, but who will only reveal their deficit on such a Neuropsych Battery. Then again, there are plenty of psychologists who affect the Neuro-prefix because they give a WAIS, a Rorshach, and a Bender-Gestalt; their testing batteries are neither sensitive nor reliable.

The role of neurodiagnostic testing is sometimes misunderstood. It is not meant to be diagnostic; it is only meant to supplement clinical judgment. The computed tomography (CT) scan is useful for demonstrating fractures, bone fragments, missile particles, intracranial fluid collections, hydrocephalus, and other clinical features that are important for the acute management of the head trauma victim. It is a fast test, too, so it is especially useful in the acute care setting. NMRI, on the other hand, is a long test that requires the patient to sit still in a claustrophobic tube as the machine clicks and whirs; it is not appropriate to the acute care setting, and it is not tolerable to the acutely agitated patient who is hard to sedate. On the other hand, it will demonstrate subtle lesions, especially in the white matter, that do not show up on CT, and this is where the neuropathic correlates of TBI are often to be found. The NMRI, therefore, is the test of choice for the stable TBI patient, for whom the aim is to define the location and extent of the lesion or to acquire a baseline for future comparison (e.g., against the development of hydrocephalus or cortical atrophy, late after the injury).

The EEG may show diffuse slowing, compatible with CHI but not very specific, or focal slowing that localizes a lesion; or paroxysmal discharge, that is compatible with (but not diagnostic of) epilepsy. Sleep deprivation may enhance the value of an EEG by evoking an epileptiform focus, but nasopharyngeal leads do not necessarily generate additional knowledge. A baseline EEG is good to have in the TBI patient.

The most sensitive instrument in the initial evaluation of the TBI patient is a good neuropsychiatric history and examination, as outlined here; if that is absolutely normal, it is extremely unlikely that a significant abnormality will show up on neuropsychological testing, NMRI, or EEG. What one looks for is consistency in the clinical picture: from the nature of the trauma to location of the lesion to symptoms to findings on examination to course and the trajectory of recovery. In mild TBI cases, one has, most of the time, only a few of these elements.

For serial evaluation of the TBI patient, for example, in measuring change over time, or in measuring the response to specific treatments, the best instruments are a selective (preferably, a computerized) neuropsychological examination, and a Neurobehavioral Rating Scale.

CHAPTER 2

Delayed Neurobehavioral Sequelae of Traumatic Brain Injury

Head injury and its natural sequelae are not necessarily the worst thing, or to put it another way, they are not the only worst thing. New problems develop in people who have had traumatic brain injuries (TBI), sometimes many years down the road. These are clinical problems that can be as debilitating as any consequence of the injury itself, but they may arise after a year, or after several years, or after many years. They are usually insidious in onset, in contrast to the catastrophic arrival of neurological deficit following TBI, so they may be overlooked and thus go untreated.

The delayed neurobehavioral sequelae of TBI are not only the result of exhaustion after years of debilitation and neglect, nor are they the simple accretion of clinical elements that finally emerge above the threshold of detection. They are probably the consequence of unique pathophysiological processes set in motion at the time of injury.

There are five delayed neurobehavioral sequelae of TBI:

1. Affective disorders, especially depression, especially in the first year or two after injury
2. Memory deficits that may arise *de novo* after about 2 years
3. Posttraumatic epilepsy
4. Posttraumatic psychosis, which seems to arise with similar frequency as posttraumatic epilepsy, and usually within the first 10 years of injury
5. Dementia, which is a long-term proposition.

It appears that TBI increases the risk over basal rates for the general population to this degree: for depression, by a factor of 5 or 10; for seizures, by 2 to 5; for psychotic disorders, by the same factor; and for dementia, by 4 or 5. Severe TBI, or injuries with special characteristics, may increase the risk of delayed sequelae even further.

Other problems arise in TBI patients with the passage of time, but the five listed here are the major clinical neurobehavioral issues. Posttraumatic headache, in contrast, usually begins within the first few days or weeks after TBI, and although

---

Sections of this chapter are scheduled to appear, in substantially modified form, in the journal *Brain Injury* in 1991.

the nature of headache may evolve over time and may well be a long-term problem, it is not usually delayed in onset. The appreciation of sexual dysfunction or of anosmia may not come for many months, or even years after an injury, but that is more a question of detection; the problem was always there, but no one thought to inquire about it, and the patient never related it to the injury.

It is important to consider the delayed neurobehavioral sequelae of TBI in their own right, because patients deserve to know, and so do their families. Estate planning for severely injured individuals also requires at least some appreciation of long-term risks. Physicians and psychologists should also have these data in hand, for reasons that are obvious.

Affective Disorders

More has been written on this topic than any of the others and there is also an extensive literature about depression in association with other neurological disorders, such as stroke, Parkinson's disease, and multiple sclerosis; useful information, for purposes of contrast and comparison. In fact, the comparison is more pertinent, because depression after TBI is about as common as it is in other severe neurological disorders.

The prevalence and incidence of affective disorders, in general, will naturally be influenced by the diagnostic categories and the diagnostic criteria that are being used at the time, and by the ascertainment criteria and the sampling method of the particular survey. There is no statistic that is universal for any of the affective disorders such as there is for schizophrenia, which occurs at the same rate across the boundaries of continents and appears always to have occurred at the same rate over the years. The frequency of occurrence of the various affective disorders is usually found to vary with sex, race, and culture, and there has even been comment to the effect that the prevalence of affective disorder, especially depression, is increasing in modern times. One may read that 13% or 20% of the general population in this country will have at least one clinically significant depressive episode at some time in their life (Blazer et al., 1988). The number will be much smaller, however, if one refers to the most severe forms of affective illness, like bipolar disorder, affective psychosis, or melancholia (1.9%–3.5%; Blazer et al., 1988).

Affective disorders in general and major affective disorders in particular are clearly associated with significant morbidity, and they are a major public health problem around the world. They also carry significant mortality. *The lifetime risk of suicide may be as high as 15% for patients with major affective disorder* (Black et al., 1987). Depression and related affective disorders also contribute to mortality from other causes such as accidents and natural diseases. The standardized mortality ratio (SMR) is increased in people with depression or anxiety disorders. *The SMR for such patients is 1.5, a 50% increase over the mortality rate of the general population; 2.1 for men, 1.2 for women* (Murphy et al., 1987).

The most recent definitive statement concerning the epidemiology of affective disorder is based on the NIMH Epidemiologic Catchment Area (ECA) Program in which 18,571 people were interviewed in five U.S. cities: New Haven, Baltimore, St. Louis, Durham, and Los Angeles. The prevalence of affective disorders was determined within a specific time frame: over 1 month, 6 months, and a lifetime. The three categories were manic-depression (bipolar disorder, MDi), major depressive disorder (MDD), and dysthymic disorder (depressive neurosis, Dysth). For the total U.S. sample, the following prevalence rates were determined:

	1 month	3 months	lifetime
MDi	0.4	0.5	0.8
MDD	2.2	3.0	5.8
Dysth	3.3	3.3	3.3

The prevalence rates for North Carolina, as you might expect, were among the lowest:

	1 month
MDi	0.2
MDD	1.5
Dysth	2.2

that is, about one-half or two-thirds of the national averages (Regier et al., 1988).

One may therefore assume, for the sake of argument, a lifetime prevalence rate for major depressive disorder at about 5% for the general population, and about 3% for dysthymic disorder. It is clear, then, that major insults to the central nervous system, like TBI or stroke, carry a significant increase in the probability of occurrence.

For example, McKinlay et al., (1981) reported that more than half their patients with TBI complained of depressive symptoms at 3, 6, and 12 months after the injury. Levin et al., (1987) reported that the prevalence of depressive symptoms in a three-center study of patients who had sustained mild head injury was 34%–39%, but the rate must be higher for patients who have sustained a moderate or a severe head injury, since it is known that the severity of the injury is directly related to the severity and the prevalence of residual affective disorder (Levin and Grossman, 1978). *The suicide rate for wartime victims of TBI has been reported at 14% over 18 years (Vauhkonen, 1959), a statistic that is equal to the suicide rate of patients with major depression.* The frequency of bipolar disorder, on the other hand, may not be increased by TBI (Grant and Alves, 1987). *Even if one were to grant the weakness of these surveys, from an epidemiologic and a diagnostic perspective, one is compelled to concede an increase in the liability to affective disease in TBI patients by a factor of 5 or 10.*

If anything, patients who have sustained a cerebrovascular accident (CVA) are at higher risk for developing affective symptoms than TBI patients. This may be a function of age, because the latter are, as a rule, younger, or on concomitant medication; stroke patients may be on antihypertensive medications, for example, which can by themselves cause depressive symptoms. For example, in one survey it was found that 60% of stroke patients had clinically significant depression, compared to only 20% of TBI patients (Robinson and Szetala, 1981). In another study, 50% of CVA patients developed clinically significant depressive symptoms, and 25% developed major depression (Robinson et al., 1984).

The depressive conditions associated with stroke appear to be particularly difficult to treat. The duration of poststroke depression is at least 7 to 8 months, on the average, and there is an increase in the prevalence of depression even in the second year after CVA (Robinson et al., 1983a). This phenomenon may not necessarily be confined to stroke. Berrios and Samuel (1987) compared the outcome of 83 neurological patients with depression to 44 neurological patients without depression and to 43 depressives who had no neurological disease. The neurological patients with depression were less likely to respond to antidepressive treatments than the depressed patients, and they did less well than the pure neurological patients, in terms of their medical outcome. The authors described the combination of depression and neurological disease in general as a "particularly lethal combination" (Berrios and Samuel, 1987).

The association between depression and neurological disease is not limited to stroke and CVA by any means. Depression in conjunction with Parkinson's disease (PD) is something that was noted by James Parkinson himself (Mayeux et al., 1981). Brown and Wilson reported a 52% rate of clinically significant depression in PD patients. Mayeux et al. (1981) reported a depression rate of 47% in PD; 31% of the depressions were mild, 13% moderate, and 4% severe.

Mayeux et al. also reported that depression was more likely in patients with severe intellectual impairment, suggesting a connection between the dementia of PD and the affective symptoms (Mayeux et al., 1981; Huber et al., 1988). On the other hand, intellectual impairment is not necessary for the development of depression, and the latter can certainly develop even when there is no sign of cognitive deterioration (Taylor et al., 1986). Patients with severe PD are more likely to be depressed than patients with mild or moderate manifestations of the syndrome (Santamaria et al., 1986), a pattern that also seems to hold for TBI and for stroke. Depression may be more likely an accompaniment of the form of PD that is associated with rigidity and bradykinesia than the form that is primarily characterized by tremor (Huber et al., 1988).

The prevalence of affective disorder is also higher (42%) in multiple sclerosis patients (Joffe et al., 1987). So, it appears that depression after TBI follows a pattern that is established for other severe central nervous system (CNS) disorders. The prevalence rate is increased dramatically; the condition is longstanding; it is difficult to treat; and its presence confers a negative influence on the course of the medical condition.

Whether affective disorder is more common after stroke, or after TBI, one cannot really say. Perhaps it is best to consider the Morbidity Ratio as 5 or 10 times higher in these patients, compared to the population at large. When this is computed on the basis of prevalence rates in the general population, one may estimate a 25% to 50% rate of major depression after TBI or stroke, and a 15% to 30% rate of dysthymia.

There have been attempts to relate the occurrence of affective symptoms following brain trauma with a specific lesion site, although the results of such attempts have not been conclusive. There is the long-standing belief that symptoms of depression, dysphoria, anxiety, and sadness relate to functional alterations in the frontotemporal regions of the right hemisphere (Flor-Henry and Koles, 1980), and this has been attributed to the functional organization of the right hemisphere for the "modulation of affective components of language and behavior" (Ross and Rush, 1981). The studies of Robinson and his co-workers have not agreed with this formulation, and they have actually alluded to a left hemisphere predominance in terms of poststroke depression (Robinson et al., 1983a). They have also suggested that poststroke depression may be related to lesion proximity to the frontal poles bilaterally (Robinson and Szetala, 1981). Starkstein et al. (1988c) have found that patients with poststroke depression were likelier to have evidence of subcortical atrophy. Cummings and Mendez (1984) have asserted that the focal lesions most commonly associated with secondary mania are diencephalic, while others have asserted that damage to orbitofrontal structures in the right hemisphere seems to be associated with secondary mania (Starkstein et al., 1988a). There really does not seem to be a cerebral localization to the problem of poststroke depression.

The high frequency of affective symptoms following TBI may well be a consequence of damage that is done to anterior frontal and temporal lobe structures, or to damage that is done to subcortical structures, or to both.

It is not possible to identify a particular group of TBI or of CVA patients who are likelier to develop affective symptoms or major affective disorder, which is why the failures of the anatomic model are so disappointing. One may assume, however, that the problem of posttraumatic depression will be more serious in women compared to men, in older patients, in patients who have to take medications that are potentially depressive, and in patients with preexisting affective disorders or with family histories of affective disorders. One might also expect to see more serious problems with depression in patients with more severe injuries, in patients whose residual handicaps are more severe, in patients with subcortical as well as cortical damage, and in patients whose psychosocial support systems are less effective.

Nor is one able to say that there is a peak period during which affective disorders are likeliest to develop and after which the risk necessarily subsides. On the basis of clinical observations and of surveys, the prevalence of affective disorder is very common in the first 2 years after TBI, just as it is following stroke. The studies of Vauhkonen (1959) and of Robinson et al. (1983a) suggest that the risk is carried for a long time further after the insult.

Delayed Amnesia

Disorders of memory are some of the most common deficits following mild or moderate or severe head injury. Anterograde amnesia, dense or patchy, is usually a problem that one attributes to the effects of the initial blow. That should not be surprising, especially after closed head injury, considering the pathological anatomy.

It is usually assumed that memory deficits will recover, at least to a degree, after TBI, and various psychological treatments and medications have been brought to bear to effect a more efficient return. The TBI victim therefore may hope to achieve at least some degree of improvement in memory function, or, if an impairment is resistant to therapy, then the adoption of specific compensatory strategies.

What the TBI victim does not usually consider, nor do his doctors, is the possibility of delayed deterioration in memory. This new concept has evolved from the longitudinal neuropsychological studies of TBI victims from the National Coma Data Bank. What is developing is the entirely novel idea that some TBI patients actually lose cognitive function, especially memory, at about 2 years after injury. This appears to be a specific effect, not a dementing condition, and it is not the function of some other delayed sequelae like depression, psychosis, or epilepsy (Gualtieri and Cox, in press).

Posttraumatic Epilepsy

Seizures that arise in the first 24 hours after TBI, or in the first 7 days, are the result of acute trauma. The fact that a patient has had one such seizure, or even several, does not mean that he has posttraumatic epilepsy. EEG abnormalities in the first year after TBI are not necessarily predictive of posttraumatic epilepsy, although persistence of an epileptiform EEG may well be meaningful (Aicardi, 1986).

Patients who are recovering from TBI, even a mild injury, may have "spells" during the first year during which they may experience focal weakness, or paroxysms of abnormal movement, or sudden unusual sensations; these may be indistinguishable from a focal seizure. These "spells" do not necessarily recur, nor do they necessarily develop into overt epilepsy.

The onset of true posttraumatic epilepsy may be in the first year, but it may come later. In the study by Salazar et al. (1985), the onset of posttraumatic epilepsy in Korean war veterans who had penetrating injuries was 57% in the first year, 18% after 5 years, and 7% after 10 years. Caveness et al. (1979) reported that 50% to 80% of the cases of posttraumatic epilepsy following wartime brain injury arose during the first 2 years.

The incidence of epilepsy after penetrating injuries is much higher than it is after closed head injuries (CHI). *The overall prevalence of posttraumatic epilepsy in the study of penetrating injuries by Salazar et al. (1985) was 53%, while the prevalence of epilepsy after closed head injury is from 2%* (Annegers et al., 1980a) *to 5%* (Jennett, 1979). *Severe CHI may have a higher rate: 7.1% at 1 year, 11.5% after 5 years* (Annegers et al., 1980a). McQueen, (1983) reported the incidence of posttraumatic epilepsy after severe head injury to be 7% in the first year and 10% after 2 years. In children, the data are higher: the incidence of epilepsy is 9.8% after severe TBI, and most patients have their first seizure in the first year (Young et al., 1983).

By way of comparison, the frequency of epilepsy following stroke is 6.5%–9%–13% (Olsen et al., 1987; Faught et al., 1989).

In terms of predictive factors, posttraumatic epilepsy following penetrating injuries is said to be related to the depth of dural penetration and to injury in the region of the central sulcus (Caveness et al., 1979); to the presence of focal neurological signs, especially hemiparesis and aphasia, and to the size of the lesion (Salazar et al., 1985); but not to the family history of epilepsy or to the patient's premorbid IQ (Salazar et al., 1985). For CHI, the predictive factors are coma duration and duration of posttraumatic amnesia; evidence of focal cortical injury associated with a mass lesion or depressed skull fracture; presence of focal neurological signs; and seizures in the first week after injury (Jennett, 1979). The occurrence of early fits raises the prevalence of posttraumatic epilepsy to about 25% (Jennett and Teasdale, 1981). Stroke patients who develop seizures are much more likely to have a cortical lesion; in one study, no fewer than 50% of stroke patients with persisting paresis and a specific cortical lesion developed epilepsy (Olsen et al., 1987).

An algorithm has been developed to estimate the probability of posttraumatic epilepsy (Feeny and Walker, 1979). The predictive elements, and their relative weight, are

Centroparietal lesion	0.25
Dural penetration	0.20
Hemiparesis or aphasia	0.20
Hemorrhage	0.20
Early seizures	0.15
Temporal lesion	0.15
Depressed skull fracture	0.10
Persistent EEG abnormality	0.10
Prefrontal lesion	0.10
Occipital lesion	0.10
CNS infection	0.10
LOC, PTA > 1 hour	0.05
Linear skull fracture	0.05

An algorithm for predicting epilepsy following penetrating head injury has been published by Weiss et al. (1986). Although there is no consensus among neurosurgeons on this issue, it does not appear that anticonvulsant prophylaxis is likely to diminish the likelihood of posttraumatic epilepsy (McQueen et al., 1983; Salazar et al., 1985; Young et al., 1983).

Young children seem likelier to develop posttraumatic epilepsy than children above the age of 2 years, but in children, it appears that the latency to seizure onset is delayed even further, compared to adults. For children 2 or younger, the latency to onset is up to 13 years; for children 3 to 14, 6 years; and for children older than 15, 3 years on average (Manaka et al., 1981).

The follow-up studies of posttraumatic epilepsy suggest that half the patients cease having seizures after 5 or 10 years (Caveness et al., 1979; Salazar et al., 1985). These are studies of penetrating injuries, however, which generally have a good prognosis; there are no epidemiologic data on the outcome of posttraumatic epilepsy following closed head injury.

Other problems may arise, however, as a consequence of epilepsy. Complex-partial seizures are the most common form of epilepsy after brain trauma, and lesions of the temporal lobe or limbic cortex are frequently involved. The long-term psychiatric consequences of temporal lobe epilepsy have been covered extensively in the literature (e.g., Bear and Fedio, 1977), but the most elegant epidemiologic study is that of Lindsay et al. (1980), published over two years in *Developmental Medicine and Child Neurology*. In their 13-year follow-up of 100 children with temporal lobe epilepsy, 5 had died; 33 were living independently and were seizure free; 32 were more or less independent, but not seizure free, on anticonvulsants; 30 were completely dependent and severely handicapped. Only 15% had been completely free of psychological problems. The most common psychiatric problems were attention deficit/hyperactivity, explosive rage attacks, and antiso-cial personality. No fewer than 10% developed an overt psychosis (Lindsay et al., 1979).

People with posttraumatic epilepsy have shorter lives than the general population or TBI victims without epilepsy. The death rate (death from any cause) of men with posttraumatic epilepsy is higher at all ages, but especially after age 45 (Walker and Blumer, 1989). As these men age, they are prone to increasing disability from their original physical handicaps, and they are also prone to early dementia (Walker and Blumer, 1989).

The final element of risk that is introduced by the occurrence of posttraumatic epilepsy are the neurotoxic effects of long-term anticonvulsant treatment, especially phenytoin, associated with encephalopathy, dementia, benign intracranial hypertension, and cerebellar atrophy (Masur et al., 1989; Kalanie et al., 1986; Reynolds, 1975) and barbiturates, associated with depression (Brent et al., 1987) or rheumatism, of all things (Taylor and Posner, 1989). For women, there is the problem of teratogenesis, a dilemma that is posed by use of any of the anticonvulsants.

If one assumes, therefore, a basal rate for epilepsy in the general population at less than 1%, a mild-to-moderate CHI may be conservatively estimated to increase the risk of epilepsy by a factor of 2 to 5; a severe head injury or a stroke will increase the risk by a factor of 10; a severe stroke or a penetrating brain injury will increase the risk by a factor of at least 50. If posttraumatic epilepsy develops, there is a 50% probability that the disorder will not remit. If the seizure disorder involves a temporal or a limbic focus, there is a 33% risk that severe psychiatric sequelae will develop.

Psychosis

Psychosis is, without doubt, the most severe and devastating outcome of brain injury. It may not be so dehumanizing as dementia, or so dangerous as epilepsy or depression, but there is nothing that is so destructive to the human personality or to the essential relationships one has with family and friends. There are drugs, to be sure, that can control at least some of the severe manifestations of a psychotic disorder, but they are not pleasant drugs to take; the side effects are cumulative over the years, and most of the time the drugs are only partially successful.

It is known that psychosis immediately following TBI occurs during states of delirium, in which orientation and anterograde memory are also impaired (Cummings, 1985). Such psychotic symptoms may be accompanied by hallucinations, poorly systematized delusions, agitation, combativeness, and marked fluctuations in the mental state. This form of psychosis occurs in patients in the early stages of recovery from coma, and it is not necessarily germane to the problem of late-onset psychosis.

After the coma-recovery stage, but within the first few months of coma recovery, patients with a clear sensorium may develop psychosis. These psychotic symptoms are not, as a rule, related to acute perceptual and orientation deficits. Delusions, for example, have been reported in patients with lesions in the basal ganglia (Cummings et al., 1983; Bogerts and Meertz, 1985), thalamus (Cummings, 1985; Krauthammer and Klerman, 1978), mesencephalon (Trimble and Cummings, 1981; Trzepacz et al., 1985) and various limbic structures (Nasrallah et al., 1983). In these cases, the delusions involve referential thought, persecutory beliefs, fears of illness and death, and jealousy. The complexity and organization of these more systematized delusions are related to the level of general cognitive and intellectual functioning of the patient (Trimble and Cummings, 1981; Cummings et al., 1983).

The psychosis of the coma-recovery stage is associated with delirium, confusion, and cerebral disorganization. Postrecovery psychosis is attributed to the effects of specific cortical or subcortical lesions. For late-onset psychosis, however, it is likely that another process must be brought to bear.

Late-onset psychosis 3 years after CHI, a case of "delayed reduplicative paramnesia" related to right hemisphere and bifrontal pathology, was described by Filley and Jarvis (1987). Delayed psychoses following stroke in one patient and CHI in another were described by Hayman and Abrams (1977), although the intervals were "contaminated" by the seizures in the first case and by alcoholism in the second. Levine and Finkelstein (1982) reported delayed psychotic reactions following right temporoparietal stroke or trauma in eight patients, seven of whom had seizures. Epilepsy, then, is a common feature but not a necessary ingredient in the development of delayed psychosis following cerebral insult.

Barnhill and Gualtieri (1989) reported two cases of late-onset psychosis following CHI: one was a young woman whose condition developed abruptly after 3 years and the second was a young man whose condition developed abruptly after $3\frac{1}{2}$ years. Although in both cases there were elements suggestive of the psychosis of temporal lobe epilepsy, in neither case was there clinical evidence of seizures. Both patients were severely aphasic, and it is likely that left temporal lobe damage was one element of the diffuse injuries they had sustained. It is possible that they also sustained damage to deep temporal lobe structures, and that the kindling phenomenon could be held to explain the late development of psychosis (Furgerson and Rayport, 1984). In both cases, at least a measure of relief came from treatment with carbamazepine.

In Thomsen's survey (1984, 1987) of 40 patients in Denmark followed up 10 to 15 years after severe CHI, the incidence of posttraumatic psychosis was 20%. Six of the eight psychotic patients had a late-onset condition; none had a preexisting psychiatric condition, and none were said to have seizures.

Most studies of the neurobehavioral sequelae of TBI have come from wartime patients with penetrating CNS injuries. In the follow-up study of 3552 Finnish war veterans with TBI, the prevalence of psychosis was 8.9% (Achte et al., 1967). In Lishman's review (1968) of 670 TBI patients 1 to 5 years post injury, significant psychiatric sequelae were described in 144 patients (21.5%). Risk factors for neurobehavioral symptoms related to localization and extent of the penetrating injury; the degree of subcortical involvement; duration of coma; and emergence of posttraumatic epilepsy. Pertinent neurological findings included severe cognitive deficits, sensorimotor impairments, dysphasia, and visual field deficits to confrontation. In general, the severity of psychiatric disease correlated with the extent of the CNS lesion (Lishman, 1968; Levine et al., 1987).

Although there have been no epidemiologic studies of sufficient strength to establish clear incidence and prevalence rates for delayed or late-onset psychosis, it is reasonable to surmise a prevalence that is similar to that of posttraumatic epilepsy: 2% to 5% following mild or moderate injuries, and 10% or more, after severe TBI.

Dementia

Senile dementia is the antepenultimate resting place for many of us, so we all take an interest in the elements that may occasion an increased likelihood of that condition. There are three: none can be foreseen or prevented. With respect to Alzheimer's disease, the only clinical factors that appear to increase one's risk are a family aggregate of Alzheimer's or of Down's syndrome; or, alternatively, a record of TBI earlier in life (Amaducci and Lippi, 1988). Other than that, we have only the incidence of dementia with every passing year beyond the age of 65, and that has been estimated in the past to be about 1% (Henderson, 1986); the prevalence of dementia in people above the age of 65 is 3.5%, and the prevalence of Alzheimer's disease in the same age cohort is 2% for men and 2.7% for women (Kokmen et al., 1989). More recent epidemiologic studies, however, suggest that the prevalence of Alzheimer's disease is much higher: 3% of people aged 65 to 74; 19% of people aged 75 to 84; and 47% (sic) 85 and older (Evans et al., 1989).

After a dementing condition like Alzheimer's is diagnosed, the outcome is first dependence and then death. Five years after Alzheimer's is first diagnosed, 73%

of patients will be in nursing homes, and 30% will have died. After 7 years, 84% will be in nursing homes, and 44% will have died (Berg et al., 1988).

The odds ratio, that is, the degree to which TBI will increase one's risk of developing a dementing condition, has been estimated at 4.5 (French et al., 1985); or 5.3 (Heyman et al., 1984); or 2.4 (Shalat et al., 1987). The last figure is too low by far, because the entry criteria for that survey actually tried to exclude patients who had TBI (Shalat et al., 1987). Henderson (1986) reported that 15% of Alzheimer's patients had a previous history of TBI, but only 3.8% of controls. The TBI patients who go on to develop dementia are more likely to have had a severe injury, or more than one head injury, or a concurrent illness like alcoholism or atherosclerosis (Violon and Demol, 1987). Older TBI patients, for example, people who are older than 60 years, are also more likely to develop a posttraumatic dementia.

One should place the morbidity ratio, therefore, at 4 or 5 for dementia following TBI. *That is to say, a person who has sustained a severe brain injury is four or five times likelier to develop a dementing condition later in life, and the problem is likely to arise at an earlier age.* If the prevalence of dementia in the population at large is 3.5%, then the prevalence of dementia in the brain-injured population should be 14% to 17.5%. That is less than the prevalence of dementia associated with Parkinson's disease (20%–40%) (Brown and Marsden, 1984; Mortimer et al., 1985a), but comparable in order of magnitude.

It is not likely that such a diverse range of outcomes will be given to any unitary explanation, nor is one necessary to end the discussion. It is sufficient to reflect on the number of neurological conditions that are given to late transformation, in addition to conditions just described: the weakness, fatigue, and pain of postpoliomyelitis syndrome (Cashman et al., 1987); postencephalitic Parkinson's disease; early dementia in people who are mentally retarded by virtue of viral encephalitis (e.g., Townsend et al., 1975); Alzheimer's disease in Down's syndrome; the neuroleptic-induced tardive syndromes (see Chapter 10, this volume); epilepsy in autism (see Chapter 9, this volume); brain atrophy following leucotomy (Pakkenberg, 1989); the psychosis of temporal lobe epilepsy, and the intellectual decline of epileptic patients (see Chapter 5, this volume). It is as if late transformation following a serious insult to brain were the rule, not the exception.

CHAPTER 3

The Psychopharmacology of Traumatic Brain Injury

Advocates insist that the clinical needs of traumatic brain injury (TBI) patients are different from those of other patients. In this contention, they are probably correct. TBI patients are not like stroke patients, or cerebral palsy (CP) patients, or developmentally handicapped patients, or psychiatric patients; they are different, and they are unique. Physicians and therapists who were originally trained with other patient groups soon discover that major adjustments in therapeutic approach are necessary when the sequelae of TBI are at issue. So it is, too, when pharmacological approaches are brought to bear.

Neuropharmacological treatment for TBI patients may be directed to the alleviation of specific neurological symptoms such as spasticity, headache, and posttraumatic epilepsy. It may be aimed at correcting neuropsychological deficits in attention, memory, arousal, or executive function. It may be aimed at specific psychopathological symptoms, because virtually any psychiatric symptom or syndrome may occur in a TBI patient as a direct consequence of brain injury, or as the indirect consequence of having to cope with a life of handicap, dependence, and isolation. Such a division is only a platonic ideal, however, because it is impossible to treat one dimension of the TBI patient without influencing some other facet. Drugs that are brought to bear on behalf of one system may also affect other systems. Drugs that reduce spasticity may cause mental depression; drugs for seizures or depression or anxiety may impair memory and motor performance. The practice of neuropsychiatry in head injury patients must therefore be a synthesis of knowledge from many different fields—from neurology, epileptology, neuropsychology, physiatry and psychopharmacology.

While it may be true that TBI patients are different from other neuropsychiatric groups, the study of neuropharmacology and of psychopharmacology in TBI will only be advanced if one remains attentive to advances in treatment for other special populations: patients with senile dementia, mentally handicapped patients, epileptics, and children with neuropsychiatric disorders. The process is one of extrapolation and inference; some people might think it is less than ideal, but is an efficient process. If lithium is effective as an antiaggressive drug in psychiatric patients and

Parts of this chapter appeared in substantially modified form in *Brain Injury* 1988; 2(2): 101-129.

in retarded patients, why should it not be an effective antiaggressive drug for TBI patients? The burden of proof would seem to devolve upon a person who contended that it was not.

The process also allows a certain degree of cross-fertilization of ideas among the different specialists concerned with neuropsychiatric patients. The clinical characteristics of several patient groups are known to resemble those of TBI patients (for example, young patients with attention deficit/hyperactivity, or specific learning disabilities (MBD)). Principles of pharmacological treatment developed for hyperactivity and learning disabilities are relevant also to treatment and research in TBI. To a large extent the same drugs are prescribed and the same measures used to evaluate the efficiency of treatment. To a large extent, the problems of "MBD" patients are similar to the clinical problems of mild TBI cases.

Progressive principles for behavioral neuropharmacology have also evolved in the treatment of severe behavior and emotional problems in autistic and mentally retarded people. In these patients, psychotropic medications are prescribed around specific symptoms, such as emotional outbursts, stereotypies, or aggressiveness. Psychotropic medications and anticonvulsants are prescribed with a critical eye to the potential neuropsychological toxicity and their impact on the client's overall habilitative program.

The study of nootropic and neuronotropic drugs is developing primarily among geriatric patients and people with dementia. There has always been an interest in cholinergic treatment for TBI patients, but the major work in this area now is being done in patients with dementia of the Alzheimer's type. The fact that TBI patients may be at increased risk of developing Alzheimer's disease in later life makes this area extremely important.

Principles of Treatment

Medical therapeutics are, ideally, rational and disease specific. That is, they arise from an understanding of the etiology and pathophysiology of a particular disease state. Pharmacological intervention is targeted to some specific central element of the disease process. This model is not salient, however, to most disorders involving the central nervous system (CNS). Because our understanding of the etiopathogenesis of brain disorders is necessarily limited, diagnostic categories are never more than descriptive or phenomenological. Pharmacotherapy that is based on descriptive diagnosis is necessarily imperfect.

The clinical indications for a specific drug may be diverse; the possible treatments for a specific disorder may include drugs from a number of drug classes, and a specific drug may be used to treat a wide range of disorders. The antidepressant imipramine may be used, for example, to treat panic attacks, enuresis and encopresis, attention deficit/hyperactivity, and explosive disorder. The anticonvulsant carbamazepine may be prescribed for affective disorders, neuralgia, aggression, hyperactivity, schizophrenia, and the Kluver–Bucy syndrome. Attention deficit disorders may be treated with stimulants, antidepressants, or neuroleptics. This is not exactly what the textbooks say, but it is the truth. The point is that therapeutics in neuropharmacology are rarely specific or rational.

Instead, therapeutics in neuropsychiatry are symptomatic, functional, or hypothetical. Treatments are symptomatic if they are directed to the suppression or alleviation of a particular symptom, such as depression; functional, if they are designed to augment or improve a specific physical function, for example, attention or memory; or hypothetical, if they are based on some reasonable hypothesis concerning the central mechanisms of aberrant behavior.

Rational pharmacotherapy is aimed at connecting a known pathophysiological derangement; the only real example in neuropharmacology is L-dopa for parkinsonism, based on the demonstration of diminished levels of the neurotransmitter dopamine in basal ganglia of afflicted patients. There is no rational therapy for the chronic neurobehavioral sequelae of TBI, but there is a hypothetical treatment based in part on the observation of diminished monoamine metabolites in the cerebrospinal fluid (CSF) of TBI patients, especially the metabolites of dopamine and serotonin (van Woerkum et al., 1977; Bareggi et al., 1975; Vecht et al., 1975)—thus the hypothesis that monoaminergic drugs in general, or dopaminergic drugs in particular, may comprise a "rational" treatment. Treatment with L-dopa seems to have promoted coma recovery (Vecht et al., 1975), amphetamine treatment has enhanced recovery in brain-lesioned rats (Feeny et al., 1982) and monoamine infusions are known to promote cortical plasticity in kittens (Kasumatsu and Pettigrew, 1979; Kasumatsu et al., 1981). This experimental rationale is the basis for treatment of TBI patients with drugs that selectively and specifically enhance monoaminergic neurotransmission; it is also the basis for one's prejudice against drugs, like the neuroleptics, that impede the activity of monoamines.

Another hypothetical treatment uses drugs that affect the endogenous opioid system, which is known to achieve an intense level of activity following CNS trauma (e.g., Faden, 1986). Thus, treatment with opiate antagonists may ameliorate the effects of brain injury and improve the state of consciousness (Baskin and Hosobuchi, 1981; Symons et al., 1982).

Usually, however, treatment is neither rational nor hypothetical, but symptomatic and functional. Practice is guided not by diagnosis but by an empirical approach based on trial and error. This should not be construed as an inferior method; it is simply a method stated honestly and carried out with no excess baggage.

The following sections are organized by drug classes. Each section is devoted primarily to the symptomatic and functional uses of the drugs at issue; only occasionally is a hypothetical basis for drug treatment put forth. Because the TBI literature is so small, most of the references are to other patient groups whose problems are germane to the treatment of TBI patients and also, on occasion, to the preclinical literature.

Throughout the following discussion, however, the author has been guided by a couple of simple rules. A drug is considered to be "relatively contraindicated" for TBI patients if there is any evidence that it is neurotoxic (e.g., fenfluramine) or that it may retard the course of cortical recovery (e.g., neuroleptics); if it is epileptogenic (e.g., maprotiline), if it is a depressant (e.g., benzodiazepines), or if it is known to have significant cognitive or behavioral toxicity (e.g., every other neuropharmacological compound).

Psychostimulants

The psychostimulant drugs are methylphenidate (MPH, Ritalin), amphetamine (AMP, Dexedrine), and pemoline (PEM, Cylert). There are several reasons to believe that drugs in this class might improve the clinical state of TBI patients:

1. Stimulants are known to improve symptoms of inattention, distractibility, disorganization, hyperactivity, impulsiveness, and emotional lability in children and adults with attention deficit–hyperactivity disorder (AD/HA). Many TBI patients have similar symptoms and respond well to low or moderate doses of stimulant drugs. This has been established over the short term (Evans et al., Patterson, 1987b) as well as in longer term studies (Gualtieri and Evans, 1988).
2. Stimulants are known to improve symptoms of hypersomnia, apathy, anergia, and hypoarousal in narcoleptic patients, in patients with the Kleine–Levin syndrome (Orlosky, 1982) and in "senile apathy". TBI patients who are afflicted with similar symptoms may respond favorably to low-to-moderate doses of stimulant drugs.
3. Stimulants appear to improve long-term memory in AD/HA patients through a direct mechanism, dissociated from medication effects on attention or fatigue (Evans et al., 1986b). They appear to have similar effects in TBI patients (Evans et al. 1987b).
4. Stimulants are known to improve perceptual-motor function in AD/HA children (Golinko et al., 1981), to improve fine motor speed, accuracy, and steadiness (Gualtieri et al., 1986a) and (in normals) to alleviate the perception of fatigue that accompanies strenuous exercise (Novick, 1973). Some of these effects have also been reported in TBI patients (Gualtieri and Evans, 1988).
5. It has been suggested that stimulant drugs exercise a therapeutic effect by modulating or by enhancing dopaminergic neurotransmission to rostral brain structures, especially in the frontal neocortex (Gualtieri and Hicks, 1985a). They may be particularly useful for TBI patients whose deficits are attributable to frontal lobe damage; these deficits include diminished flexibility, inability to execute complex behavioral programs, poor planning, lack of initiative, and poor impulse control, in addition to the "hyperactive" and the "anergic" elements listed in items 1 and 2.
6. Profound deficits in monoaminergic neurotransmission are seen in TBI patients, presumably as a consequence of shear damage to axial brain structures where the cell bodies of neurons that synthesize monoanomines are concentrated. The administration of monoaminergic drugs such as stimulants is, in this context, "rational pharmacotherapy"; that is, drug therapy intended to correct an underlying neurochemical deficit.

Stimulants are comparatively easy to use, and positivé effects, when they occur, are apparent within days—or hours—after an optimal dose is achieved. Methylphenidate (MPH) and dextroamphetamine (DEA) are the stimulants most frequently prescribed for AD/HA, narcolepsy, Kleine-Levin syndrome and senile apathy, and probably also for TBI. Pemoline (PEM) is a third alternative, but not a very good one.

Stimulants are not hard to monitor for side effects; anorexia and insomnia are amenable to dose or dose-schedule adjustments; headache and dysphoria, irritability, and "on-off" and "rebound" reactions usually respond to minor changes in prescription. The stimulant side-effect profile is, in fact, a model of clarity: Acute toxic effects are clear and apparent, and they resolve quickly as soon as the drugs are withdrawn. But once the hurdle of initial sensitivity is past there is no long-term toxicity, no secret effect that will come along after months or years of treatment. Stimulants have the enormous advantage of being "yes-no" drugs; they either work or they don't, and when they do work, positive effects are readily apparent.

This is not to suggest that stimulants can be administered freely, or that they can be prescribed by inexperienced physicians. Stimulant therapy is perfectly safe in the hands of a knowledgeable and responsible practitioner; but stimulants are complex drugs, and acute toxicity is not an insignificant matter. Adults, for example, seem to be very sensitive to stimulants, and very low doses may be sufficient for a 70-kg male (Gualtieri et al., 1982). Higher doses may cause cognitive overfixation, stereotyped thinking, perseveration, or palilalia. High doses may actually impair memory and clear thinking (Wetzel et al., 1981). A patient who is sensitive to stimulants may become anxious or disorganized, fearful, agitated, paranoid, or frankly psychotic. Somatosensory hallucinations may occur. Patients can develop increased spasticity, choreic and athetoid dyskinesias, and motor and phonic tics. Patients may become intensely dysphoric, irritable, and prone to rage attacks. Although stimulants may alleviate the symptoms of posttraumatic headache, or enhance the effect of analgetic agents, they may also cause headache or precipitate migraine. This is not a trivial list by any means, and it speaks to the need for careful monitoring.

Although stimulant treatment can be stopped abruptly in AD/HA patients with no withdrawal symptoms at all, even after years of treatment, TBI patients seem to be different. In TBI patients, abrupt stimulant discontinuation may lead to a severe withdrawal reaction, with symptoms of depression, anergia, or agitation. Thus a clinical trial should never be undertaken lightly in a TBI patient, because the medication cannot be withdrawn suddenly without risking the additional problem of rebound depression. No TBI patient should be treated with stimulants unless there is a physician experienced in the use of the drugs in close attendance, and unless the patient and his family fully understand the attendant risks.

Research has not advanced to a point at which it is possible to predict *which* TBI patients should be treated with stimulant drugs. It is the author's clinical impression, however, that the best response occurs in relatively high-level, mildly to moderately impaired patients, with relatively circumscribed deficits in attention, memory, and organization, or initiative. More severely impaired subjects, especially those with severe motor impairment, seem less likely to respond, and they also seem to be more prone to acute toxic effects and to withdrawal reactions. This parallels the clinical experience of child psychiatrists and developmental physicians: AD/HA children are less likely to respond to stimulants if they have associated emotional, behavioral, or cognitive problems; mildly to moderately retarded children are more likely to respond to stimulants than the severe-to-profoundly retarded.

There is evidence from animal experiments that stimulants may influence the cortical recovery process in some way, conceivably by correcting the monoaminergic deficits that accompany TBI. There is a new preclinical literature concerned with pharmacological effects on the growth and recovery of nervous tissue: compounds reported to be beneficial, in addition to the stimulants, include naloxone and thyrotropin-releasing hormone (TRH) (Faden, 1984). This is an incipient literature, however, and none of the animal research has yet proven useful for human beings with brain or spinal cord injury. Nor is it even clear how clinical studies should be designed to demonstrate the utility of a compound on the cortical recovery; this remains a moot point, and one that is not likely to be resolved soon.

Stimulants are currently indicated for TBI patients who have these prominent symptoms:

a. attention deficit/hyperactivity, listed in previous item 1
b. anergia/apathy, listed in previous item 2
c. the frontal lobe syndrome, previous item 5

Stimulants may also be used in some patients with symptoms of emotional incontinence ("catastrophic reactions"), emotional inability, or rage outbursts, although the usual treatment for this syndrome is a serotonergic antidepressant or carbamazepine (see Chapter 1, this volume). They may some day be indicated as a kind of "tonic" to improve the pace of cortical recovery after TBI, although this is at present only speculation, and the routine use of stimulants for asymptomatic TBI patients, in hopes of improving the rate of recovery, cannot be recommended.

There is no absolute contraindication to stimulant therapy, except perhaps in the case of patients with a prior history of drug abuse or addiction. Stimulants have very few untoward interactions with other drugs. They are likely to raise, not lower, the seizure threshold in epileptic patients, physicians' desk reference (PDR) to the contrary (Feldman 1989); although it is true that very high doses may be epileptogenic (Alldredge et al., 1989). In low doses the cardiovascular effects of psychostimulants are minimal.

Side effects of stimulants may include agitation, disorientation, emotional lability, cognitive perseveration, increased spasticity, tremor, and dyskinesia, especially in patients with severe motor sequelae of TBI. Abrupt stimulant withdrawal in TBI patients may lead to severe symptoms of depression, agitation, or suicidal ideation. For this reason the prescription must never be allowed to lapse; the fact that MPH and Amphetamine (AMP) are schedule II drugs, that prescriptions can only be written for a month at a time, and that prescriptions cannot be refilled by phone, mean that a greater degree of vigilance is required in follow-up.

The contention that psychostimulants may exercise some benefit against symptoms of inattention, abulia, and anergia is hardly controversial; one would be surprised if such were not the case. The idea that stimulants are the treatment of choice for many of the depressive syndromes that accompany TBI requires a small degree of imagination, but it is not a staggering inferential leap. There is, however, a third area of speculation, and this does require the most critical scrutiny, because it speaks to the effect of stimulant drugs on the very process of cortical recovery.

There is, as we have mentioned above, at least suggestive evidence from the preclinical literature that stimulant treatment may advance the recovery of brain-injured animals (e.g., Feeny et al., 1982). There is the clinical evidence from experience with AD/HA children on stimulants, who require treatment only for a couple of years, on the average, because they appear to mature and to acquire more stable patterns of relating to their environment after a course of treatment with stimulants. And, finally, there is evidence from controlled studies of TBI patients on stimulants that the drugs may exercise lasting effects, even after they have been discontinued (Gualtieri and Evans, 1988). The issue is whether this particular pharmacological intervention is capable of actually accelerating the recovery process, that is, whether it restores a lasting balance to neuromodulatory monoamine systems that have been upset by traumatic injury.

The issue will probably not be settled for a long time, but it carries sufficient weight at this point to lend impetus to clinical trials in appropriate patients.

Amantadine

Amantadine (1-adamantamine) is a water-soluble acid salt that can penetrate all cell membranes, including those of the CNS. It has been used therapeutically: as an antiviral agent, in the prophylaxis of infection with influenza A; as a dopamine agonist, in the treatment of Parkinson's disease; and, in the same vein, as a treatment for some neuroleptic side effects, including pseudo-parkinsonism, dystonia, akathisia, and neuroleptic malignant syndrome. There have been indications, however, of efficacy for a wider range of neuropsychiatric disorders, and it is at the present time the drug of choice for certain conditions in TBI patients.

Amantadine derivatives were first prepared in 1954, and its antiviral effects were first studied during the 1960s (Herrman et al., 1960). Its efficacy in Parkinson's disease was discovered serendipitously by Schwab et al., in 1969 when the drug was given for influenza prophylaxis to a woman with Parkinson's disease. As an anti-parkinsonian agent, it appears to exercise a more potent effect than the anticholinergic drugs, and with fewer side effects (Harvey, 1986). For example, anticholinergic drugs are known to impair memory performance, and this is an important consideration in the treatment of elderly patients. Amantadine, compared to benzotropine, does not impair memory in young, normal volunteers (Van Putten et al., 1987), or in normal volunteers who are elderly (McEvoy et al., 1987). It is as effective as the anticholinergics for the acute side effects of neuroleptic treatment, but it is free of any atropine-like side effects, and so may be preferable in many if not most clinical situations (Stenson et al., 1976; Borison, 1983).

The neuropsychiatric effects of amantadine are presumably related to its effect on the neurotransmitter, dopamine, but it is not really known exactly what that effect is. It is generally accepted that amantadine acts presynaptically to enhance dopamine (DA) release or inhibit DA reuptake without any direct effect on DA receptors (Gianutsos et al., 1985). On the other hand, there is additional information to suggest a direct, postsynaptic effect; perhaps to increase the density of postsynaptic dopamine receptors (Gianutsos et al., 1985), or to alter the conformation of the dopamine receptor (Allen, 1983). Stone noted a specific inhibitory effect of amantadine on cortical and striatal neurons when applied microiontophoretically (Stone, 1977). In various animal models, amantadine appears to behave as a competitive blocker of the receptor effects of apomorphine and amphetamine (Allen, 1983). It would seem, therefore, that the dopaminergic effects of the drug represent a combination of direct (postsynaptic) and indirect (presynaptic) influences. The relative weighing of such effects for the various dopamine agonists would account, then, for their overlapping but not necessarily identical clinical profiles (Schneiden and Cox, 1976). Although the dopaminergic effect of amantadine is multifaceted and complex, there is no convincing evidence that it exerts any meaningful influence on the behavior of other neurotransmitter systems (Allen, 1983).

Amantadine has been shown to antagonize neuroleptic-induced prolactin secretion (Siever, 1981), indicating an effect on hypothalamic (or pituitary) dopamine receptors. It has been claimed that amantadine has a selective affinity for striatal dopamine receptors, without affecting mesolimbic or mesocortical dopamine systems (Allen, 1983), but this kind of information requires more convincing demonstration.

The rationale for clinical trials of amantadine in diverse groups of neuropsychiatric patients is based on the premise that not all dopamine agonists are the same. The important distinction between presynaptic agonists like methylphenidate and L-dopa and postsynaptic agonists like bromocriptine and lergotrile was drawn first by Ross and Stewart (1981) in their discussion of the treatment of a 36-year-old man with akinetic mutism from an anterior hypothalamic tumor. The patient responded to the latter class of dopamine agonists, but not to the former. The lesson is that pathological anatomy should guide neuropharmacological treatment, insofar as that is possible; and that pathological differences among patients will mandate the adoption of different neurochemical strategies. Thus amantadine, with a neurochemical profile that is different in all probability from any other dopamine agonist, will be effective for some patients, and in those patients no other agonist will work as well.

The question is, which patients? There have been only clinical reports and small clinical studies to suggest that amantadine is useful for neuropsychiatric conditions other than those mentioned in the beginning of this chapter.

Amantadine for Neuropsychiatric Patients

Parkinsonian patients with symptoms of rigidity and akinesia are the ones most likely to respond to amantadine (Harvey, 1986). Among amantadine responders, there will often be a moderate decline in clinical efficacy during the first months of treatment (Schwab et al., 1972). The drug has stimulating properties, and amantadine patients report that they feel more lively and alert on the drug (Schwab et al., 1972). The major side effects of the drug are stimulant like: irritability, agitation, disorganization, or psychosis. These four elements are reflected in the wider clinical profile of the drug.

In the treatment of neuroleptic-induced extrapyramidal disorders, amantadine is most effective for pseudo-parkinsonism, bradykinesia, abulia, rigidity, and akinesia, and relatively less effective for dystonia and akathisia (Kelley and Abuzzahab, 1971; Ananth et al., 1977; Gelenburg and Mandel, 1977; Borison, 1983). Its use as a neuroleptic companion is compromised by the occasional occurrence of behavioral toxicity. (Its unavailability in parenteral form is another limiting factor.) It has been used successfully to treat the neuroleptic malignant syndrome (Lazarus, 1984).

The activating properties of amantadine have led to trials for patients with "negative" symptoms of schizophrenia (withdrawal, abulia, bradykinesia), and in this application the drug has about as much success as the other dopamine agonists (Angrist et al., 1980; Davidoff and Reifenstein, 1939; Kornetsky, 1976). It is occasionally effective in catatonia (Baldessarini, 1977; Neppe, 1988). It is found to be effective for fatigue and depression that accompanies multiple sclerosis (Murray, 1985).

It has been natural to consider amantadine for dementia and the neuropsychiatric sequelae of stroke or head injury: first, because the behavioral symptoms that occur in these conditions are sometimes similar to those we know to improve in parkinsonian patients; and second, because dopamine agonists are believed to enhance at least some aspects of cortical recovery from (or accommodation to) a neuropathic process (Gualtieri and Evans, 1988). The clinical work that has been done in this area, however, has not been enlightening. The results of clinical trials of amantadine and of memantine, a closely related derivative (Reiser et al., 1988; Meldrum et al., 1986), have not been encouraging, but that may have to do with patient selection; there have been reports of reduced agitation and improved alertness and function in demented patients treated with amantadine (Muller et al., 1979) but therapeutic effects have been compromised by the frequent occurrence of behavioral toxicity.

We originally reported reduction of agitation and assaultive behavior with amantadine in two patients with frontal temporal lesions following closed head injury (Chandler et al., 1988); the patients were young men whose difficulties arose during the transitional stage of coma recovery.

Amantadine is effective for the treatment of one cerebral dysmaturation syndrome, nocturnal enuresis (Ambrosini and Fried, 1984), but its effect in another, AD/HA, is equivocal (Mattes, 1980).

Schwab described seizures as a high-dose side effect of amantadine (Schwab et al., 1969, 1972), and we have observed the same association in clinical experience with head injury patients. On the other hand, dopamine agonists are usually associated with a higher seizure threshold, and one influential report has claimed benefit for amantadine in the treatment of refractory epilepsy in childhood (Shields et al., 1985).

Toxicity

The toxicity profile for amantadine is quite favorable, especially when it is compared to alternative treatments. As an antiviral agent, it has had wide use and little serious toxicity in children, elderly adults, and the mentally handicapped (MMWR, 1987; Atkinson et al., 1986).

Behavioral toxicity has been the most important side effect, and it appears to have limited the use of amantadine in some patients who need it the most. Behavioral symptoms include insomnia, vivid dreams, anorexia, hallucinations, irritability, nervousness, agitation, disorganization, psychosis, hyperactivity, aggression, delirium, and depression. The symptoms remit when the dose is lowered or when the drug is discontinued.

Abrupt discontinuation of amantadine in patients on neuroleptics may precipitate severe toxicity, including neuroleptic malignant syndrome (Hamburg et al., 1986) and neuroleptic-induced catatonia (Brown et al., 1986).

Amantadine overdose is associated with cardiac arrhythmia (Sartori et al., 1984) and the interaction with phenelzine may cause severe hypertension (Jack and Daniel [sic], 1984). Amantadine may cause livido reticularis and it may also cause pedaledema.

Pharmacokinetics

Amantadine is almost completely absorbed (the site has not been determined) and peak plasma concentrations occur one to four hours after ingestion (Wu et al., 1982; Aoki and Sitar, 1979; Montanari et al., 1975; Aoki and Sitar, 1985; Aoki and Sitar, 1988). Distribution is through all the tissues of the body, including the CNS.

Rationale for Neuropsychiatric Treatment

On earlier occasions, we have written about the use of dopamine agonists and their effect on cortical recovery, and their indications for patients with neurobehavioral sequelae of TBI (Evans 1987b; Evans and Gualtieri, 1988; Gualtieri, 1988). We developed an extensive clinical experience with the presynaptic agonists, methylphenidate, amphetamine, and L-dopa, in patients with TBI, and we frequently observed beneficial effects on behavior, mood, and neuropsychological performance. But improvement was limited, in large part, to patients with relatively good outcomes, and was best for patients with relatively mild postconcussion syndromes. Patients with more extensive injuries, a lower level of general arousal, and a greater degree of motor impairment had little or no response to stimulants or L-dopa, or, if they did respond, the effect was lost within a short period.

The idea was not that dopamine agonist therapy was irrelevant in such cases, but that the presynaptic dopamine neuron was so severely damaged in low-level cases that the effects of a presynaptic agonist could not be sustained. In other words, there was no substrate upon which such drugs could exercise their effect. The next logical step was to try a dopamine agonist that possessed a mixed direct-indirect profile, and thus the choice of amantadine for the two cases described in Chandler et al., (1988). The dramatic success of these first two treatment cases—men with severe problems who had failed to respond to conventional medications—led to further treatment trials in other patients with TBI. The idea was that high-level patients who did not have extensive subcortical damage would respond well to presynaptic agonists, but that lowlevel patients, with more extensive subcortical injury, would respond better to amantadine. It was an easy hypothesis to test, at least on a preliminary basis.

We selected a group of patients in the acute stages of coma recovery—Rancho levels 4 and 5—who usually experience symptoms of agitation, disorientation, disorganization, confusion, and emotional lability. For most patients these symptoms are mild and transitory, and they are handled behaviorally. For others, however, the symptoms can be severe, with violence, wandering, negativism, severe agitation, screaming, sleep disturbance, and self-injurious behavior. In some unfortunate patients, these problems can persist for weeks or months, and in such cases psychotropic drugs are usually prescribed. It appears that amantadine has a success rate in such patients that is better than 50%, and that treatment may be continued for several months, if necessary, without serious side effects (Gualtieri 1989).

The advantage of amantadine for such patients, in contrast to the conventional psychotropic drugs, is that it is an easy drug to try. The dose range is narrow (100–400 mg/day), the onset of therapeutic action is relatively quick (4 days at each dose increment), the side-effect profile is favorable, monitoring is a simple task, and there are not a lot of troublesome drug interactions to worry about. Amantadine is not a sedating drug, an important consideration at this stage of coma recovery. If behavior toxicity develops, the effect is readily reversible when amantadine is withdrawn.

The successful treatment of postcoma agitation with amantadine is consistent with the theory that subcortical dopaminergic neurotransmission is severely impaired at this stage of recovery, and that direct stimulation of striatal and cortical dopamine neurons can lend a degree of higher regulatory support; it is possible to improve cognitive processing and alleviate confusion and dismay with amantadine treatment, and thus reduce the occurrence of severe target behaviors like agitation and assaultiveness.

The treatment of agitation, however, does not reflect the cardinal indications for amantadine in Parkinson's disease, which are akinesia, abulia, rigidity, and low arousal. We have also had the opportunity to test the efficacy of amantadine for head injury patients who had neurobehavioral symptoms that fit this template; it appears to be equally successful in this group of TBI patients, and it is a suitable alternative to the psychostimulants, especially for patients with more extensive injuries (Gualtieri et al., 1989).

Having established a degree of success with amantadine in some difficult patients, we were encouraged to investigate its utility for a second group of neuropsychiatric patients, developmentally impaired individuals; another group prone to behavior difficulties, and for whom neuroleptics had long been a mainstay. The problem of neuroleptic treatment for mentally handicapped people is, of course, a matter of record (see Chapter 12, this volume). The continued use of neuroleptics, however, is very much a function of a dearth of alternatives.

It is remarkable how the clinical situation is analogous to that for TBI patients. We have described success with developmentally handicapped patients with symptoms of abulia, bradykinesia, and withdrawal, and also in patients whose behavioral difficulties may be operationally described as "hyperactive-disorganized"; this included symptoms of aggression, screaming, agitation, noncompliance, destructiveness, emotional lability, and tantrums (Chandler and Gualtieri, 1990).

The therapeutic profile of amantadine has thus expanded considerably with the inclusion of four patient groups who had not been previously considered: head injury victims with symptoms of agitation and of abulia; and mentally handicapped individuals with analogous symptom pictures. These preliminary observations require further development, of course, under controlled circumstances, but the proper design of controlled studies can only come after a period of clinical observation and the necessary accumulation of basic information about the drug, its likely indications, problems with treatment, and the consequences of long-term treatment.

We have mentioned some of the practical advantages of amantadine treatment, but it is appropriate to list a few more at this point. First, it is a "yes-no" drug; it either works or it doesn't, and when it does work, the effects are usually dramatic. It is not simply a mild tranquilizer that "takes the edge off" a troublesome behavior pattern. If the patient is not substantially improved, there is no reason to continue the drug at all. Thus, there should be no difficulty in detecting the positive effects of treatment using more systematic measures than the clinical observations we have relied on.

Second, therapeutic effects come quickly, within a matter of days, and dose increments, from 50 bid to a maximum of 400/day, can be made at weekly intervals. Thus, it should not be long before the effects are apparent.

Third, toxicity is overt, not covert, as it is for drugs like the neuroleptics and phenytoin, for example. The major side effects are behavioral toxicity and seizures. They are reversible when the drug is discontinued, and it may be discontinued abruptly if that is necessary.

Fourth, the drug is not sedating. It does not confer behavioral improvement at the expense of cognitive impairment. In fact, patients appear to be more alert and attentive in therapies of various sort. Nor is there any apparent motor impairment.

The design of a placebo-controlled, double-blind study of amantadine effects with objective measures of behavioral and neuropsychological improvement should not, then, be difficult. Such a study should necessarily include a prolonged follow-up period for amantadine responders, because there is an occasional fall-off in effect over the months, as there is on occasion among patients with Parkinson's disease.

There is the obligate apology one must make for speculating about the mechanism for drug action, when one's impressions are entirely anecdotal and so much more must be determined about the parameters of amantadine treatment. The extreme heterogeneity of the patient groups in our four tables should warn one away from idle speculation or theorizing.

One is impelled, however, by the arguments made in favor of direct dopamine agonists in the treatment of neuropathic patients with subcortical lesions. In certain classes of patients it is reasonable to surmise that the presynaptic neuron is incapable of supporting the action of an indirect agonist, while the striatal or the cortical neuron retains at least a limited capacity to respond to the agency of direct stimulation. This is an inference borrowed from the therapeutic physiology of Parkinson's disease, and its validity would not be proven even if the clinical observations contained herein were supported by controlled studies. After all, the precise nature of the dopaminergic action of amantadine is incompletely understood. But it represents, if not a testable hypothesis, at least a rationale for further investigation.

The psychopharmacological model for dopaminergic treatment is the use of stimulant drugs for hyperactivity. There is however an interesting aspect to stimulant treatment that is well established in developmental neuropsychiatry and that is germane to our reflections on amantadine and its therapeutic utility. Hyperactive children who are intellectually well endowed respond well to stimulants; as one descends the ladder, however, the response is diminished. Mildly retarded children respond less well to stimulants; moderately retarded children respond only on rare occasions; and severely retarded children respond not at all. The degree of neuropathic insult, then, measured in terms of intellectual capacity, predicts the success of treatment with a presynaptic agonist. Yet, it is among the moderate and severely retarded that we find the greatest degree of amantadine response. It would seem, then, that there is a Jacksonian hierarchy to dopaminergic therapeutics. When axial brainstem structures are impaired, whatever hope one may have of success can come only by way of directly stimulating the postsynaptic neuron.

Other Dopamine Agonists

The therapeutic effects of psychostimulants and amantadine are attributed to their neurochemical action as dopamine agonists. It is therefore reasonable to inquire whether other dopamine agonists may also be therapeutic for TBI.

In the treatment of AD/HA patients, the strategy has yielded variable results. The dopamine agonists amantadine and L-dopa have not been useful (Mattes, 1980; Langer et al., 1982), while the tricyclic antidepressants and monoamine inhibitors are very effective (Gualtieri, 1977; Zemetkin et al., 1985). The antidepressant bupropion, a dopamine reuptake blocker, is also an effective treatment for AD/HA patients (Clay et al., 1988). Along the same lines, narcoleptic patients may be treated with tricyclic antidepressants as well as stimulants (Dement and Guillemenault, 1973).

The utility of antidepressants in TBI patients is a special case, and the issue will be discussed further on. The central focus here are the dopamine agonists bromocriptine, pergolide, and L-dopa, which are not notably successful in AD/HA or narcolepsy but which may have some utility for TBI; for example, it has been claimed that L-dopa may promote coma recovery (Bareggi et al., 1975). It has also been claimed that Sinemet may advance the recovery process in TBI patients who have achieved a "plateau" in their recovery (Lal et al., 1988). Sadjapour et al. (1984) described the case of an 18-year-old male who had a left occipital lobectomy at age 9 because of an arteriovenous malformation. His residua included spastic right hemiparesis, bilateral spasticity, and expressive muteness. Following treatment with Sinemet (25/100 q, 3–4 h), the patient's motor function and expressive skills underwent a "remarkable transformation" (Sadjapour et al., 1984, p. 4); he was able to dress and feed himself, to ambulate with assistance, and to speak comparatively fluently. Tremors and dysmetria were also improved. Clinical benefits were confirmed initially in a placebo comparison; they persisted over 30 months of follow-up, and were seen virtually every day when the patient experienced an "on–off" phenomenon.

Bromocriptine is an ergot polypeptide derivative, originally characterized as a prolactin inhibitor. It decreases dopamine turnover in the median eminence and in the corpus striatum. Central dopaminergic stimulation is assumed to be responsible for its significant therapeutic action in patients with idiopathic parkinsonism (Johnson et al., 1976a). Bromocriptine is either a direct or an indirect agonist at the dopamine receptor.

Bromocriptine is currently marketed as a treatment for galactorrhoea and to arrest of physiological lactation. It is the treatment of choice for the neuroleptic malignant syndrome (Pearlman, 1986), and it is also used as a treatment for parkinsonism.

Treatment with bromocriptine has been reported to improve the level of arousal in one man with akinetic mutism (Ross and Stewart, 1981); to alleviate symptoms of neglect in two patients with right hemisphere infarcts (Fleet et al., 1987); and to improve symptoms of apathy and stereotyped behavior in a young woman with bilateral thalamic infarcts (Catsman-Berrevoets and Van Harskamp, 1988). The combination of bromocriptine and morphine was successful in controlling diencephalic autonomic seizures in a young man with diffuse brain injuries (Bullard, 1987). Bromocriptine also reversed the incapacitating effects of chronic portasystemic encephalopathy, a disorder that is believed to be related to a defect in central dopamine neurotransmission (Morgan et al., Sherlock, 1977).

Pergolide is a potent dopamine receptor agonist, an alternative to bromocriptine in patients with Parkinson's disease. There is no literature on pergolide in TBI. The stimulant pentylenetetrazol (metrazol) is formulated in combination with vitamins as a "tonic" for geriatric patients. In addition to its alleged stimulating effects, pentylenetetrazol may retard the neuromorphological correlates of aging in rats (Landfield et al., 1981). However, it is an epileptogenic drug, and this could limit its utility in TBI patients. Most geriatric physicians consider it to be an "obsolete" treatment of limited use.

It would appear, then, that the broad spectrum of dopaminergic drugs has therapeutic utility in the treatment of TBI patients, to enhance recovery or to alleviate undesirable symptoms and difficult behaviors. The same is true of animals; for example, a number of different dopamine agonists (L-dopa, amantadine, pirebedil, apomorphine) led to a "dramatic and apparently permanent abolition" of the hyperreactivity or rage syndrome that results from surgical damage to the septal nuclei of the rat forebrain (Marotta et al., 1977).

It has been suggested that L-dopa, amantadine, pirebedil, bromocriptine, apomorphine, and amphetamine are examples of a spectrum of drugs acting on the dopamine system, but with different weightings of direct and indirect dopaminergic activity (Schneiden and Cox, 1976). The different behavioral effects of dopamine agonist may be explained on the basis of differential behavioral effects at specific classes of dopamine receptors: excitatory and inhibitory receptors, pre- and postsynaptic receptors, and D_1 and D_2 receptors (Gianutsos and Moore, 1980).

There is, however, no clear guide to the choice of a dopamine agonist beyond the simple rule that has already been advanced (Gualtieri et al., 1989): the psychostimulants are better for high-level patients, with comparatively mild symptoms of apathy, anergia, inattention, and amnesia; and the other dopamine agonists are better for lower level patients with a wider variety of behavioral symptoms and more diffuse and severe injuries.

Antidepressants

There are three classes of antidepressants: one that is defined chemically (the tricyclic antidepressants, TCA); one that is defined pharmacologically (monoamine oxidase inhibitors, MAOI); and one that is defined historically (the 'novel antidepressants'). The first group, the TCA, is the most venerable and the most popular; but for all practical purposes, all the antidepressants are more or less equal for treating depression, anxiety, and panic. The proper choice of an antidepressant is based on subtle differences in the pharmacological activity of the drugs, on even more subtle differences in their clinical response profiles, and on major differences in their side-effect profiles.

The TCA are composed of two groups: the "tertiary" or the dimethylated amines [imipramine (IMI), amitryptiline (AMI), doxepin (DOX), chlorimipramine (CMI)] and the "secondary" or monomethylated amines [desipramine (DMI), nortyptiline (NOR), protrypiline (PRO)]. You can tell the difference by holding a tablet up to the light and counting the number of methyl groups on the side chain. This structural difference confers special pharmacological effects. Tertiary amines, for example, are more potent blockers of norepinephrine reuptake (Svensson, 1978). It is possible that this structural difference accounts for the relative potency of tertiary amine TCA in agitated depressives, because it may confer a sedative effect.

The sedating effects of a given TCA may also be a function of its anticholinergic and antihistaminic properties. The relative anticholinergic potencies of commercially available TCA are (in descending order): AMI-DOX-PRO-IMI-NOR-DMI (Richelson, 1979). This list is extremely important for TBI patients, because an anticholinergic drug may have negative effects on memory and motor performance (Wetzel et al., 1981). Thus, NOR and DMI may be better choices for the TBI patient than more anticholinergic TCA such as AMI, DOX, or IMI. On theoretical grounds, one is led to prefer secondary amines because they are less anticholinergic. In individual cases, however, such theoretical differences may be less salient; clinical success may be won with tertiary amine TCA, and behavioral improvement may occur without overt evidence of cognitive/motor compromise (e.g., Jackson et al., 1985).

The relative antihistaminic potencies of the TCA are (in descending order): DOX-AMI-NOR-IMI-PRO-DMI (Richelson, 1979). On this count, then, DMI ought to be the first-choice drug for depressed TBI patients when sedation is not a desired effect. In TBI patients it hardly ever is. On the other hand, DOX or AMI might be better choices for the depressed TBI patient with severe insomnia; in some instances, the importance of restful sleep may outweigh the theoretical disadvantage of negative memory and motor effects. Trazodone, however, is usually preferred for such indications. One advantage to AMI is that it is said to be the TCA least likely to lower the seizure threshold (Clifford et al., 1985), which may or may not be true.

All the TCA are toxic in overdose situations. In an adult, as little as 800 mg of IMI, for example, can be fatal; suicide is always a risk in TBI patients, and the TCA are the most lethal of all psychoactive drugs.

The MAOI have not been used very frequently in North America because physicians were afraid of the hypertensive crisis that can attend the consumption of tyramine-rich foods (Chianti, beer, aged cheese, broad beans). Patients in turn are often reluctant to forgo such delicacies, especially broad beans. That is probably an excess of zeal, however, because a tyramine-induced hypertensive crisis is not a common sequela to MOAI treatment, and the drugs are extremely effective antidepressants, with stimulant-like effects and hardly any known negative neuropsychological effects (Zametkin et al., 1985). They are barely anticholinergic (Comfort, 1982), and they may be particularly useful in the "atypical depressions" that TBI patients are wont to suffer (Robinson et al., 1978). On the other hand, Saran (1985) did not have much success in depressed TBI patients treated with the MOAI phenelzine.

Representatives of this class of antidepressants include phenelzine (Nardil), tranylcypromine (Parnate, Eutonyl), and isocarboxazid (Marplan). All these are competitive inhibitors of MAO-A, so patients who take them are vulnerable to the "cheese effect." Deprenyl, which will be discussed later on, is an inhibitor of MAO-B, so patients who take it do not have to worry about dangerous cheese.

MOAI should not be used in combination with stimulants or carbamazepine, or with sympathomimetic or tricyclic antidepressant drugs.

Stimulants are occasionally useful as antidepressants, but only occasionally (Keaton and Raskind, 1980). In a TBI patient who has memory/attention problems, hypoarousal, apathy, and depression, it might be better to begin treatment with a stimulant in hopes that depressive symptoms will also lift as other symptoms clear. Failing that, an MAOI (Deprenyl) might be tried, or a heterocyclic antidepressant like trazodone or a monomethylated TCA like DMI.

Carbamazepine (CBZ, Tegretol) is an antidepressant in theory but only rarely in fact; more than simple depression is required to indicate a trial of CBZ (see following). Lithium is not a very good antidepressant, but it may serve to *augment* the TCA response in refractory depressives (Heninger et al., 1983), and it may prevent the recurrence of depressive episodes (Gerbino et al., 1978). If CBZ or lithium were indicated for other symptoms in a TBI patient, for explosive episodes for example, one would not be surprised if an antidepressant effect were also observed. But it may not happen. Temporal lobe epileptics, for example, are usually treated with CBZ, but they are terribly vulnerable to depressive episodes in spite of it.

One should never forget that psychotherapy may be an extremely effective treatment for mild-to-moderate depressions; or that the first treatment for any depressive disorder ought to be to alleviate life situations that may lead to frustration, bitterness, alienation, and demoralization. There is no reason to propose extreme treatments such as ECT or combined TCA–MAOI treatment for refractory TBI depressives.

Even in the face of losses and handicaps that may aggravate depressive feelings, it is not unlikely that the prevalence of dysphoria and depression in TBI patients is related to the monamine derangements they suffer as a result of brain injury. This neurochemical origin to their difficulties should impel research in the direction of neuropharmacological correctives. Comparative treatment studies for TBI patients should be a high priority. The antidepressant effects of stimulants, MAOI, trazodone, and DMI are well worth careful clinical investigation. Physicians who treat TBI patients deserve to be guided by information carried from research with TBI patients, not only by information from other clinical groups.

Deprenyl, Selegeline, or Eldepryl

The new name is Selegeline, but for a long time it was called L-deprenyl. It was an orphan drug in the United States, but it has been used in Europe since 1985 as an adjunct in the treatment of Parkinson's disease and as an antidepressant. It is a monoamine oxidase inhibitor (MAOI), a selective and irreversible inhibitor of MAO-B. Because this is the primary enzyme that metabolizes dopamine in the brain, treatment with deprenyl increases the availability of endogenous and exogenous dopamine, thus its anti-parkinsonian and antidepressant effects.

Because deprenyl is only an inhibitor of MAO-B, it is free of the "cheese effect," the sympathetic crisis produced by ingestion of tyramine, levodopa, or other amines

(Golbe, 1988). That is a function of antagonism of MAO-A, which is located primarily in the periphery (i.e., outside the brain) and which catabolizes serotonin, norepinephrine, and tyramine. Because deprenyl is only an MAO-A inhibitor at high doses, the risk of hypertensive crisis is small, except perhaps in overdose situations. But what you have to do is overdose on deprenyl and cheese, too.

Deprenyl was synthesized and developed in Hungary as a novel MAO-inhibitor antidepressant. When L-dopa was introduced, people began to use deprenyl as a supplement, and the current indication is to augment the effect of L-dopa in advanced cases of Parkinson's disease (Golbe, 1988).

Maximum plasma levels are achieved within 30 to 120 minutes after oral administration, and a decline in platelet MAO-B activity is apparent, in most subjects, after 2 hours. The elimination half-life averages 39 hours (range, 16-69), and after the drug is discontinued MAO-B activity returns to baseline levels in 2 or 3 weeks (Golbe, 1988). Because of the long half-life, a once-per-day dose is possible, although it is usually given twice daily to Parkinson's patients. The usual dose is 5 mg bid. Inhibition of MAO-A probably does not begin until a dose of 40 mg/day has been achieved (Golbe, 1988; Tariot et al., 1987).

Deprenyl is metabolized to amphetamine and metamphetamine, although it is not clear whether its therapeutic effects are related to the amphetamine metabolites. The toxicity profile is quite favorable, with no observed cardiovascular effects such as orthostatic hypotension. Peptic ulcer disease may be reactivated by deprenyl, and mild and usually transient elevations of hepatic enzymes have been noted.

The importance of deprenyl is more than its adjunctive behavior with L-dopa and its unique status as a safe MAO-inhibitor antidepressant. There have been reports to suggest that it may prolong the life of parkinsonian patients with advanced disease, and that it may delay the requirement to initiate treatment with L-dopa in patients with beginning symptoms of Parkinson's disease (PD). It may delay the death of striatal dopaminergic neurons. The experimental model was a unique experiment of nature, the development of PD in a group of heroin addicts who had been exposed to the neurotoxic contaminant. The conversion of MPTP to a neurotoxic metabolite, 1-methyl-4-phenylpridinium ion (MPP^+), is blocked by MAO inhibitors, including deprenyl. The idea is that striatal death may be delayed in parkinsonian patients by preventing the formation of pyridinium species (Tetrud and Langston, 1989).

The alternative is the oxidation hypothesis: oxidation of dopamine by MAO results in the formation of oxygen-derived species, such as hydrogen peroxide and hydroxyl radicals, that can be toxic to dopaminergic neurons. As neurons die, turnover of dopamine is increased in the neurons that remain, and there is even more production of neurotoxic oxygen radicals. Deprenyl is thought to be prophylactic in PD because it moderates oxidative stress by preventing the oxidation of dopamine by MAO-B. This may have some importance on the physiology of normal aging, a process that is associated with an inexorable depletion of dopaminergic neurons even in the absence of PD. Indeed, deprenyl has been discovered to prolong the life span of laboratory rats who do not have PD (Sonsalla and Golbe, 1988; Tetrud and Langston, 1989).

If deprenyl does exercise some sort of "prophylactic" effect in PD, or if it does attenuate one of the natural degenerative processes associated with aging, one should ask whether it can also be useful in slowing the course of deterioration in other neurodegenerative conditions like Alzheimer's disease. There have been reports of symptomatic improvement in Alzheimer's patients treated with deprenyl, over the short term (Tariot et al., 1987), so it is not unreasonable to test the hypothesis in longer term trials.

Deprenyl is, at least, an alternative dopaminergic drug for TBI patients, and the possible indications are the same as they are for other dopaminergic drugs. If, however, there is any chance that it exercises some kind of effect against neurodegeneration, it may well become the dopaminergic drug of choice for TBI patients. Clinical experience to date, at the Neuropsychiatry Clinic, has been entirely favorable.

Bupropion (BP)

Bupropion is a unique antidepressant (a "phenylaminoketone" or a "monocyclic phenylbutylamine"). It is not serotonergic or noradrenergic, like all the other antidepressants; it has no cholinergic effects, and it is not an inhibitor of monoamine oxidase (MAO) (Stern et al., 1982). It is possible that its activity is mediated by an obscure but significant effect on dopaminergic neurotransmission (Dufresne et al., 1984). The chemical structure of BP bears some resemblance to amphetamine and other central stimulants, although it does not have amphetamine-like abuse potential (Griffin et al., 1983).

BP has several advantages over the tricyclic antidepressants: It has no anticholinergic side effects, it does not cause tachycardia or orthostatic hypotension (Chouinard et al., 1981), there is no tendency to weight gain, it does not have an additive depressant effect with alcohol, and it is not lethal in circumstances of overdose (Stern et al., 1982). It also does not have an adverse effect on memory or motor performance. Indeed, it may improve neuropsychological performance in some patients (Clay et al., 1988).

Peak levels are achieved within 3 hours of an oral dose, and the elimination half-life is 10 to 20 hours. The manufacturer's recommended dose is 300 mg/day and the recommended maximum is 450 mg/day. Dosing is recommended at tid, although a bid schedule is usually satisfactory.

The efficacy of BP for depression is about equal to the other antidepressants, although there appears to be a class of patients who respond to BP and not to other antidepressants. BP is also an effective treatment for patients with attention deficit/hyperactivity; in these, positive behavioral effects may be complemented by positive effects on attention, memory, and motor performance (Clay et al., 1988). It may be that BP is effective prophylaxis against cyclic mood disorders (Wright et al., 1985; Shopsin, 1983).

The side-effect profile is quite favorable. Skin rash occurs in about 3% of patients. There are no associated laboratory or EEG changes (Van Wyck Fleet et al., Hart-Truax et al., 1983). The major side effects are neuropsychiatric. BP may evoke vivid dreams, increased emotionality, increased intensity of sensory experience, and alteration of time perception (Becker and Dufresne, 1982). Some of the subjective effects may be positive, like the feeling of improved attention and memory (Becker and Dufresne, 1982), but subjective side effects that are really bothersome are nervousness, agitation, and excitement, even to the point of frank psychosis (Golden et al., 1985).

BP was withheld from the market because of an apparent high frequency of generalized tonic-clonic seizures in certain patient groups. This was a difficult problem to evaluate, because virtually all the antidepressants have been associated with occasional seizures; the association appears to be dose related (Peck et al., 1983). The incidence can only be estimated, although 0.5% to 1.0% is the usual range that is given. It is not clear that any existing antididepressant is better than another for the patient who is prone to seizures, although some clinicians recommend doxepin, and others, amitryptiline.

The manufacturer says that the incidence of seizures in patients treated with BP is 4 in 1000, which is the same as the rate for all the other antidepressants, maprotiline excepted. At doses greater than 450 mg/day, the risk of seizures may be higher. Seizures are said to be more likely to occur with BP if the patient has a predisposing factor, for example, a history of head trauma, a history of drug or alcohol abuse, or concomitant treatment with other drugs that lower the seizures threshold. But that is conjecture. The association between BP and seizures may simply turn out to be one of those spurious associations, like carbamazepine and agranulocytosis, that will cloud the reputation of the drug for years.

This is a shame, because BP would appear to be one of the ideal antidepressants/dopamine agonists for head injury patients and for other neuropathic groups such as demented and parkinsonian patients. A physician who prescribed BP to such patients, however, would be flying in the face of the most stern admonitions from the FDA.

On the other hand, high doses of psychostimulants and of dopamine agonists like amantadine may also lead to occasional seizures, but that has not prevented their prescription to neuropathic patients. Nor has the problem of seizures limited their clinical utility. Low doses of BP may turn out to be perfectly all right, but it will take very careful surveillance before one can address that issue with confidence.

Trazodone

Trazodone (TRZ) is a phenylpiperazine derivative of triazolopyridine. It is the sole representative of a unique class of antidepressant drugs. It has been used in Europe since 1974, and in the United States since 1982.

TRZ is a competitive inhibitor of serotonin reuptake into the synaptosome, with little effect on the uptake of norepinephrine or of dopamine. It is less potent than chlorimipramine in terms of serotonin reuptake, but more selective in terms of effect on other monoamine neurotransmitters (Riblet et al., 1979).

TRZ is well absorbed from the gastrointestinal tract, and absorption may be enhanced by food. The elimination half-life of the unchanged drug is about 6 hours, and for total drug and metabolites about 13 hours (Brogden et al., 1981). The therapeutic dose range is very broad; the minimum effective dose may be as low as 50 or 100 mg/day; and the maximum is 600 mg/day. The average adult dose for depressive illness is 150 to 400 mg/day.

TRZ is an antidepressant, of course, and the primary indication is treatment of unipolar depression. It may be particularly good for depression with anxiety or for depression with severe insomnia. Because it is a serotonergic antidepressant, however, it is also considered as an alternative treatment for neuropsychiatric disorders that are customarily treated by other serotonergic antidepressants. An example is obsessive-compulsive disorder (OCD), although fluoxetine (FXT) and chlorimipramine (CMI) are usually better choices. Some OCD patients, however, develop akathisia on FXT and CMI and thus are better treated with TRZ. Amitrypitiline and FXT are prescribed for chronic pain patients and for patients with dysesthesia of thalamic origin; TRZ is another alternative there.

One's real interest in TRZ is with TBI patients. In a review of antidepressant prescription at the Neuropsychiatry Clinic, it was the drug most commonly used for brain injury patients with agitated depression, and with postconcussion syndrome with severe insomnia.

TRZ has been effective in the treatment of sleep apnea associated with olivopon-tocerebellar degeneration (Salazar-Grueso et al., 1988). It has also been effective in two severe cases of essential tremor that failed to respond to propanalol (McLeod and White, 1986). It has been used effectively to control aggression and self-injurious behavior in mentally handicapped patients (see Chapter 7, this volume).

The singular advantage of TRZ is its relative lack of cardiovascular and anticholinergic side effects, which makes it a good choice, for example, for the geriatric depressed patient (Gerner 1980; Gershon, 1984). It is however very sedating. This might be an advantage for patients with severe insomnia, but excessive daytime sedation is its major limitation.

Sedation is the most common psychological side effect of TRZ, but there have also been reports of delirium (Damlouji and Ferguson, 1984) and mania (Warren and Bick, 1984). It may increase the libido (Gartrell, 1986) and there have been a couple of fabulous reports of women who took TRZ and experienced spontaneous orgasm whenever they yawned.

The catastrophic effect of TRZ is priapism, a prolonged and usually painful penile erection unrelated to sexual activity. It is estimated that some degree of increased penile tumescence occurs in 1 of 7,000 male users of TRZ, and that the problem may be so severe that surgery is required in 1 of 23,000 male users (Hayes and Kristoff, 1986). The catastrophic result of priapism is permanent impairment of erectile function or impotence. Some of the reported cases had reported abnormal or unusual erections before priapism developed; patients on TRZ should be advised to discontinue the medication if this occurs (Hayes and Kristoff, 1986).

Priapism has also been associated with drugs like chlorpromazine, thioridazine, mesoridazine, molindone, thiothixene, phenelzine, guanethidine, hydralazine, prazocin, heparin, ethanol, and marijuana, but much less commonly than with TRZ. The pathogenesis is probably related to peripheral $alpha_1$-adrenergic blockade and/or central serotonin agonism (Kogeorgos and de Alwis, 1986; Yeragani et al., 1987).

The most common symptoms of TRZ overdose are drowsiness, ataxia, nausea/vomiting, and dry mouth. In some cases, CNS depression may progress to coma, but this is more likely if TRZ is taken with alcohol or with other CNS depressant drugs. There have been no reported cases, to date, of death from overdose of TRZ (Coccaro and Siever, 1985).

TRZ has fallen from favor among psychiatrists, whose patients may be sedated to an excessive degree as a consequence of treatment, and who tend to prefer the newer serotonergic antidepressants like FXT. It remains a favorite, however, among physicians who treat TBI patients especially for insomnia.

Fluoxetine

Fluoxetine (FXT) and its demethylated metabolite, Norfluoxetine, are chemically distinct from the tricyclic antidepressants (TCA) and from the monoamine oxidase inhibitors (MAOIs) (FXT is substituted propylamine). Neither FXT nor its active metabolite inhibits norepinephrine reuptake; neither blocks cholinergic (muscarinic), alpha-adrenergic, histaminergic, or serotonergic$_2$ (5-hydroxytryptophol, 5-HT$_2$) receptors. They are, however, potent inhibitors of serotonin reuptake (Byerley et al., 1988). FXT is more potent than TRZ, but it may not be as potent a serotonergic compound as chlorimipramine (CMI); the latter has noradrenergic properties that FXT does not have, so FXT may be a more "selective" drug. In this respect, it is similar to two other antidepressants, zimelidine and fluvoxamine, but they are not commercially available at this time (Lemberger et al., 1985).

FXT is well absorbed after oral administration, and peak plasma concentrations occur in 6 to 8 hours; absorption is not affected by food. The parent drug (FXT) has a half-life of 2 to 3 days, and Nor-FXT has a half-life of 7 to 9 days. The recommended starting and maintenance dose of FXT is 20 mg/day, and daily doses as high as 80 mg/day have been used.

The common side effects are nausea, nervousness, insomnia, headache, tremor, anxiety, drowsiness, dry mouth, diaphoresis, and diarrhea (Ayd, 1988), but it is really quite remarkable how seldom side effects occur with the drug, especially at the ordinary dose of 20 mg/day. Because it is free of anticholinergic side effects, has no cardiovascular side effects, and is a very effective antidepressant, it has become quite popular. In contrast to the TCA, it does not cause weight gain, which is a very desirable aspect; in fact, it may often work as an appetite suppressant. Patients on FXT may actually lose weight. For adult patients at least that is even more desirable (Fuller and Wong, 1989), but for children it may be problematic.

FXT, like TRZ, has been associated with the bizarre concatenation of yawning, clitoral engorgement, and spontaneous orgasm (Modell et al., 1989). It is only a matter of time, then, before a case of priapism or of nipple priapism is also reported.

Akathisia is a clinically significant side effect of FXT. It has also been known to cause or to aggravate extrapyramidal symptoms. These have been, thus far, only transient reactions, and there is no reason to be afraid of long-term side effects like tardic dyskinesia.

One may speculate that FXT, as a cationic amphiphilic drug, can lead to intracellular accumulation of phospholipids. This is probably only a theoretical risk, and its clinical significance may be small. But it is something to consider in patients who are forced to take the drug for long periods of time. In such patients one may consider periodic (annual) slit-lamp examinations, chest x-rays, and measures of renal, adrenal, and hepatic function.

No clinically significant drug interactions have been reported with FXT. There are no clinical laboratory tests that seem to be affected by FXT treatment. There are no clinical data on teratogenic effects yet, but animal studies in doses as high as 15 mg/kg/day have shown no mutagenic or teratogenic effects. No deaths have been reported, thus far, from overdose of FXT. Doses in the range of 1 to 3 g have been noted to cause seizures, blurred vision, tachycardia, emesis, and ST segment depression (Somni et al., 1987). The problem, however, of FXT-induced suicidal preoccupation, or thoughts of violence, is extremely disturbing information (Teicher et al., 1990). It is likely to limit the extraordinary popularity of this new antidepressant. It certainly changes the nature of the warning one has to give the patient, and people have come to be wary of the drug.

The major use of FXT, of course, is as an antidepressant. As a serotonergic antidepressant, one may expect it to be useful for cases of OCD, and indeed it is (Levine et al., 1989). It has been effective in at least one case of self-injurious behavior in a mentally retarded child (see Chapter 7, this volume). Physicians have begun to prescribe FXT as an appetite suppressant, a weight-loss drug. The first clinical trials are being done, apparently, for members of their families.

Neurologists have begun to use the drug for pain syndromes and for thalamic dysesthesias, and it may prove to be the drug of choice for poststroke emotionalism. The absence of anticholinergic side effects and the absence of risk in circumstances of overdose make it an interesting drug, indeed, for TBI patients, and there have been preliminary reports of efficacy in the literature (Cassidy, 1989).

Lithium

In the nineteenth century, lithium salts were added to patent medicine formulations, perhaps for their mild sedating properties or more likely as just one more inert substance. Lithium, as it occurs in natural springs, for example, has no biological activity at all; if an old country spa was named "Lithium Springs"—and there are a few, in North Carolina and Tennessee—some other medicinal element must have contributed to the success of the place.

At one point lithium was marketed as a salt substitute; it is an element just above sodium on the periodic table. There was a time when people would actually flavor their food with the salty crystals of lithium chloride, and there were a few deaths that resulted from that practice. This unhappy experience may have contributed to the initial skepticism that greeted the introduction of lithium as a psychotropic drug. In spite of the signal work of Mogens Schou, a Danish psychiatrist, lithium was not approved by the FDA until 1970, for acute mania, and not until 1974 as a prophylactic in manic-depression. (In Japan, lithium was not available until the late 1970s, this is what led Okuma to investigate carbamazepine as a possible treatment for bipolar disorder.)

Lithium salts were once a treatment for gout. The lithium salt is the most soluble of the urate compounds, and lithium was prescribed for its uricosuric effects. It was this property that led Cade, an Australian psychiatrist, to examine the protective effects of lithium against urea toxicity in guinea pigs; why Cade was interested in the subject of urea toxicity is a mystery to the author.

With lithium, the guinea pigs became "lethargic and unresponsive" (Cade, 1949). Although "it may seem a long distance from lethargy in guinea pigs to the excitement of psychotics," Cade treated 16 chronic psychotic patients with remarkable results, especially in manics. This inferential leap still leaves one breathless. It led to the lithium era, one of the most important chapters in the history of psychiatry. Cade's genius was inspired, by the way, not only by his experiments in lower animals. He cited, incidentally "the waters of certain wells (with) special virtue in the treatment of mental illness ... Very likely proportional to the lithium content of the waters."

Lithium today is prescribed for bipolar affective disorder and for the prophylaxis of recurrent manic or depressive psychosis. The prophylactic effect may also be felt in recurrent unipolar depression (Gerbino et al., Gershon, 1978). The drug may also be useful for people with severe mood swings; patients who are "cyclothymic," but not given to extremes of mania or depression. It is extremely effective in some —but not all—patients with explosive rage attacks or aggressive outbursts (Worrall et al., 1975). It may augment the treatment of depression in patients who are refractory to antidepressant treatment (Heninger et al.,1983) and in obsessive-compulsive patients who are refractory to the effects of fluoxetine or chlorimipramine (Rasmussen, 1984).

Lithium has two major therapeutic advantages: it is a "yes-no" drug; that is, it works either very well or not at all. It is rarely difficult to decide whether a lithium trial has been successful, especially if therapeutic blood levels are maintained, and so long as the positive effects of drug treatment—over several months in some cases—are allowed to unfold.

The second advantage of lithium is its unique toxicity profile. A low therapeutic index is sometimes thought to be a disadvantage, but a drug that makes the patient sick when toxic levels are approached has some real advantages for monitoring. High (but not dangerous) levels of lithium are associated with nausea, vomiting, diarrhea, irritability or sedation, and tremor or muscle rigidity. When this occurs the medication can be stopped until the blood concentration falls to a safer level, and serious toxicity can be averted. A simple examination for hyperreflexia will usually reveal mildly elevated lithium levels. On the other hand, tremor, polyuria, and polydypsia are side effects that may occur within the therapeutic range.

Although lithium toxicity can be catastrophic, it can be avoided by exercising the most elementary precautions. The cost is minor, because acute toxicity is probably the only toxicity the drug has. There are no subtle, long-term side effects that can sneak up on you. At one point people were afraid that long-term lithium treatment was nephrotoxic, and this is true, on a microscopic level. But it does not lead to functional renal impairment, even after 20 or 30 years of treatment (Jenner, 1979).

Lithium may be sedating in normal subjects (Reisberg and Gershon, 1979) and also in patients. This may be troublesome for head injury patients, but the drug would never be prescribed to such a patient unless there were severe behavior problems or emotional instability against which a modicum of sedation, if it occurred, would be an acceptable price to pay. On the other hand, sedation is not an inevitable lithium effect. Neuropsychological effects of lithium are reported to be nonexistent (Henry et al., 1973) or in the direction of impaired performance. Negative effects have been noted in digit symbol and trials in normal subjects (Judd et al., 1977); in tactual performance, finger-tapping, block design, and digit symbol, trials, form board, and verbal comparison in psychotic patients (Friedman, et al., 1977); in short-term memory in depressives (Kusumo and Vaugn, 1977; Christodoulo et al., 1981); and in aggressive children (Platt et al., 1981).

Lithium has been said to lower the seizure threshold (Brumback et al., 1975), but that is probably a canard, and it is more likely that lithium treatment will actually raise the seizure threshold (Jus et al., 1973). In epileptic patients who have psychiatric disorders for which lithium may be indicated, carbamazepine and valproate are suitable alternatives, but lithium is not by any means contraindicated.

When should lithium be considered in a TBI patient? When there is a traditional psychiatric indication. Not necessarily for "classical" affective disorders, because these are not very common in TBI patients. Rather for its "secondary" indications, for conditions characterized by extremes of emotional instability, such as explosions of rage or violence. If these attacks are not epileptic in origin, lithium is the drug of choice; if there is any indication at all of an epileptic focus, carbamazepine is the drug of choice.

Lithium was the first psychotropic drug found to possess specific antiaggression properties. The evidence is very strong. It will induce Siamese fighting fish to live together harmoniously in the same tank; it will reduce territorial aggression in mice and hamsters, too (Weischer, 1969). Isolation-induced aggression and footshock-induced aggression decreases in lithium-treated rats (Sheard, 1970b), and the hyperaggressive and hypersexual behavior of cats and rats treated with *p*-chlorophenylalanine is inhibited by lithium in doses that do not inhibit motor activity (Sheard, 1970a). The effect of lithium in reducing aggressive behavior of coyotes against sheep is not a pharmacological effect, however; it is a taste-aversion effect, because lithium tastes so bad (Smith, 1977).

Lithium has reduced aggressive behavior in assaultive prisoners (Sheard, 1975) and in aggressive mentally retarded people (Worrall et al., 1975) and in self-injurious retarded people (Cooper and Fowlie, 1973). The site and mode of therapeutic action of lithium for aggression, or, indeed, for any of its psychiatric indications, are unknown. Presynaptic effects include adenylate cyclase inhibition, prostaglandin E1 synthesis inhibition, enhanced reuptake of serotonin and norepinephrine and nerve terminals, and a functional decrease in dopamine. Lithium may also decrease dopamine and norepinephrine effects at postsynaptic receptors. It blocks the release of thyroid hormone and it may interfere with testosterone synthesis (Jefferson et al., 1983).

Lithium, by substituting for various cations, and possibly by stabilizing cell membranes, can alter the properties of excitable tissue. Lithium can also inhibit the final dephosphorylation step of inositol synthesis, and inositol lipids play a major role in cell signaling by functioning as precursors of second messengers, which release intracellular calcium (Berridge, 1989). This may account for its teratogenic effects as well as its diverse neuropsychiatric effects.

There are no controlled studies of lithium in TBI patients, but there is an extensive literature on its use in other patient classes with 'organic' brain problems. Lithium trials have been reported to be successful in one TBI patient with agitation, confusion, and belligerence (Haas and Cope, 1985); in "organic brain syndrome" of "diverse etiology" (including TBI) characterized by affective instability (Hale and Donaldson, 1982); and in one patient who became hypomanic following CVA and surgical trauma to the temporal lobe (Levine et al., 1986). Lithium carbonate and behavioral treatment were said to benefit two severely damaged TBI adults who had demonstrated unrelenting assaultive, destructive, and self-injurious behavior of several year's duration (Rosenbaum and Barry, 1975). Lithium will probably find its niche for severely disturbed TBI patients for whom neuroleptics might at one time have been prescribed.

There is probably not much point in mounting efficacy studies of lithium in TBI patients; the burden of proof would be on someone who proposed that lithium *did not* work in TBI patients who were manic, cyclothymic, or explosive. The important research questions are exactly *how* effective lithium is in TBI patients, in *whom* is it most effective, whether any *cognitive* or *motor* impairment accompanies the treatment, and how it compares to its major alternative, carbamazepine.

Most of the Western world's supply of lithium comes from Gastonia, North Carolina, where it is dug out of the earth with steam shovels; there is an outlet store at the plant.

Neuroleptics

Neuroleptics (major tranquilizers, antipsychotics) are unsurpassed for the treatment of the acute psychosis, agitation, disorganization, or assaultiveness in patients with a wide range of mental disorders. Long-term neuroleptic treatment is indicated for many (but not all) schizophrenic patients, for some Tourette's syndrome cases, and for cases of severe agitation or psychotic disorganization. Neuroleptics have been used for untold millions of patients around the world, but their extraordinary clinical utility is almost equaled by a troublesome side-effect profile and a tendency to be overprescribed in certain clinical settings. All too often, the short-term benefits of neuroleptic treatment are translated into long-term treatment of limited utility.

The following is a typical neuroleptic scenario for TBI patients: a patient is treated with intramuscular and then oral haloperidol, to control agitation and assaultiveness during emergence from coma. The drug is continued for months after the patient is discharged. Then the patient appears for evaluation at a rehabilitation facility, anergic, depressed, and apathetic, with fine and gross motor coordination problems and deficits in attention, memory, and emotional control. The neuroleptic is withdrawn, and there is immediate improvement.

This is a typical example of short-term benefit for an appropriate indication— acute agitation—turning into inappropriate long-term treatment. The more intelligent course would have been to gradually taper the neuroleptic after the patient's emotional state had been stable for a couple of weeks. Neuroleptics should usually be tapered, by the way, not withdrawn abruptly; abrupt withdrawal from neuroleptics may precipitate seizures (Itil and Soldatos, 1980), and can also be the occasion of prompt relapse of severe behavior problems. Stepwise reduction by 25% decrements over 4 to 8 weeks usually averts such problems.

Agitation, explosiveness, emotional instability, disorganization, and psychosis in TBI patients are not necessarily confined to the immediate postrecovery period; they may be persistent symptoms of TBI. In such instances neuroleptics may be indicated, although they are not always effective. Relatively short trials of two or three neuroleptics, in succession, should be sufficient to determine whether treatment is going to be successful, and if it is not successful it is common sense to withdraw the patient from neuroleptics, reestablish a baseline, and try some other approach. Low-to-moderate doses are usually sufficient to establish whether a neuroleptic will be useful. High-dose treatment is rarely if ever necessary. It seems trite to warn against long-term treatment with an ineffective medication, but with neuroleptics the pattern is too common to ignore.

Tourette's syndrome may be the consequence of TBI, and low-dose neuroleptics are occasionally helpful. Low-dose neuroleptics may actually *enhance* cognitive performance, for example, in attentional tasks (Gualtieri and Hicks, 1985b); this is probably a presynaptic stimulant-like effect (Gualtieri and Patterson, 1986).

Neuroleptics may be divided into "low-potency" and "high-potency" classes. The low-potency neuroleptics are thioridazine (THD, Mellaril) and chlorpromazine (CPZ, Thorazine); they tend to be sedating, and THD in particular is a strongly anticholinergic neuroleptic. It also appears that the neuroleptic CPZ may impair short-term memory at dosages less than those required to cause motor impairment (Johnson, 1983). Such drugs probably should be avoided in TBI patients. The "high-potency" neuroleptics are less sedating and are preferred when a neuroleptic is required. Representatives of this class include fluphenazine (FPZ, Prolixin), trifluoperazine (TFP, Stelazine), and haloperidol (HDL, Haldol). HDL commonly causes dysphoria, however. High-potency neuroleptics are more likely to cause acute extrapyramidal reactions and neuroleptic malignant syndrome.

Neuroleptics can lower the seizure threshold. Pimozide and fluphenazine are the two neuroleptics least likely to do so, and HDL and THD are among those most likely to lower the seizure threshold (Itil and Soldatos, 1980; Oliver et al.,1982).

Do neuroleptics compromise the recovery process for TBI patients? Yes, if one extrapolates from the pre-clinical studies of Feeny et al. (1982). Perhaps, if one extrapolates from human studies and animal studies of neuroleptic-induced anhedonia (Wise, 1982), dysphoria (Caine and Polinsky, 1979), and cognitive and motor impairment (Killian et al., 1984). Yes indeed, if one is guided by the prevailing belief that deficits in dopaminergic neurotransmission are central to the pathophysiology of TBI. One is thus inclined to consider neuroleptics relatively *contraindicated* in TBI patients.

That is, as long as one excepts TBI patients with neuroleptic-responsive psychosis, hallucinosis, mania, Tourette's syndrome, assaultiveness, and agitation. The key in such cases is to determine whether the symptoms are indeed 'neuroleptic-responsive'; that is, that the drugs exert dramatic clinical effects when no other treatment will work as well; that their efficacy is established at a "minimal effective dose"; and that their continued clinical utility is assessed at reasonable intervals, perhaps every 6 months or so, by gradually tapering the dose. There is nothing "rational" about neuroleptic treatment for TBI patients; if anything, the treatment is "irrational" and something that should be assiduously avoided.

The issue is not even the negative cognitive or motor effects of neuroleptics, or their tendency to blunt the personality of treated patients. It is only partly influenced by their serious side effects: dysphoria, pseudo-parkinsonism, dystonia, tardive dyskinesia, hyperthermia, and the 'neuroleptic malignant syndrome'; photosensitivity, cholestatic jaundice, hypotension. It is in its largest dimension defined by their limited utility in the long-term management of TBI patients, and the superior effects to be won by more carefully selected psychotropic drugs. The key issue is that there usually are more effective treatments. Neuroleptics may be the best and only drug treatment for schizophrenia, but they are usually a poor third to carbamazepine and lithium for patients whose symptoms are a consequence of organic brain disorder. Perhaps the only unequivocal indication for neuroleptic treatment in neuropathic patients, aside from schizophrenia, is the psychosis that sometimes occurs in temporal lobe epileptic patients; in such cases it is often necessary to augment the effects of carbamazepine or valporate with low doses of a neuroleptic such as fluphenazine or pimozide.

Preexisting brain damage is sometimes listed as a risk factor for tardive dyskinesia. The clinical evidence is equivocal on this point, but the research is suggestive (Kane & Smith, 1982). Long-term neuroleptic treatment requires careful monitoring for tardive dyskinesia.

Metaclopramide

Metoclopramide is a special case, a dopamine antagonist that is not supposed to be a psychoactive drug at all; in fact, as a treatment for psychosis, it is an utter failure. But as an inadvertent cause of typical neuroleptic toxicity, like tardive dyskinesia, it is a thoroughgoing success.

Metaclopramide is a procainamide derivative, the first of a new class of dopamine antagonists with pronounced effects on the gastrointestinal tract (altered motility and antiemetic effects) (Harrington et al., 1983). It is not uncommonly prescribed for TBI patients in coma to alleviate some of the problems attendant on gastrostomy and gastric tube feeding, like esophageal reflux and gastric distension, because it decreases gastric emptying time. It is important to remember, however, that metaclopramide is also a centrally acting dopamine blocker, with particular affinity to the D2 receptor; that it is, in essence, an neuroleptic, with all the problems that drugs of this class may hold for TBI patients; for example, extrapyramidal effects, tardive dyskinesia, sedation, and possibly delayed or diminished recovery (Albibi and McCallum, 1983).

The prescription of metaclopramide may be unavoidable, at least for a short period of time, but it should not be an automatic choice; efforts should be made, first, to discover whether an H2 antagonist like famotidine, or a thoroughly innocuous substance like sucralfate (Carafate), will suffice for the clinical problem at hand.

The Psychotropic Anticonvulsants

The first question is whether an antiepileptic drug is necessary; the incidence of posttraumatic epilepsy is very low, lower in closed head injury patients, and higher in patients with penetrating head wounds. A seizure or two immediately post trauma does not spell the need for continued anticonvulsant treatment, and there is no evidence that "prophylactic" anticonvulsant therapy has any value at all (Salazar et al., 1985). Nevertheless, a large number of TBI patients present to rehabilitation centers on maintenance doses of anticonvulsants, usually phenytoin (dilantin). (Phenytoin is the ideal anticonvulsant to use in the neurosurgery ICU because it can be administered parenterally.) Maintenance anticonvulsants may be continued by inadvertence for months or even years after head injury. Not only is such treatment unnecessary, more likely than not, but it may contribute to depression, memory problems, and motor coordination difficulties.

The second question is, if an anticonvulsant is necessary, which anticonvulsant? Phenytoin and the barbiturate antconvulsants are perfectly effective for seizure control in patients with complex-partial seizures, focal seizures, or posttraumatic epilepsy. But they should be considered second- or third-line drugs, after carbamazepine (CBZ) and valproic acid (VPA).

The superiority of CBZ is based on three important elements:

1. It will suppress not only the electrical spread that emanates from an epileptic focus, but also the abnormal electrical activity of the focus itself (Wada, 1977). Thus, it may be an "anti-kindling" drug, one that prevents the long-term sequelae of focal epilepsy, especially temporal lobe epilepsy (Taylor, 1975).

2. It is an effective psychotrope, with a wide range of therapeutic uses, especially for depressed patients, bipolar patients, and patients with emotional instability, rage attacks, or assaultive or aggressive behavior (Evans and Gualtieri, 1985). Thus, it is the ideal treatment for epileptic patients with concomitant psychiatric difficulties.

3. The neuropsychological effects of CBZ are highly favorable when compared to other, more sedating anticonvulsants such as phenytoin, phenobarbital, and primidone. We have reviewed the comparative neuropsychological effects of CBZ on an earlier occasion (Evans and Gualtieri, 1985); in contrast to other anticonvulsants, CBZ effects on attention, memory, and motor performance are much less pronounced. That is not to imply that CBZ is perfectly benign in these respects, because it is not. It is not by any means a stimulant, which usually *improves* function in these areas (Evans et al., 1987b). But it is vastly preferable to the usual alternatives.

The psychotropic anticonvulsants CBZ and VPA are discussed in Chapter 6.

The behavioral problems of TBI patients that may respond to CBZ are similar to the current psychiatric indications for the drug:

1. mania, hypomania, recurrent affective disorders
2. emotional inability, emotional incontinence, 'catastrophic reactions', 'cyclothymic personality'
3. aggression and assaultiveness, especially of the episodic type.

Practicing psychiatrists have learned that some drugs—notably CBZ and VPA— are effective for a wide range of patients with severe, but diagnostically non-specific, disorders. Thus, they may be prescribed for virtually any severe psychiatric problem that proves refractory to conventional therapies. They may also be effective in *combination* with other psychotropic drugs: in combination with lithium, for refractory bipolar patients; in combination with neuroleptics (especially fluphenazine), for psychotic patients; and in combination with stimulants or amantadine for patients with concomitant attention or memory problems. Not only is CBZ the "universal second choice psychotrope" for refractory patients, it may also be a helpful adjunctive drug for patients who enjoy only a partial response to first-line medications.

Some TBI patients experience a dramatic change in behavioral status 1, 2, or 3 years after the original injury. The late development of severe psychopathology in a TBI patient is a rare and peculiar phenomenon. Although it may be analogous to the late psychosis of temporal lobe epilepsy patients, presumably the result of kindling, the actual mechanism is unknown. The fact that CBZ is sometimes effective in such patients supports the kindling hypothesis.

Physicians who treat TBI patients usually learn that CBZ is an extraordinarily useful treatment for a wide range of severe behavior problems. Although it is a routine second-choice psychotrope for severe psychiatric disorders, it is probably a first-choice treatment for TBI patients, and its range of therapeutic efficiency is dramatic. Failure to achieve success with low CBZ blood levels—4 to 8 ng/ml—

may simply require raising the dose to higher levels—10 to 15 ng/ml—so long as toxic effects do not intervene.

CBZ has the annoying proclivity, in some patients, of *inducing* or aggravating many of the problems for which it was originally prescribed. There is a class of epileptic patients, for example, whose seizures are worse on CBZ (Snead and Hosey, 1985). Irritability, agitation, and assaultiveness may be CBZ side effects, especially at high blood levels (Snead and Hosey, 1985). And although the neuropsychological profile of CBZ is generally favorable, there are occasional patients who may be sedated by the drug, and it can occasionally impair memory or motor performance. CBZ can also cause depression (Gardner and Cowdry, 1986).

Sodium valproate (VPA, valproic acid, Depakene, Depakote) is a relatively new anticonvulsant effective for many kinds of epilepsy, especially those characterized by absence seizures. It is known to block at least two enzymes that degrade the inhibitory neurotransmitter GABA (gamma-aminobutyric acid), and its net GABAergic effects have inspired a series of studies to explore its therapeutic potential in psychiatric disorders. As an anticonvulsant-psychotrope, it is second in importance only to CBZ. It is effective in the treatment and prophylaxis of mania (Emmrich et al., 1981), and it may also be beneficial in the treatment of schizophrenia (Emmrich et al., 1981; Linniola et al., 1976).

A short review of the psychological effects of VPA was written by Reisberg et al. (1983). Several authors have described beneficial psychological effects in epileptic patients on VPA; they are perceived as "more active, alert, cooperative" (Haigh and Forsyth, 1975; Jeavons and Clarke, 1974; Volzke and Doose, 1973). Others have reported positive effects on psychological test performance, or at least no decrement in performance, compared to placebo (Thompson and Trimble, 1981).

It is possible that the spectrum of psychiatric uses for VPA will come to resemble that of CBZ. That would be an interesting development, because VPA does not bear the same structural resemblance to neuroleptics and to tricyclic antidepressants that CBZ does. The side-effect profile of VPA is similar to that of CBZ, and behavioral toxicity is more often in the direction of excessive "activation" rather than sedation. It is said that sedation may be a VPA side effect; in neuropathic patients, it is more likely insomnia.

Benzodiazepines

The benzodiazepines (BZ) do not have a strong history of prescription for special populations, and that is just as well, because they are a troublesome class of drugs, and they never seem to have worked very well. Once in a long while, you will see a TBI patient who had insomnia, or agitation, or anxiety or panic, and who did well on one of the BZ without any subsequent difficulties, but this is rare. The party line is that the BZ tend to impair memory, and that is true (Block and Berchou, 1984;

Tinklenberg and Taylor, 1984; Romney and Angus, 1984); that they may be disinhibiting, like alcohol and the barbiturates, which is also true (Gualtieri, 1988). This may account for why they are rarely preferred drugs in TBI. But neither problem represents an invariant effect, and there is no need to take that occasional BZ responder off a successful drug simply because of a possible side effect.

Further, taking the patient off the drug may not be that easy. BZ withdrawal has proven to be the major difficulty of long-term treatment—rebound anxiety or panic, restlessness, insomnia, apprehension, dizziness, nausea, tremor, and seizures (Power et al., 1985). It is a familiar story; it is hard to know what is rebound from preexisting symptoms, and what is new and entirely withdrawal induced.

BZ withdrawal may be very important, though, in a patient who shows signs of depression, psychomotor retardation, cognitive or motor impairment, or failure to progress satisfactorily in therapy. Depression, anergia, and lack of motivation are some of the most troubling side effects of prolonged treatment. They may be more likely to occur in patients on long-acting BZ, because the drugs will tend to accumulate, especially in elderly patients, or in patients on concomitant therapy with cimetidine (Greenblatt et al., 1984).

There are several BZ to choose among, if one is inclined to choose one at all. The various compounds are usually differentiated on the basis of metabolism—whether psychologically active metabolites are formed from the parent compound, and what the half-life of the drug is. The reason why clonazepam (Klonapin) and lorazepam (Ativan) are currently in such favor as acute anxiolytics is that they have no active metabolites whose metabolism and elimination may be extremely slow. The elimination of lorazepam and cloanzepam is intermediate, neither fast, like triazolam (Halcyon), nor slow, like diazepam (Valium) or chlordiazepoxide (Librium). Thus, there is not the danger one faces, with diazepam for example, of gradual accumulation over time; or the danger one faces with triazolam, with early-morning insomnia or rebound anxiety (Greenblatt et al., 1983). Lorazepam also has the advantage of prompt and reliable action with intramuscular injection (Greenblatt and Shader, 1978). Clonazepam has the special advantages of antimanic activity, and of antiepileptic activity in the oral form.

The relatively new BZ, alprazolam (Xanax), is equal to diazepam as an anxiolytic and equal to imipramine as an antidepressant and an antipanic drug. For a short while, it was the perfect drug, and a mainstay of outpatient psychiatric treatment. Then it turned out to be even more difficult to get off of than the other BZ, with the problem of rebound panic and, occasionally, seizures (Breier et al., 1984; Lydiard et al., 1987).

The other new BZ was triazolam (Halcyon), a fabulous sedative with an amazingly short onset of action and a short duration of action that rendered it free of morning hangovers. Short-acting BZ like triazolam and alprazolam, however, may be more likely to induce rebound symptoms, because they are eliminated quickly; longer acting BZ, eliminated more slowly, may be less likely to cause rebound (Noyes et al., 1985). There have also been reports of transient global amnesia with triazolam, especially when it is taken with alcohol (Morris and Estes, 1987).

Both alprazolam and triazolam have been associated with severe disorganizing side effects, such as depression (Lydiard et al., 1987), mania (Pecknold and Fleury, 1986), and paroxysmal excitement (Strahan et al., 1985). The clinical problem is something akin to akathisia with neuroleptics. It is too easy for the clinician to mistake BZ-induced excitement or agitation for a recurrent symptom of what the drug was originally prescribed for, so the dose is raised, the problem grows worse, the patient is finally judged to be psychotic, and a neuroleptic is prescribed. It is the kind of vicious circle that leads to unnecessary hospitalization, misdiagnosis, and long-term "treatment" for an iatrogenic disease.

There is a small role for BZ in TBI patients, especially for patients with associated cervical injuries and patients with spasticity; aside from such patients, however, the BZ will only enjoy a small role, and there is no reason to encourage it to grow. Buspirone is probably the anxiolytic of choice in this population, at least for now.

Buspirone

Buspirone, or, as it is commonly known, 8-[4-[4-(2-pyrimidinyl)-1-piperazinyl]-butyl]-8-azaspiro[4.5]-decane-7,9-dione, has been introduced as an anxiolytic, but it is an azaspirodecanedione, not a benzodiazepine. It is as effective as diazepam as an anxiolytic, or at least they say it is, but it is nonsedating, nonaddictive, and does not seem to have any unfavorable neuropsychological effects. Its effect is not additive or synergistic with alcohol, overdose is not lethal (Kastenholz and Crismon, 1984; Staughan and Conradie, 1988), and it is not a respiratory depressant (Garner et al., 1989) These are very important differences.

Buspirone is an anxiolytic, and it is prescribed by physicians who are concerned with the potential toxicity of benzodiazepines and antidepressants, the alternative treatments for generalized anxiety disorder. Because the onset of action is over a few weeks, however, it is not like taking a Valium or a belt of whiskey for tensionanxiety. It seems to have a different kind of effect on anxiety, and indeed the mechanism of action is quite different from the benzodiazepines.

Buspirone does not exert an anxiolytic effect by directly occupying the benzodiazepine receptor, although it may exert an indirect effect at this locus (Skolnick et al., 1984). There may be a GABAantagonist aspect to its action, in contrast to the benzodiazepines, which are GABAmimetic (Eison and Temple, 1986).

Buspirone does seem to exercise pharmacological effects on serotonin, norepinephrine, and dopamine systems, although the nature of these effects, and their relationship to the clinical actions of the drug, are still not clear. It increases the activity of noradrenergic neurons that originate in the locus coeruleus, an event that is consistent with the absence of sedation or psychomotor impairment but hard to reconcile with its action as an anxiolytic (Skolnick et al., 1984).

It is a specific dopamine antagonist at the presynaptic receptor, and it also has some postsynaptic dopamine blocking effects, such as reduction of apomorphine-induced stereotypy (Eison and Temple, 1986). But it also increases the firing rate of midbrain dopamine neurons, and it is capable of reversing neuroleptic-induced catalepsy with more potency than amantadine (Goa and Ward, 1986). So, it may be one of those mixed dopamine agonist-antagonists. There is one report on its efficacy in the treatment of attention deficit disorder (Balon, 1990), a finding we have confirmed in our Clinic.

Although buspirone has been claimed to be a serotonin agonist at the 5-hydroxytryptophol$_{1A}$ (5-HT$_{1A}$) receptor (Goa and Ward, 1986), administration will reduce the firing rate of serotonin neurons in the dorsal raphe, decrease striatal serotonin concentration, and decrease the number of serotonin-binding sites in the frontal cortex (Eison and Temple, 1986). It is possible that the effect of buspirone in reducing neuroleptic-induced catalepsy is a function of its antiserotonin effect; this paradigm may also explain its clinical usefulness in the treatment of akathisia.

The ambiguity of its neurochemical profile is a measure of one's clinical uncertainty about what exactly buspirone is good *for*. No doubt it is an effective treatment for generalized anxiety disorder, and its many advantages over the benzodiazepines guarantee its place in the formulary of useful psychotropic drugs. But its neuropsychiatric indications may be much broader, and it may prove to be a very important drug for some clinical problems that so far have been resistant to pharmacotherapy.

Buspirone has been effective in the treatment of agitation associated with dementia (Colenda, 1988) and head injury (Levine, 1988); this is a therapeutic effect that comes on almost immediately, in contrast to the 2-week latency of its anxiolytic effects. It has been reported to be effective in controlling aggression, self-injurious behavior, and psychosis in mentally retarded patients (Ratey et al., in press; Sovner and Parnell-Sovner, in press), and aggression and hyperactivity in autistic patients (Realmuto et al., 1989). We have had positive effects in the treatment of akathisia, anxiety, and depression following head injury, and it appears to be particularly effective in higher level patients with temporal lobe symptoms, like somatic preoccupation, hypochondriasis, nervousness, and the peculiar kind of turgid self-concern one learns to associate with temporal lobe lesions. It is fast becoming the drug of choice for PCS patients with these symptoms. We have not been especially impressed, however, with its positive effects on agitation during the coma-recovery phase following TBI.

Considering the extremely favorable side-effect profile of buspirone, the possibility of positive effects on neuropsychological performance, and its general profile as a stimulant of monoaminergic activity, it should be an important compound to investigate further for TBI patients. It works quickly, the dose range is narrow, and the initiation of treatment does not require intensive medical monitoring, as do carbamazepine, lithium, and the beta blockers. The trick is to discover which patients buspirone is good for. The second trick will be to figure out exactly how it works.

Because we have claimed that the side effects of busipirone are very mild, it is necessary to add that they may be intolerable. Because the benefit of drug treatment comes on slowly, and usually after a latent period of several weeks, and the side effects come on early, people will stop the drug and throw it away: "It didn't work, and it made me light-headed (or, dizzy)"—the two most common side effects. The others are headache, nervousness, diarrhea, paraesthesia, excitation, and sweating/clamminess (Newton et al., 1986). The side effects of dizziness, lightheadedness, and headache will limit its appeal to some patients with the postconcussion syndrome.

Beta-Adrenergic Blockers

The beta blockers are indicated for hypertension, angina pectoris, cardiac arrhythmias, essential tremor, and prophylaxis of migraine. They are also an extremely important class of drugs for neuropsychiatric patients, although the list of indications is not nearly so concise.

The beta blockers are classified in the following ways:

1. By selectivity, that is, selective affinity for the B_1 receptor. Atenalol, then, is "cardioselective," while propanalol and nadalol have "mixed selectivity" because they block both the B_1 and the B_2 receptors.
2. By relative degree of lipophilia/hydrophilia; a "lipophilic" beta blocker like propanalol will cross the blood-brain barrier quite readily, and a "hydrophilic" drug like nadalol will cross very slowly, if at all. There is some disagreement on this point. Some physicians maintain that the actions of hydrophilic beta blockers like nadalol are entirely peripheral, while others maintain that its psychotropic actions are explicable in terms of a central effect, an effect that may be slower in onset, but which is nevertheless real.
3. By "intrinsic sympathomimetic activity" (ISA), that is, the capacity to act as a partial agonist at the beta receptor. Pindalol, a drug with ISA, may not cause the same degree of bradycardia and hypotension as the other beta blockers. On the other hand, it may have behavioral toxicity in the way of excitement and agitation; this is unusual for beta blockers, which are more often associated with depression. For some reason, by the way, beta blockers with high ISA are the only ones with no proclivity to raise blood lipid levels (Roberts, 1989).
4. By elimination half-life. Propanalol, for example, has a very short half-life, and unless the "long-acting" form is used, the patient with anxiety or akathisia may experience a disconcerting "on-off" phenomenon. Nadalol, in contrast, is a very long acting drug, so once-daily dosing is entirely feasible.

In 1966, Granville-Grossman and Turner reported relief of the somatic symptoms of anxiety in patients who were treated with propanalol, and the first studies of propanalol as a psychotropic drug concentrated on the treatment of anxiety. It was thought that propanalol might be a superior anxiolytic for patients whose symptoms were largely "somatic"; for example, tremor, tachycardia, palpitations, diaphoresis, and urge to micturate (Granville-Grossman and Turner, 1966; Noyes et al., 1981). The beta blockers are the drugs of choice now for musicians, for example, who are afflicted with performance anxiety, because the symptoms are relieved with no detectable effect on memory or motor performance (Lockwood, 1989).

The next indication was schizophrenia, and there was a time when propanalol was advanced as an antipsychotic drug (Atsmon et al., 1972). It may only serve, however, to raise plasma concentrations of neuroleptics administered concomitantly (Peet et al., 1981a; Peet et al., 1981b). Beta blockers may have a specific effect on aggressive behavior in chronic psychotic patients, just as they do in other classes of patients (Sorji et al., 1986).

Beta blockers have been recommended for other neuropsychiatric disorders, including alcohol withdrawal (Jefferson, 1974), benzodiazepine withdrawal (Tyrer et al., 1981), opiate withdrawal (Jefferson, 1974), narcolepsy (Kales et al., 1979), and phantom limb pain (Ahmad, 1979).

Elliott (1976, 1977) was the first to describe the effectiveness of propanalol for belligerence during coma recovery in brain injury patients, and his findings have been extended to a wide range of patients with episodic rage and violent behavior due to a number of causes, including infectious encephalopathy (Schreier, 1979), temporal lobe epilepsy, Wilson's disease, mental retardation (Yudofsky et al., 1981), the late sequelae of closed head injury (Mansheim, 1981), and dementia (Petrie and Ban, 1981). These findings have been replicated in large-scale reviews (Williams et al., 1982), and it has always been encouraging that beta blockers have been effective even when more conventional therapies have failed. The usual dose of propanalol is about 160 mg/day, but the range of effective doses is quite broad, from 50 to 960 mg/day (Williams et al., 1982).

Propanalol has been successfully prescribed to treat temper outbursts in patients with AD/HA (Mattes, 1986). In AD/HA patients who are only partially controlled with stimulants or tricyclic antidepressants, beta blockers have been noted to augment the therapeutic effect (Ratey et al., 1990).

In 1967, Strang described success in treating the restless legs syndrome (RLS, or Ekbom's syndrome) with propanalol. In fact, it was not Ekbom who first described the RLS, it was Joseph Babinski.

It was Lipinski, on the other hand, who extended this work to the treatment of neuroleptic-induced akathisia with propanalol (Lipinski, 1983), and this was a signal advance, because there have been several subsequent studies of beta blockers in the treatment of neuroleptic-induced akathisia, and they tend to be very favorable, even for the hydrophilic beta blockers (Adler et al., 1989). Even clonidine, another adrenergic antagonist, albeit at the alpha receptor, has been effective in reducing symptoms of neuroleptic-induced akathisia (Zubenko et al., 1984a; Adler 1987b). This is interesting information, indeed, because it suggests that adrenergic mechanisms may be at play in the development of akathisia (Adler et al., 1987a). The alternative treatment, with benzodiazepines, is posited on a more conventional model, that GABAmimetic drugs will serve to dampen dopamine neurotransmission in striatal neurons.

Treatment with beta blockers should be undertaken only with a clear understanding of its influence upon peripheral beta receptors. Beta blockers are contraindicated in patients with asthma, sinus bradycardia, conduction defects, and brittle diabetes (because they may mask the symptoms of hypoglycemia), and in patients on concomitant adrenergic drugs like the MAOI.

The psychological side effect that is most commonly associated with beta blockers is depression (Petrie et al., 1982), and this is a significant factor that has diminished their utility in general medicine. On the other hand, it is not unreasonable to suggest that the hyperaroused neuropsychiatric patients who are likeliest to respond to beta blockers may be relatively inured to this effect.

Other negative effects include acute delirium with or without psychotic features (Peters et al., 1978; Fraser and Carr, 1976; Gershon et al., 1979; Voltolina et al., 1971), hallucinations (Shopsin et al., 1975), and vivid nightmares. Propanalol has been reported to cause transient spatial orientation disorder (Belin and Larmande, 1985). It is not entirely clear whether beta blockers that are highly lipophilic are more likely to cause neuropsychiatric impairment than the less lipophilic compounds (McNeil et al., 1982; Gengo et al., 1987).

The efficacy of the beta-blocking drugs for neuropathic patients, for example, TBI victims, or mentally handicapped individuals, has called forth a number of speculations concerning the mechanism of action of this drug class. A number of hypotheses have been offered, including central beta blockade, nonspecific membrane stabilization effects, presynaptic noradrenergic effects, serotonergic effects, and the attenuation of peripheral feedback via a number of different possible routes. The last idea has given rise to an interesting hypothesis about the mechanism of drug action, apart from the obvious one, having to do with central adrenergic blockade at the beta sites. It is raised by the interesting observation that beta antagonists that do not cross the blood-brain barrier, like nadalol for example, are often as effective, and sometimes more effective, than beta antagonists like propanalol that enter the CNS quite readily.

The concept of "noise," in this particular regard, refers to the relative inability of the neuropathic patient to "filter" or to "screen out" irrelevant signals from their internal or their external environment. The stimuli that all of us receive are necessarily composed of signals, or useful information, and noise, or meaningless information. The patient with diffuse brain injury, congenital or acquired, is postulated to process information with a low signal-to-noise ratio. In response to a given stimulus, the patient receives a signal that is less clear than a normal person does, and he receives more noise or clutter too (Sands and Ratey, 1986).

A normal person who is exposed to severe static in a telephone conversation, or to a channel of distracting information in a dichotic listening task, is likely to experience annoyance, frustration, and irritability. A person who receives such a noisy stimulus, and then has to decode it with a mental apparatus that is already compromised by injury, experiences double the frustration. The attention deficit of the schizophrenic patient, for example, may be attributable to a defective filter that allows irrelevant intrusions to overwhelm normal cognition (Maher, 1966; Rappaport, 1968; Shakow, 1962).

The result of experiencing a signal that can neither be intelligibly perceived nor correctly integrated may produce stimulus overload, and then internal chaos, personal distortions, impulsivity, hypervigilance, increased physiological stress, and aggression (Glass and Singer, 1972; Sands and Ratey, 1986; Miller, 1959). When the stimuli one receives over a long period of time, from the external environment as well as from one's own body, is chaotic and uncontrollable, one may be reduced to responding rigidly and sometimes very intensely in an attempt to organize the stimuli (Goldstein, 1948).

To such a patient, novel stimuli are perceived as threatening, and the response is stereotyped:

> The CNS seems to react to any overwhelming threatening and uncontrollable experience in a consistent pattern. Regardless of the precipitating event, traumatized people continue to have a poor tolerance for arousal. They tend to respond to stress in an all-or-nothing way: either unmodulated anxiety, often accompanied by motoric discharge that includes acts of aggression against the self and others, or else social and emotional withdrawal (Krystal, 1978).
>
> —*van der Kolk and Greenberg, 1987, p. 64*

Theoretically, at least, treatment with peripheral beta blockers may reduce the noise level in a patient's incoming stimuli. Nadalol, for example, may reduce anxiety in the patient by relaxing the skeletal and striate musculature. This may decrease the somatic contribution to the noise level that a patient experiences and increase the signal-to-noise ratio, thus alleviating the chaotic internal environment and allowing the patient to experience a greater degree of disorganization (Ratey and Gualtieri, 1990).

This is a compelling theory, but it is posited on two requirements: (1) peripherally active beta blockers do not cross the blood-brain barrier at all (Tyrer, 1980); and (2) they are equally effective, or more effective, with a more benign side-effects profile, than the centrally active beta blockers (El-Mallakh, 1986; Lader, 1988; Ratey et al., 1987). There is reason to believe that both these requirements have been met. On the other hand, there is also reason to think that a combination of central and peripheral actions may account for the unique clinical utility of the beta antagonists, even for the ones that are supposed to stay on the outside.

Alpha Agonists

The prototype of alpha agonists, in terms of behavioral effects, is clonidine, a centrally acting alpha$_2$ agonist that binds predominantly to presynaptic receptors or "autoreceptors," that is, receptors on the soma, dendrites, and terminals of a neuron that are responsive to its own transmitter (Hoehn-Saric et al., 1981). At lower doses, the effect of presynaptic receptor stimulation is to diminish the release of norepinephrine across the synaptic junction, and thus to lower the concentration of norepinephrine in the brain. However, at higher doses clonidine may act as a postsynaptic stimulant of the alpha$_2$ receptor. It does not have any other direct effects on monoamine neurotransmission, although it may also be a serotonin inhibitor by virtue of its negative effect on adrenergic activity (Hoehn-Saric et al., 1981).

Clonidine is one of those drugs that seems to be partially effective for a wide range of neuropsychiatric conditions. ("Partially effective" means partial response in most patients, or good therapeutic response for only some patients, or effective, but only for a while.) The list includes: anxiety disorders (Hoehn-Saric et al., 1983); obsessive-compulsive disorder (Knesevich, 1982); bipolar disorder (Zubenko et al., 1984b); tardive dyskinesia (Nishikawa et al., 1984); Tourette's syndrome (Bruun, 1984); and attention deficit/hyperactivity (Hunt et al., 1985). The current use that has received the most recent attention is clonidine, especially in the form of a transdermal patch, to control the autonomic and the psychological symptoms of opiate and cocaine withdrawal (Gold et al., 1980; Charney et al., 1981).

Clonidine has been reported to raise the seizure threshold in one patient who was treated with ECT for depression (Elliott, 1983). In fact, clonidine is capable of an anticonvulsant effect on seizures induced by a wide variety of stimuli, including electric shock, sound, decapitation (sic), and convulsant compounds like picrotoxin, strychnine, pentylenetetrazol, and glycine (Elliott, 1983). The effect can be blocked by yohimbine, an alpha$_2$-adrenergic antagonist.

Clonidine is also known to stimulate the release of growth hormone (GH) from the anterior pituitary, an effect that is presumably mediated by its action on the alpha$_2$ receptors in the hypothalamus; thus, it accelerates growth in children with impaired GH secretion (Pintor et al., 1985).

More to the point, clonidine has been found to ameliorate the cognitive deficits of aged primates (Arnsten and Goldman-Rakic, 1985) and also in patients with Korsakoff's psychosis (McEntee and Mair, 1980). Presumably, this is because it may be an adrenergic stimulant at certain doses. Clonidine treatment has also been associated with functional restoration of the traumatically injured spinal cord in laboratory animals, and there is preliminary evidence that it may reduce spasticity in humans resulting from cervical or thoracic transverse myelopathy, perhaps by stimulating alpha$_2$ receptors in the cord and thus inhibiting gamma and alpha motor neurons (Naftchi, 1982).

The developing indications for clonidine in neuropsychiatric patients may include the syndrome of hypervigilance-hyperreactivity that is sometimes seen in association with severe orbitofrontal lesions and which has been described in Chapter 1, this volume. (Bakchine et al., 1989; Bougousslavsky et al, 1988). This posttraumatic syndrome may be reflected in developmentally handicapped patients, particularly autistic patients who may also be hypervigilant-hyperreactive, and who also may be given to stereotypies, compulsive rituals and perseverative behavior, and motor and phonic tics. This is addressed in the Autism chapter (see Chapter 9). In both clinical conditions, the therapeutic effect of clonidine is probably mediated by its net effect in reducing adrenergic stimulation from brainstem and midbrain nuclei; it may be augmented, if necessary, by concomitant therapy with beta-adrenergic blockers. It may take several weeks for the full therapeutic effect to mature, however, so one should go very slowly before adding a second drug to a clonidine regime.

Such patients must be observed very carefully for signs of hypotension and bradycardia. In fact, the toxicity profile of clonidine is hardly favorable, and there are several other things to look out for. The common side effects of clonidine in psychiatric patients include sedation or, conversely, sleep disturbance, dry mouth, inattention, irritability, decreased sexual interest, and impotence (Hoehn-Saric et al., 1983) dizziness, lightheadedness, depression, delirium (Schaut and Schnoll, 1983), hyperactivity, mania, and paranoia (Ahsanuddin, 1982). Abrupt withdrawal from clonidine is well known to cause hypertensive crisis; it may also lead to severe psychiatric decompensation, even to a state of acute psychosis, in vulnerable patients (Adler et al., 1982).

The therapeutic utility of an alpha$_2$ antagonist like clonidine may, in theory at least, be limited by the reciprocal association of adrenoreceptors of the alpha and beta type. For example, drugs that lower the synaptic availability of norepinephrine and serotonin (e.g., clonidine) may cause supersensitivity in the beta receptor, whereas increased responsiveness in the alpha receptors may lead to beta receptor downregulation (Janowsky and Sulser, 1987). The net effect on adrenergic neurotransmission may be zero, if alpha blockade leads to beta supersensitivity while beta blockade does the reverse. It is a theoretical concern, but it may explain why the beneficial effects of clonidine or of the beta blockers are only partial, or transient, and it may predict that some patients with behavioral conditions charac-terized by diffuse adrenergic hyperactivity require cotreatment with clonidine and with a beta blocker.

In such cases, a beta blocker with intrinsic sympathomimetic activity may be required to preserve cardiovascular integrity as the central effects of noradrenergic hyperactivity are managed. On the other hand, the combination of beta blockers and alpha agonists has been used in the treatment of refractory hypertension with no increased risk of cardiovascular side effects (Weber et al., 1978; Vanholder et al., 1985), although there are individual case reports of hypertensive crisis when clonidine was abruptly discontinued while treatment with beta blockers continued (Jounela and Lilja, 1984).

Calcium Channel Blockers

This new class of psychoactive drugs is only beginning to reveal its therapeutic potential. Clinical experience and research are only beginning.

Calcium antagonists operate on a new level of therapeutic understanding, and the physiology of their effect deserves a brief discursion. Ionic calcium plays a critical role in regulating the function of excitable cells. Extracellular calcium enters cells, neurons, for example, or smooth muscle cells, through glycoproteins, which are functional pores or 'calcium channels.' Voltage-dependent channels "open" in response to membrane depolarization, thus coupling electrical stimula-tion of an excitable cell with diverse physiological responses, including neurotransmitter release or muscle contraction (Snyder and Reynolds, 1985). Drugs that block this functional pore tend to diminish the excitability of the target cell, and thus alter its physiological response.

The three "calcium channel blockers" currently available in the United States have been proven effective in the treatment of cardiovascular disease, where the excitability of smooth-muscle cells is at issue. Calcium blockers such as verapamil, nifedipine, and diltiazem are prescribed for angina and hypertension (Snyder and Reynolds, 1985). Other vascular disorders for which the drugs may be prescribed include migraine (Greenberg, 1986) and Raynaud's phenomenon (Roddenheffer et al., 1983).

Psychiatric interest in calcium channel blockers was originally stimulated by the fact that several psychoactive drugs, most notably lithium, are calcium agonists (Giannini et al., 1984) and also by the fact that altered calcium metabolism seems to characterize certain psychiatric disorders (Dubovsky, 1986). There are several reports to suggest its efficacy in bipolar affective disorders (Giannini et al., 1984; Gitlin and Weiss, 1984), and verapamil, in particular, is said to be well tolerated by demented patients (Giannini et al., 1984). Calcium blockers may also be effective in depression (Hoschl, 1983), panic disorder (Klein and Uhde, 1988), refractory schizophrenia (Bloom et al., 1987), and also in Tourette's syndrome, of all things (Berg, 1985; Walsh et al., 1986).

Childs (1986, unpublished) described two severely disturbed individuals who responded very well to verapamil. One had severe aggression and self-injurious behavior; he was a TBI victim. The other was an impulsive, aggressive adolescent.

This diversity of clinical effects is consistent with the fact that calcium channel antagonists may modify dopaminergic neurotransmission in brain; the caudate nucleus, for example, is among the brain areas with the highest density of specific binding sites for such compounds (Fadda et al., 1989). Calcium channel blockers are also known to induce acute extrapyramidal side effects, such as oculogyric crisis and akathisia (Singh, 1987).

The clinical study of calcium channel blockers may prove to be an important new chapter in neuropsychiatry unless they simply prove to be a new variant of neuroleptic, in which case they will simply reiterate an old chapter. But that view is overly lugubrious. The calcium channel blockers have a relatively favorable side-effect profile, and they may be even better tolerated, in some patients, than lithium (Giannini et al., 1984). They are not sedating; the major effects are, in fact, somewhat stimulating. It is appropriate to explore their clinical usefulness for TBI patients for problems as diverse as agitation, depression, assaultiveness, emotional instability, and posttraumatic headache.

Calcium channel blockers are even likelier to capture the imagination of psychopharmacologists as new compounds become available. For example, funarizine may be effective not only as an antimigraine drug but as supplemental treatment in cases of refractory epilepsy (Caers et al., 1987).

Nimodipine has recently been approved by the FDA for use in improving neurological outcome in patients who have suffered a subarachnoid hemorrhage. It is a calcium channel antagonist that is highly lipophilic and crosses the blood-brain barrier quite readily, and it is selective for vascular smooth muscle. Thus, it is capable of reducing cerebral arterial spasm, which is one of the primary causes of neurological deficits in patients who survive a subarachnoid hemorrhage. This is a delayed effect that occurs within 4 to 21 days after the initial hemorrhagic event, and because nimodipine will prevent or reverse the event, it can improve the survival rate and prevent neurological deficits in stroke patients (Gelmers, 1987; Pickard et al., 1989). It is one of those unique drugs that is worth its weight in gold, and the manufacturer thinks so, too, because the pharmacy cost of 21 days of treatment is about $1210.

Nimodipine is also effective in migraine prophylaxis (Stewart et al., 1988) and episodic cluster headache (de Carolis et al., 1987).

After some German neurologists noted that stroke patients who were treated with nimodipine seemed to recover some earlier learning losses, neuroscientists investigated the effect of the drug in attenuating the learning decrement that occurs with aging, an effect that may be due to accumulation of intraneuronal calcium, kind of an ossification of the brain. In elderly rabbits, it seemed that nimodipine treatment improved learning on an eyeblink task, and their performance equaled that of young rabbits (*Science*, February 10, 1989). This is the kind of information that elicits strong interest among neuropsychiatrists, the families of closed head injury victims, and Alzheimer's patients, and any person, in fact, who wakes up in the morning to find a crust on the inner lining of his neurons. On the other hand, the retail cost of nimodipine is in excess of $400 a week; if people were really worried about their brains getting fossilized, they wouldn't watch TV.

Opiates

There is preclinical evidence to suggest that some aspect of the endogenous amnesic mechanism is mediated by opioid peptides; the evidence is that opiate antagonists cause memory facilitation, and the opiate agonists, in particular opioid peptides, cause amnesia (Izquierdo et al., 1980). The relevant experiments in rats used the short-acting, parenterally administered opiate antagonist naloxone. Were similar experiments to be attempted in humans, the long-acting, orally administered antagonist naltrexone would be more amendable to extended clinical evaluation. Naltrexone is currently studied as a treatment for autistic (Campbell et al., 1988) and retarded children (Herman et al., 1987), with marginal results. Clinical experience with drugs of this class has been extensive, and the long-term side-effect profile is not unfavorable (Kleber, 1977). This fact, and the fact that opiate antagonists may promote recovery in certain CNS-injury paradigms (see foregoing discussion), increases the importance of clinical experiments in TBI patients.

Because endorphins and enkephalins may impair memory, it was natural to try opiate antagonists in the treatment of memory disorders—dementia of the Alzheimer's type (DAT), for example. Although there have been preliminary reports of improvement in DAT patients with intravenous naloxone, subsequent experience has not corroborated the finding, either with naloxone or with orally administered naltrexone (Serby et al., 1986).

The positive cognitive effects of naloxone have been attributed to nonspecific behavioral effects rather than to a direct 'nootropic' action (Tariot et al., 1985).

The argument can be made against any nootropic drug. It should not discourage clinical research on the subject.

Childs reported improvement in four head injury patients with bulimia who were treated in open trials with naltrexone (Childs, 1986). The rationale was derived from clinical experience with Prader-Willi patients, who have compulsive hyperphagia, food stealing, and extreme obesity, and who sometimes respond to opiate antagonists.

Other Neuropeptides

In addition to their specific endocrine functions, the pituitary peptide hormones adrenocorticotropin (ACTH) and melanocyle-stimulating hormone (MSH) exert a "trophic" influence enhancing the metabolic activity and the viability of their target cells. These effects include enhanced blood flow in the target region and stimulation of macromolecular (RNA/protein) synthesis (Gispen et al., 1986). The brain and behavior effects of the melanocortins (ACTH, MSH) probably result from peptide effects on neurons and or glial cells that are similar to the peptide-target cell interactions (previously described) that are known to occur in peripheral tissues. The idea that the melanocortins may enhance adaptive neural responses to injury has been tested, and has won at least a measure of support, in preclinical studies employing the following preparations: peripheral nerve damage, hippocampal plasticity, recovery from brain damage, and 'behavioral plasticity' (Gispen et al., 1986).

Some neuropeptides, notably ACTH, MSH, and vasopressin, have been shown to affect the learning process, particularly in animals. Subsequent work demonstrated that the heptapeptide ACTH 4-10, a peptide fragment common to both the ACTH and the MSH molecular structures, was responsible for the learning effects of these compounds (Reisberg et al., 1981). For example, both the stimulant pentylenetetrazol (metrazol) and the peptide ACTH 4-9 can retard the development of neuromorphological and behavioral correlates of aging in rats (Landfield et al., 1981). In human volunteers a synthetic function of ACTH (ACTH 4-10) seemed to improve visual memory, enhance alertness, and increase motivation—all without the hormone's usual endocrine effects (DeWied, 1976). Human studies with ACTH 4-10 have not, however, confirmed its clinical utility (Frederiksen et al., 1985; Rigter and Van Riezen, 1978).

Vasopressin is a posterior pituitary hormone with well-defined effects on the kidney and on blood pressure. There have been extensive studies of vasopressin and other pituitary hormones, because hypophysectomy is known to improve requisition in a variety of learning paradigms (Jennekens-Schinkel et al., 1985). Thus, the idea of vasopressin, like ACTH 4-10, may modulate some aspect of the learning/memory process (DeWied, 1976). Oxytocin, another posterior pituitary hormone, is also known to facilitate learning in laboratory animals (Legros et al., 1978). The long-term effects of vasopressin-like peptides on acquisition and extinction of behavior suggest that these peptides facilitate memory consolidation.

However, it has not been possible to extend the results of laboratory research to the clinical arena. Well-constructed clinical studies of neuropsychiatric patients, including TBI cases for example, have not supported the idea that vasopressin improves memory performance (Tinklenberg et al., 1982). On the other hand, elderly patients treated with vasopressin performed better in tests involving attention, concentration, and motor speech, and better in tests of memory (visual retention, recognition, and recall) (Legros et al., 1978). It is possible, however, that vasopressin peptides exercise positive effects on psychological performance, not through any direct nootropic effect, but indirectly, by improving mood, motivation, or alertness.

The tripeptide thyrotropin-releasing hormone (TRH) has been shown to improve long-term neurological outcome following experimental spinal cord injury in cats (Faden and Jacobs, 1985). Because TRH can only be given as continuous infusion, pharmacological analogues with a longer half-life and the potential for oral administration will be required before clinical trials may be run (Faden, 1986). TRH has been successful in improving recovery from experimental brain injury in cats (Fukuda et al., 1979). DN-1417, a TRH analogue that is long acting, and not as potent in stimulating the endocrine system, has been shown to promote recovery from concussive head injury in mice (Miyamoto et al., 1981).

Nerve growth factor (NGF) is a protein of known sequence and structure, a neurotrophic factor for central cholinergic neurons (but not for central catecholaminergic neurons). In animal studies NGF is known to "preserve" cholinergic neurons from lesion-induced degeneration, and to improve learning in rats, for example, with cholinergic septohippocampal lesions (Hefti and Weiner, 1986). NGF has not been tested in human patients with brain disorders associated with cholinergic deficits, such as DAT, and human research will be limited by the fact that the protein cannot cross the blood-brain barrier. Nevertheless, the therapeutic potential of the protein is well worth exploring, and it is possible that compounds exercising NGF-like effects may at some point be a rational treatment for TBI patients.

Cholinergic Drugs

The earliest attempt to correlate recovery of cortical function with cholinergic stimulation was made in 1928 when Chavany advocated the use of acetylcholine in the treatment of hemiplegia (Chavany, 1928). Positive effects with acetylcholine injections in hemiplegic patients, aphasics, and other neuropathic cases were at first attributed to cerebral vasodilation. Subsequent research was conducted by Luria (Luria et al., 1968) and by Ward and Kennard (1942) at Yale, during the Fulton era.

This venerable treatment is still current. Indeed, it is central to pharmacological research in DAT; not as a vasodilator, but as a rational treatment aimed at correcting what is thought to be the fundamental deficit in DAT in the cholinergic cells of the median forebrain (Coyle et al., 1983). Because acetylcholine is an important neurotransmitter in the physiology of memory, and because deficits in acetyl-choline systems are found in amnestic patients, it has been appropriate to explore the potential utility of cholinergic drugs in treatment. Because memory impairment is a major element of TBI, cholinergic treatments have been brought to bear in that group as well, with positive effects in at least one study (McLean et al., 1987).

Luria's favorite cholinergic drug for TBI was "gallanthamine," a long-acting acetylcholinesterase inhibitor that is not available in the United States (Luria et al., 1968). Commercial availability is not the only limiting factor in the study of cholinergic treatments for amnestic patients. The clinical utility of available cholinergic drugs is also limited by their (1) extremely short half-life; (2) lack of specificity to CNS; (3) poor passage through the blood-brain barrier; (4) high incidence of adverse side effects; and (5) extremely narrow therapeutic window (McLean et al., 1987). The problem of cholinergic treatment, then, has been logistic: to find a drug that can be administered conveniently over the long term, has central rather than peripheral effects, and can be used safely. Various strategies have been used to achieve this end, thus far with little success.

The clinical utility of cholinergic drugs has been explored extensively in patients with Alzheimer's disease and other dementing conditions associated with diminished levels of acetylcholine in certain areas of brain. However, "despite several years of clinical attempts to improve geriatric cognition, no *therapeutically* useful results have been demonstrated with cholinergic agents" (Bartus et al., 1986, p. 427). Neither acetylcholine (ACH) precursors, nor acetylcholinesterase in-hibitors nor direct muscarinic receptor agonists have shown therapeutic utility. On the other hand, novel treatment strategies could change this dim picture. It is possible, for example, that combined treatment with an ACH precursor and a cholinesterase inhibitor would have more utility than treatment with either com-pound by itself (Jorm, 1986; Catsman-Berrevoets et al., 1986). The availability of more effective drugs may enhance the success of this strategy.

Tetrahydro-9-aminoacridine (THA) is a potent central-acting anticholinesterase that can be administered orally; it has a longer duration of action and a more favorable therapeutic index than physostigmine (Summers et al., 1986). Long-term treatment of 12 DAT patients with THA was associated with significant improve-ment in general clinical status and learning; it is a potential palliative treatment that alleviates some of the symptoms of DAT without, unfortunately, altering the ultimate course of the disease (Fitten et al., 1990).

Intracranial infusion may be an effective means for delivering cholinergic drugs (e.g., bethanecol) to brain tissue, bypassing the blood-brain barrier, and achieving continuous therapeutic drug levels (Harbaugh et al., 1984). The technique is in its infancy, however, about as far along as neural cell transplants insofar as the actual treatment of patients is concerned.

McClean's work with physostigmine suggests that stimulating the cholinergic system may effect positive changes in learning and memory in TBI patients even after the direct pharmacological action of the drug is passed. That is encouraging news, but it is more heartening to learn of new advances in cholinergic drug delivery and the therapeutic potential of THA.

Nootropes

'Nootrope' is a neologism that was coined to describe a class of drugs that improve "higher cognitive function." The term was invented by Guirgea, who developed Piracetam ('Nootropyl,' UCB), the alleged "memory drug," described as the first of a new class of nootropic psychoactive drugs. Piracetam has been reported to facilitate learning in animals, limit the decline in human performance associated with cerebral hypoxia, and improve cognitive performance, alertness, fatigue, and psychomotor retardation in aged subjects (Simeon et al., 1983). It may improve verbal learning in normals (Dimond and Brouwers, 1976) and in dyslexics (Wilsher and Melewski, 1983). In addition, the combination of lecithin and piracetam may ameliorate specific memory deficits in some patients with DAT (Smith et al., 1989). Clinical trial of piracetam for dyslexic children were conducted in the United States, and although there were some indications of treatment success (Helfgott et al., 1984), the evidence was not sufficiently strong to convince the FDA and there are no current plans to market the drug here. Based on the author's experience with piracetam, however, it is unlikely that the drug will be missed, and there is no reason to send one's patients to Mexico or to Belgium to obtain a supply; the therapeutic benefits or piracetam have probably been overstated (Evans and Gualtieri, 1986, unpublished). It is possible that one or more of a family of nootropes structurally related to piracetam will prove more effective than the "parent compounds," and studies of aniracetam and pramiracetam, for example, are proceeding.

Pramiracetam is a unique new "cognition activator," which, in various behavioral modes, in the quantitative electroencephalogram and in other studies, has been found "superior" to other drugs marketed for cognitive disorders in the elderly (Pugsley et al., 1983). Pharmacologically it appears to be cholinergic and a dopamine agonist, but an indirect one, because it does not bind the dopamine receptor. However, its precise mode of action, for example in improving the rate of complex learning in rhesus monkeys, is not known. Single-unit studies show an increase in the firing rate of cholinergic neurons in the medial septal nucleus and the ventral globus pallidus, an effect that is not observed, for example, with piracetam (Poschel et al., 1983). Pramiracetam is well tolerated and apparently successful in improving the affective and behavioral symptoms of DAT: learning/memory, motivation, depression, anergia, and the ability to perform activities of daily living (Branconnier et al., 1983). Apparently successful, it is important to emphasize.

Cranial Electrostimulation (CES)

The following discussion is adapted from Kellaway (1971).

People have been experimenting with electricity for many centuries, to cure disease or to raise the dead or for some other gainful purpose. The Egyptians were familiar with the electric catfish (*Malopterurus electricus*), although they did not necessarily know that he was electric. The Greeks knew that the torpedo fish and some other fish with electric organs could deliver a stinging sensation, and one name they used was "narke", which was also their word for "numbness." Thus, the etymology of two words in current usage.

The ancients understood that the numbing force of the electric fish had a biological purpose, for defense, for example, or predation, but the nature of the force was not understood until Averroes (twelfth century) compared it to the effect of a lodestone on iron. This, of course, is remarkably close to the truth of the matter.

The use of electric fish for medicinal purposes, was a contribution of Roman physicians, who recommended the torpedo fish for a number of therapeutic purposes including headache, gout, excess of venery, or alternatively as an aphrodisiac. Scribonius, who may be considered the father of cranial electrostimulation therapy, or at least of electroichthyology, applied the electrical discharge of the black torpedo fish as a form of galvanic headache therapy. Galen, who is the father of every other branch of medical practice, had his doubts.

Because medical history is always biased in favor of the Western world, it is necessary to report that people in ancient Nigeria and of Abyssinia used the discharge of electric fish as a remedy for various purposes. We may thank these peoples for keeping traditions alive during an era that medical historians have referred to as the "Dark Age of Electroichthyology."

Then the Europeans, who had been influenced more by Galen than Scribonius during this long dark age, began to experiment with the Leyden jar around 1745. The similarity between the shock it delivered and the discharge of the electric fish was soon pointed out, and there was renewed clinical interest in electroichthyology. In 1761, Frans van der Lott performed one of the first preclinical trials of a therapeutic agent when he threw a chicken into a barrel containing a live conger eel (*Gymnotus*). He thus cured a problem the bird had with cramps in the feet.

Then van der Lott took an inferential leap as breathtaking as that of Moniz, who developed psychosurgery on the basis of one chimpanzee experiment (Valenstein, 1986). He repeated the experiment with an Indian slave who was paraparetic, and effected a dramatic cure. Barrel immersion cum conger eel became an established treatment thereafter at least for slaves, for headache and other neurological disorders.

With this sort of pedigree, therefore, one can only wonder why electrotherapy is currently limited to the few psychiatrists who treat refractory depressive disorders (electroconvulsive therapy, ECT), and to physical therapists who treat nonspecific pain syndromes (transcutaneous electrical nerve stimulation, TENS). The answer doubtless lies in the checkered history electrotherapy has enjoyed in Western medicine since the days of the Leyden jar, a topic that has been described on numerous occasions in monographs more discursive even than this (Valenstein, 1986; Ellenberger, 1970).

So perhaps we ought to be surprised by the reintroduction of electrostimulation therapy for neurological disorders, or at least we should greet the news with a mixture of skepticism, deja vu, and curiosity. Of course, we are familiar with the utility of electrical stimulation in the form of motor-evoked potentials for diagnostic purposes. Now it appears that magnetic stimulation, which uses the same principles but is less painful than electrical stimulation, may be helpful for cases of multiple sclerosis, amyotrophic lateral sclerosis, and degenerative ataxic disorders (Hallett and Cohen, 1989). (This from the NIH, no less.)

Cranial electrostimulation therapy (CES) refers to the delivery of very small "doses" of alternating current (0.001 amp), about 100 times per second in a sine wave burst. There is a device currently marketed in the United States (by Neuro Systems, Inc.) called the "Relax-Pak" or the "Neuro-Tone" that uses a couple of 9-volt flashlight batteries. The idea is to deliver a subthreshold current to the brain via electrodes placed on the mastoid processes for 20 to 40 minutes. The procedure is not painful at all; treatments may be administered daily or twice daily.

The treatment was recommended by Russian investigators in the 1950s who coined the term electrosleep, or electronarcosis. That is a misnomer, because it does not appear that the beneficial effects of EST are necessarily mediated by the induction of sleep (Ryan and Souheaver, 1977;). Of course, what it is, precisely, on a physiological level that does mediate the effect of CES is not known; that is, assuming that the treatment has any effect at all. Naturally, there have been speculations that CES stimulates alpha-wave production, that it increases the secretion of endogenous opiate neurotransmitters or biogenic amines, that it alters CNS "reactivity," or that it is an active placebo (Briones and Rosenthal, 1973; Amassian et al.,1987; Empson, 1973).

On the other hand, the proposition that CES has been beneficial has not been addressed to clinical situations where a dramatically effective and otherwise life-saving conventional treatment might be delayed by virtue of recourse to this particular treatment. It has been suggested as a way to reduce anxiety and tension, for example, in patients with mild anxiety disorders (Matteson and Ivancevich, 1985), among people who are being withdrawn from addicting drugs (Schmitt et al., 1986; Gomez and Mikhail, 1979), as a treatment for insomnia (Weiss, 1973), as a way to improve memory performance in alcoholic patients (Smith and Day, 1977), and in patients with posttraumatic amnesia (Childs and Crismon, 1988). One cannot argue with the innocence of at least a trial of CES for such patients.

Nor is it outlandish to propose that EST may be a useful nonpharmacological alternative for a variety of patients, especially people with symptoms of the postconcussion syndrome who are anxious, depressed, and insomniac, who have posttraumatic headaches and deficits in attention and memory. In fact, the author has found the treatment to be occasionally helpful in precisely such circumstances. Perhaps it is nothing more than an active placebo, but it may have a biological spectrum of activity that is similar to that of the antidepressants, stimulants, minor tranquilizers, and mild analgetics, and because it is essentially free of untoward side effects, its clinical utility is well worth exploring. It is certainly cheaper than referral to a pain clinic, a masseur, or a psychotherapist, and it does not seem to be addicting. If the effects of CES are, in fact, mediated by specific effects on neurotransmission or neuromodulation, and there is evidence that it might be (Gleiter and Nutt, 1989), so much the better. But even if it is just a placebo, it is one that works, and that is more than can be said for some of the other "treatments" that one recommends.

An alternative to cranial CES is to throw the patient into a barrel of water with a conger eel or a torpedo fish. More research is clearly needed.

Examining the Patient on Psychoactive Medication

Prudent pharmacotherapy requires a baseline examination and then serial examinations to monitor the patient for therapeutic response and for anticipated side effects. Every candidate for pharmacotherapy requires a comprehensive physical and neurological examination by the physician who prescribes the drug. It is, in the author's opinion, irresponsible to rely on the examination of another physician. It is even less responsible to prescribe without an examination at all. The fact that psychiatrists routinely administer psychoactive medications without performing a physical examination at all is indefensible. One can only compare it to the situation in some Third World countries, where pharmacists dispense what are prescription drugs in the United States on the basis of the patient's complaints and nothing more.

In addition to the physical examination, every candidate for pharmacotherapy should have a baseline complete blood cell count (CBC), liver function studies, and (BUN), creatinine, and urinalysis. The general physical and laboratory studies should be repeated yearly. Blood pressure, pulse, and weight should be measured at every clinic visit, and height (in young patients) at 3-month intervals.

These are essential practices, defined by generations of medical custom, to ensure the good health of the patient at the beginning of treatment and his continued good health as pharmacological treatments are administered. The author feels no compunction to justify this recommendation, beyond noting the high frequency of medical illnesses that are concurrent or causative in psychiatric patients (Lorrin and Koran, 1989), and reminding the reader of the amazing (recent) occurrence of eosinophilia and myalgia in association with L-tryptophan (CDC/MMWR, 1989).

The routine of regular physical examination should not obscure the rationale for a specific examination and specific blood tests for patients who have specific problems or who are taking specific medications. Every drug, and every disorder, comes with its obligate inquiries and warnings and its obligate laboratory and examination procedures.

Patients treated with stimulants and stabilized on an optimal dose should be monitored at 3- to 4-month intervals, with particular attention to pulse and blood pressure, rate of growth, mood (sedation, dysphoria, irritability), abnormal movements, tics or dyskinesias, and sleep and eating patterns. Headache (including classical migraine), abdominal pain, and dysphoria are probably the most frequent side effects of stimulant drugs. Tachycardia and hypertension are rare stimulant effects. Although paradoxical excitement may occur with stimulants, it is more common to find depression. In a head injury patient or a hyperactive child on stimulants, the greater risk is for depression, either as a consequence of drug treatment or after the drug is discontinued.

A stimulant-treated child with tics should be carefully evaluated and the necessity of drug treatment should be reassessed. Stimulants do not cause irreversible tics, but that is no reason to continue treatment in the face of an annoying side effect. Tics may be eliminated if the dose is lowered, or if an alternative drug may be found. Adding tryptophan will eliminate stimulant-induced tics. Tryptophan supplementation will also reduce the occurrence of rebound symptoms after the effects of a stimulant have worn off, and it may reduce the on–off phenomenon that often occurs with methylphenidate.

Stimulant dependence has proven to be such an uncommon occurrence in the patients at the Neuropsychiatry Clinic that no special warning is required. Depression and migraine are the important warnings to give.

The other dopamine agonists have a side-effect profile that is similar to the stimulants, and monitoring is similar. Amantadine may cause pedal edema, for some reason, and a blotchy skin rash; it is probably the only dopamine agonist that can cause a rash. Amantadine may also lower the blood levels of some anticonvulsant drugs. Patients should be warned of the risks of paradoxical excitement and of seizures, especially if alcohol is consumed.

Monitoring tricyclic antidepressant therapy is similar to monitoring stimulants, although special attention should be given to the danger of antidepressant overdose, especially for patients who are potentially suicidal (every head injury patient, during the first couple of years) and patients who have young children around the house. Baseline cardiograms are not useful, as a rule, and do not guarantee the safety of subsequent treatment. The occurrence of arrhythmias, especially conduction defects, is the major concern with tricyclics. Sinus tachycardia is the most common cardiovascular effect of tricyclic antidepressants in children; heart rate elevation above 130 to 140 requires drug discontinuation or dose reduction.

The major warning that is required for the tricyclics is that of cardiac arrhythmia and accidental overdose. Weight gain may also be a problem on the tricyclics, and patients should be warned and monitored accordingly.

Virtually all the typical stimulant side effects may occur with tricyclic antidepressants: tics, headaches (including migraine), dysphoria, and irritability. The clinical utility of antidepressant blood levels has not been convincingly demonstrated, except in special circumstances: in the geriatric population, in antidepressant nonresponders, and in people with preexisting cardiovascular disease.

The novel antidepressants are generally easier to monitor than the tricyclics, because they are less prone to cardiovascular side effects, and there is little if any danger of fatal overdose. For trazodone, the warning should be about priapism; at every visit, one should inquire after the occurrence of unusual penile tumescence (unless, of course, the patient is a woman). For maprotiline and bupropion the warning should be about seizures. The fluoxetine patient should be quizzed, and examined, for symptoms of akathisia. One should inquire about suicidal or violent ruminations.

The examination of the patient on dopamine agonists or antidepressants must include inquiries about depression and irritability as well as observations of the patient's affect and mood. One examines the heart and appraises the patient for dyskinesia, increased muscle tone, and changes in fine motor coordination. One may measure verbal memory, attention, and fluency in simple paper-and-pencil tasks. No special laboratory measures are needed beyond the routine we have described.

In contrast to psychiatry's attitude to most of pharmacotherapeutics, careful physical evaluation of the lithium-treated patient has always been de rigueur. The baseline examination requires renal and thyroid studies, and these should be done subsequently at yearly intervals. Lithium blood levels require frequent monitoring, for example, at 6-month intervals, and so does the urine specific gravity.

The patient on lithium should be examined at 3-month intervals for signs of excessive sedation, motor incoordination, tremor, dyskinesia, increased tone, thyromegaly, edema, and acne vulgaris. Lithium-induced tremor may be a necessary evil, but the occurrence of motor incoordination or dyskinesia or dystonia on lithium is a serious event.

Patients on lithium should be warned that abrupt discontinuation may be the occasion of a withdrawal-induced psychosis (King and Hullin, 1983; Mander, 1986).

Neuroleptic treatment is relatively contraindicated in neuropathic patients in general. One reason is the high frequency of serious untoward effects. Careful monitoring, therefore, at 3-month intervals at least is required. Acute extrapyramidal reactions like dystonia are easy to detect, but subtle extrapyramidal reactions like akathisia may be hard to diagnose and may be misinterpreted as failure to respond. Akathisia should be suspected in any patient who is dysphoric or hyperactive on neuroleptic treatment. Coryza, urinary incontinence, and weight gain are notorious side effects of thioridazine.

Tardive dyskinesia (TD) is not uncommon in neuroleptic-treated patients, and although most such occurrences appear to be short lived, severe and persistent cases have been observed even in children (Gualtieri et al. (1980). TD is usually characterized by choreoathetoid movements, but tics, dystonia, and akathisia may also occur. The major problem with TD monitoring is that maintenance neuroleptic treatment tends to mask early signs of the disorder, so dose reduction or neuroleptic treatment also tends to mask early signs of the disorder. A standard exam for TD, the AIMS, has been developed. It can be reliably administered to most patients, even the severely handicapped, who have a high incidence of abnormal movements and stereotypies. Neuroleptic patients should have an AIMS at 3-month intervals. They should also be examined for sedation and dysphoria, abnormalities of muscle tone, and weight gain.

The neuroleptic malignant syndrome requires a special warning that may frighten patients even more than the standard TD warning. Inquiries about rigidity and hyperthermia should be made at every visit, and they should be accompanied by an admonition to avoid strenuous exertion and dehydration.

Although cholestatic jaundice and granulocytopenia are neuroleptic side effects, periodic laboratory tests beyond those just listed are not necessarily protective. Neuroleptic blood levels have no established clinical salience (Gualtieri et al., 1984b).

Carbamazepine (CBZ) is prescribed to psychiatric patients, young and old, with increasing frequency. Monitoring CBZ requires examination for ataxia and nystagmus, sedation, dysphoria, nervousness or irritability, increased occurrence of seizures (especially absences), skin rash, easy bruising, or frequent infection. CBZ blood levels should be checked at 6-month intervals, at least, along with a CBC and LFT. The tests should be done more frequently when treatment begins. Irritability in a CBZ-treated patient may be a sign of hyponatremia.

One should mention the hematopoietic effects of CBZ when discussing the drug, but the warning does not have to be draconian. It is not at all clear that CBZ is likelier than VPA, for example, or the neuroleptic drugs, to cause agranulocytosis or thrombocytopenia.

The monitoring procedure for valproic acid is similar to that for CBZ, although serum ammonia levels may also be necessary to detect subtle changes in hepatic function. The warning about hepatic failure should never be omitted, especially in young patients and patients on concurrent drugs.

The behavioral toxicity that frequently accompanies treatment with sedating anticonvulsants—phenytoin and the barbiturates—is not usually manifest during a neuropsychiatric examination, but a psychiatrist who consults on a patient treated with archaic anticonvulsants should consider recommending alternative anticonvulsant therapy before embarking on a course of psychiatric treatment.

Patients who are treated with propranolol or other beta blockers require careful cardiovascular monitoring, because bradycardia and hypotension are not uncommon side effects. The same is true for clonidine and for the calcium channel blockers. Beta blockers are contraindicated in asthmatic patients. Patients who are smokers require a chest exam at every visit. One may want to keep track of serum triglycerides and cholesterol in patients on beta blockers. The only special warning a beta-blocker patient requires is that he may live longer by virtue of the treatment he is on.

The general physical examination is supplemented by special measures aimed at detecting specific drug side effects. Balance and fine motor coordination are easily checked in a routine physical. Verbal memory, verbal and semantic fluency, and visual-perceptual processing are easily tested with a few simple neuropsychological tests. The entire procedure may require only 5 or 10 minutes.

During this brief exam, the physician may make most of the important interpersonal assessments that are part of the mental status exam. There is the opportunity for casual banter, and for serious questions: about sexuality, depression, thoughts of suicide. Patients are far more comfortable discussing such issues with someone who behaves in a familiar, doctorly manner, who competently goes about the job of a physical assessment, and who will extend himself in a bit of small talk. The physical examination is probably the best opening to a psychiatric interview. The intimacy that comes of physical contact can extend to a patient's inner side, too.

CHAPTER 4

Inadvertent Drug Effects

Nothing is all bad. Your personal health-maintenance professional might have you believe there is no good thing at all about tobacco, but nothing could be further from the truth. Smoking, chewing, or dipping snuff, in fact, is the only way to prevent Green Tobacco Sickness. That may not mean much to you, but around where I live, it is something.

The regular consumption of tobacco may also slow the onset of Parkinson's disease, and it may help prevent that disorder, too (Kessler and Diamond, 1971; Godwin-Austen et al., 1982). The beneficial effect against Parkinson's is more complicated, even speculative. The key element in the reaction is probably nicotine, which has the properties of both acetylcholine agonist and antagonist (Whitehouse et al., 1988). Nicotine receptors are widely distributed in brain, including the striatum (Schwartz et al., 1982). Nicotine induces the release of dopamine from striatal tissue in vitro and in vivo (Giorguieff-Chesselet et al., 1979; Marien et al., 1982) and it also affects the other monoamine neurotransmitters (Jones, 1987). The same mechanisms probably account for the negative effects of tobacco consumption on tardive dyskinesia, in contrast to Parkinson's disease, a hyperdopaminergic state (Yassa et al., 1987).

This is not idle information to distract my readers, but is presented for their edification. At issue are the inadvertent neuropsychiatric effects of drugs and of compounds that we have only recently come to think of as "drugs," such as tobacco and caffeine and alcohol, and how these inadvertent effects may influence the clinical condition of patients who have sustained a traumatic brain injury (TBI).

Reflections along these lines were running through the author's mind as he was consulting with a head injury patient recently. The young man had sustained a mild brain injury several months before. There was only a brief period of posttraumatic confusion, but it was followed by a long period of difficulty in concentrating, mental "fuzziness," mild memory deficits, and problems organizing his work that was complex indeed. He was a city planner for one of the major metropolitan centers in our state, responsible for the welfare of thousands of citizens, and his

Parts of this chapter appeared in substantially modified form in C. Thomas Gualtieri. "The Neuropharmacology of Inadvertent Drug Effects in Patients with Traumatic Brain Injuries," *Journal of Head Trauma Rehabilitation* 5 (3), September 1990, Aspen Publications, Inc., Rockville, Maryland.

work with budgets, contractors, and the Board of Aldermen never permitted an idle moment or a lapse in attention. His recovery from the consequences of a mild frontal lobe injury was successful, in spite of the constant pressures of a political-administrative position. He required substantial neuropsychological nursing, but he also took his own initiatives in the service of recovery, and this included an active program of aerobic exercise. He wondered whether he should give up smoking cigarettes.

Now, any health-maintenance professional worth his or her mustard would respond in the affirmative, but not this one. After all, an answer this easy had to be half wrong. And the right answer was half wrong.

The modern American cigarette is nothing less than an efficient vehicle for the delivery of nicotine to the brain, about 1 mg of nicotine to the fag. And that makes it one of the only ways to deliver a belt of cholinergic material, and dopamine, to brain receptors that really need it. The neuropsychological importance of nicotine is in its cogent effects on vigilance attention, information processing, and acquisition and retention of new information (Jones, 1987). The beneficial effects of a dopaminergic compound are, of course, old news (see Chapter 3, this volume).

As we contend with difficult clinical problems like the treatment of Alzheimer's disease and the neuropsychological sequelae of TBI, we find ourselves at odds with the inefficiencies and the dangers of cholinergic treatments such as lecithin, physostigmine (McLean et al., 1987), and tetrahydroaminoacridine (Byrne and Arie, 1989). In fact, the major difficulty with cholinergic treatment for TBI, as we mentioned in Chapter 3, is to discover an effective way to deliver the active compound to brain.

Because the good ole American cigarette is the only cholinergic delivery system currently available, it is no surprise when TBI patients take up the habit, even when they had given it up years before their accident. In the author's opinion, it is unreasonable to expect the TBI patient to abjure the only really efficient cholinergic drug. Should head injury rehabilitation centers try to ban smoking on the premises? Well, you do not want the clients to fire the mattresses, so smoking should be discouraged; but would Nicorette be better than abstinence?

One may exercise great discretion in the prescription of psychoactive drugs, but, remember, the world is full of psychoactive drugs, and most of them are available in perfectly legitimate ways. There are three important ones, in terms of prevalence and intensity of consumption: tobacco (nicotine), caffeine, and alcohol. There are the illicit drugs of abuse, especially cannabis, cocaine, PCP, hallucinogens, and opiates. Then there are drugs prescribed for general medical (as opposed to neuropsychiatric) conditions: beta blockers, calcium channel blockers, most antihypertensives, gastrointestinal drugs, drugs for spasticity, and, of course, the anticonvulsants. Finally, there are the OTC drugs: antihistamines, decongestants, antitussives; analgetics.

This is an important issue for TBI patients. First, they are people, and everyone has some favorite recreational drug; even people whose scruples forbid the use of caffeine, nicotine, or alcohol can get an ersatz highs from sugar, khat or betel nut.

Second, they get sick. They are vulnerable to medical problems, like hypertension, headache, epilepsy, spasticity, peptic ulcer disease, and gastritis; they even get colds, and they have problems like asthma. All these problems may entail specific and medically appropriate treatment with drugs that may have inadvertent psychological effects.

Third, they have their weaknesses. They are, after all, a relatively young group of patients, and some have been given to reckless behavior. In fact, drugs of abuse play a major role in the epidemiology and etiology of brain injury. So, one should not be surprised if they continue to be at issue in the posttraumatic patient.

Licit Drugs

Tobacco/Nicotine

We have alluded to the central issues here. There are clear dangers to health and safety from smoking, but tobacco has a number of favorable psychoactive and neuropsychological effects, and these are more pronounced among tobacco addicts. Nicotine is a cholinergic and a dopaminergic drug, and cholinergic/dopaminergic treatment is one of the cornerstones of the neuropharmacological treatment for TBI and dementia.

No one should propose a study to compare the recovery from TBI in patients on Nicorette to those on Juicy Fruit gum, and no one should seriously entertain the idea of inducing an addiction to nicotine, to elicit some theoretical benefit in acetylcholine neurotransmission and brain recovery. But familiarity with the neuropharmacological properties of nicotine does lend some understanding. One might anticipate, for example, a relative weakness in the recovery of TBI patients who are also withdrawn from nicotine; one might expect to see a stronger impulse to smoke among TBI patients, and a greater degree of difficulty in withdrawing voluntarily; and one might exercise a degree of skepticism in evaluating the results of cholinergic/dopaminergic studies for neuropsychiatric patients, unless there is some control over the variable of nicotine addiction.

Caffeine

Because caffeine is a "stimulant," people got the idea that it should be a good thing for hyperactive children. In fact, it does not seem to work very well at all clinically (Klein, 1987). It does have positive effects on neuropsychological tasks that involve sustained attention but, in contrast to methylphenidate, it has no effects on memory (Judd et al., 1987).

Caffeine is not a dopamine agonist, like methylphenidate and amphetamine and pemoline, but a xanthine, and the xanthines are adenosine antagonists. Adenosine is a purinergic neurotransmitter, with modulatory effects on other neurotransmission systems including serotonin, histamine, norepinephrine, and dopamine (Williams, 1987). The stimulating effects of caffeine may be explained in terms of release from purinergic inhibitory tone (Harms et al., 1978).

To understand the behavioral effects of caffeine is in large part to understand the CNS roles of adenosine. Adenosine is a potent anticonvulsant (Dunwiddie and Worth, 1982). It can reduce food intake and decrease aggression, precisely what one would expect on the basis of the action of its antagonist, caffeine (Williams, 1987; Katsuragi et al., 1984). Carbamazepine, in contrast, is an adenosine agonist, which may account for its anticonvulsant action, its effect on carbohydrate hunger, and its antiaggression effects (Lewin and Bleck, 1977; Clark and Post, 1989).

Excessive intake of caffeine, therefore, may lower the seizure threshold (Rall, 1985), it may lead to weight loss or aggression (Williams, 1987), or it may induce a state of anxiety or agitation. This, presumably, is related to antagonism of the sedating or tranquilizing properties of adenosine, although it could have to do with a direct xanthine effect at the benzodiazepine receptor (Asano and Spector, 1979).

Even in relatively low doses, 200 to 500 mg, caffeine can produce headaches, tremors, anxiety, and irritability (Rall, 1985). Caffeine can induce panic attacks in vulnerable patients, and patients with panic disorder are known to be hypersensitive to caffeine (Boulenger et al., 1984). Caffeine can also cause akathisia, which may represent a drug interaction with one of the dopamine or opiate receptors.

All these clinical effects are salient to the diagnosis and management of TBI patients. It is appropriate to inquire about caffeine consumption as part of the patient's pharmacological history. It is also appropriate to consider limiting caffeine intake for TBI patients with certain symptoms. And it is not inappropriate to limit the availability of caffeinated beverages at TBI centers, as some have already done; that may be an extreme measure, but there is a rationale.

Alcohol

When there is too much to say, and so much of it has been said before, a list is a good idea.

1. Alcohol is related to the occurrence of TBI from single-vehicle crashes, nighttime crashes, and injuries to motorcyclists, bicyclists, and pedestrians (Baker et al., 1984).

2. People who tend to overuse or to abuse alcohol and other intoxicating drugs are overrepresented among TBI patients (Field, 1976; Kerr et al., 1971), and especially among people who have had more than one TBI (Annegers et al., 1980b).

3. Alcoholic intoxication at the time of injury may influence the accuracy of diagnosis and implementation of treatment in the emergency room or the neurosurgery ICU (Kraus, 1987).

4. The chronic abuse of alcohol and of other intoxicating substances may be more likely in patients who are in difficult social or economic circumstances, in the unemployed, and in people with depression and personality disorders. Insofar as these circumstances may be aggravated by TBI, the risk of drug and alcohol abuse may be expected to increase after TBI, although this idea has not been tested in an epidemiologic survey.

5. The idea that depression may cause alcoholism is probably naive and inaccurate (Mello, 1987). Chronic alcohol use, however, can lead to despondency (Mello, 1987). One would expect then that excessive alcohol intake can aggravate the depression that occurs in TBI patients. Alcohol is a very poor antidepressant drug, although it can cause a transient euphoria. That is one reason people drink when they are depressed. It is also a mild tranquilizer, which is why they drink when they are under stress. But it is not a good tranquilizer.

6. Chronic alcohol abuse is, by itself, associated with deficits of brain function including disorders of memory, attention, cognitive processes, and sleep (Mello, 1987). Repeated intoxication may lead to permanent brain dysfunction, such as Wernicke's encephalopathy and Korsakoff's psychosis. Chronic alcoholics may have ventricular enlargement, widening of the sulci, and diffuse cortical atrophy (Wilkinson, 1982), although the mechanism by which alcohol induces transient or permanent brain damage is not clearly known (Mello, 1987).

7. It is an intuitive surmise that the combined effects of alcohol abuse and TBI are additive; and that alcoholism may predict poor outcome from TBI, or retard in some way the cortical recovery process. There is some support for this belief (Hillbom and Holm, 1986; Brooks et al., 1989).

8. In laboratory preparations, alcohol is known to effectively suppress convulsions (induced, for example, by phenylenetetrazol), but this anticonvulsant action is followed by a period of hyperexcitability that may last for hours or days. Therefore, people who are prone to seizures are usually advised to abstain from alcohol or to use it very judiciously.

9. Interactions occur between alcohol and the psychotropic and anticonvulsant drugs. Acute alcohol ingestion inhibits the first-pass effect, increasing systemic bioavailability of drugs. On the other hand, ethanol decreases gastric emptying time and thus delays drug absorption. Acute low-dose alcohol increases hepatic blood flow, while high-dose alcohol decreases it. This would have the greatest effect on drugs with high extraction ratios. As a rule, acute alcohol inhibits drug metabolism and chronic alcohol enhances metabolism (absent liver disease). Cirrhosis spares metabolism by glucuronidation, but impairs oxidative metabolism. Hypoalbuminuria, in alcoholics with liver disease, has variable clinical effects, depending on degree of binding, hepatic extraction ratio, and binding protein (Ciraulo and Barnhill, 1986).

10. The various mechanisms of alcohol–drug interaction may be held to account for several clinical phenomena:

Alcoholics, when inebriated, are sensitive to the toxic effects of barbiturates, but they are more resistant when they have been sober. This is because alcohol first decreases, then increases microsomal enzymes.

Treatment with disulfiram increases the elimination half-life and decreases the whole-body clearance of tricyclic antidepressants, thus increasing plasma levels (Ciraulo et al., 1985)

11. There are other alcohol–drug interactions that must be explained on the basis of pharmacodynamics.

Alcohol is known to increase the negative neuropsychological effects of benzodiazepines. These are most often effects on memory and perceptual-motor function (e.g., Aranko et al., 1985; Dorian et al., 1985; Allen et al., 1988; Mamelak et al., 1987; Higgins et al., 1987; Morris and Estes, 1987; Schuckit, 1987). In contrast, the nonbenzodiazepine anxiolytic buspirone shows only slight interactions with alcohol (Erwin et al., 1986) and it has also been found to reduce ethanol craving in alcoholic patients to a significant degree (Bruno, 1989)

The deficit in manual dexterity induced by the antidepressants trazodone and amitryptiline may be increased by alcohol (Warrington et al., 1986). On the other hand, there does not seem to be any negative interaction between alcohol and the serotonergic antidepressant fluoxetine (Allen & Lader, 1989). Neither is an there an adverse interaction between alcohol and maprotiline on psychomotor performance (Stromberg et al., 1988) although alcohol may promote the development of maprotiline-induced seizures (Strawn et al., 1988).

Illicit Drugs

Cannabis

Marijuana smoking is the most common form of illicit drug use in the United States. Many people think it is a harmless vice, and that the drug has no serious medical or psychological effects. They probably are right, if the drug is used very occasionally by someone who is mature and intact, and who is seeking nothing more than a mild "high." But that does not constitute adequate rationale for legalization and commercialization, something that has been suggested on many occasions. The major problem with cannabis is its use in inappropriate or even dangerous circumstances. Insofar as legalization may be expected to increase such behavior, it may not be a very good idea.

Cannabis intoxication is inappropriate, and possibly dangerous, in people who are driving or operating machinery, in children or adolescents at school, and in someone with a preexisting psychiatric disorder.

Cannabis, or to be more accurate, delta-9 tetrahydrocannabinol, is known to affect sensory and perceptual processes, such as time perception, ocular motor tracking, and visual reaction time. For this reason, it is hazardous for people who drive, or who fly, or who operate heavy machinery (Yesavage et al., 1985). It is also known to affect cognitive processes, like short-term memory, acquisition of new information, and performance of complex cognitive tasks (Miller and Branconnier, 1983; Braff et al., 1981; Borg et al., 1975). For this reason, it is inappropriate for students.

Although the expected emotional response to cannabis is mild euphoria, it may cause untoward emotional effects, and one can become anxious or panicky or paranoid, dysphoric or akathisic, disorganized, depersonalized or disassociated. For this reason, it is inappropriate for people with preexisting psychiatric conditions, and it is dangerous for people with a tendency to psychosis (Treffert, 1978).

Cannabinoids seem to possess antiepileptic activity (Alldredge, Lowenstein and Simon, 1989), an effect that may be mediated by drug-induced release of adreno cortico tropin (ACTH). Interactions with other drugs, that is, prescribed drugs, seem to be negligible. The fact that cannabis consumption is sometimes linked to the use of alcohol and other illicit drugs raises an additional concern for its use by patients with TBI. Cannabis can complicate the assay of blood levels of tricyclic antidepressants by interfering with the chromatographic process (Devane, 1987). It is said that chronic heavy use of cannabis can lead to an "amotivational syndrome," that is, a state of relative indifference to the usual parameters that guide academic and economic achievement (Nahas, 1986). There is some controversy about this syndrome; whether, for example, it is the result or the cause of heavy cannabis consumption. But one would hardly recommend cannabis for the recreational use of a frontal lobe patient who was already indifferent, unmotivated, and abulic; of course, such a patient may not have the initiative even to acquire the illicit drug.

It is hardly necessary to iterate that TBI patients are one of those groups for whom cannabis is inappropriate, even dangerous, even if consumption is occasional and the dose is low. Nor is it necessary to say much about the interaction cannabis should be expected to have with the perceptual, motor, cognitive, and emotional deficits that exist in many if not most TBI patients. This is one case where the right answer is the easy one. Cannabis, like alcohol, should be strongly discouraged to people who have had brain injuries.

It should be absolutely forbidden to people with perceptual or mnemonic deficits, and to people who are given to emotional instability or to flights from reality.

Cocaine and Other Stimulants

People have written about the prescription of psychostimulants for some of the behavioral and neuropsychological consequences of TBI (Evans et al., 1987b; Gualtieri and Evans, 1988; Gualtieri, 1988). Cocaine is also in that family. It is not a stimulant like caffeine, it is fairly and squarely a dopamine agonist, like amphetamine. In fact, most of the toxic effects of cocaine can also occur with amphetamine.

The literature on stimulant treatment of TBI is concerned with very low doses: about 0.2 mg/kg per dose, twice or three times a day for adults, and slightly higher doses for children (Gualtieri and Evans, 1988). Higher doses of stimulants are not only unnecessary, they are toxic, and they may be dangerous. Low doses of stimulants usually raise the seizure threshold; high doses tend to lower the seizure threshold; and very high doses can cause seizures, even in people who are not prone to seize. The same is true of the dopamine agonist amantadine, which may also be used therapeutically for TBI patients (Gualtieri et al., 1989). One cannot be sure that low doses of cocaine have any effect at all on the seizure threshold, but it is certainly true that high doses can lead to seizures, and even status epilepticus. That is one reason why TBI patients should avoid cocaine.

We have written about the positive effects of stimulants on memory in TBI patients (Evans et al., 1986b), but it also appears that high doses of stimulants will have a negative effect on memory performance (Wetzel et al., 1981). Low doses of stimulants of all kinds can be expected to enhance performance, to counter fatigue, to diminish pain, and to elevate mood. Higher doses, however, can be extremely disruptive to performance and social interaction; tolerance to the euphoriant effects of the drug develops, severe aggressive behavior may occur, irritability, irrational rage, and impulsive behavior. A toxic psychosis that is virtually indistinguishable from paranoid schizophrenia may develop, and severe depression usually occurs after withdrawal (Fischman, 1987). Interaction with other drugs is not an important issue with cocaine, as it is for alcohol. Cocaine is not known to alter the disposition or metabolism of any other drug (Kreek, 1987). Cocaine may, however, complicate the assay of tricyclic antidepressant blood levels by interfering with the chromatographic extraction (Devane, 1987).

What is the major issue is the extremely disruptive effects the drug has on behavior, performance, and emotional integrity. An even more important issue is the vasculitis or vasculopathy of the cerebral vascular tree that is sometimes observed in heavy users of cocaine or amphetamine derivatives, an event that may lead to miniinfarcts or to overt stroke (Rumbaugh and Fang, 1978; Klonoff et al., 1989).

On several occasions in the past when amphetamines were freely available, there were epidemics of stimulant abuse that rivaled in severity and social disruption the present-day problem with cocaine. Considering the potential for stimulant abuse, then, and considering the devastating effects of addiction to drugs like cocaine or amphetamine, is it reasonable to prescribe methylphenidate or amphetamine to TBI patients at all?

We have had occasion to address this question, on the basis of a clinical survey at the Neuropsychiatry Clinic of 47 adults aged 18 to 38 who met diagnostic criteria for attention deficit disorder (ADD) ("residual type") and 31 adults who had neurobehavioral sequelae of TBI, and who also had problems with attention, memory, and impulsive temperamental behavior. The first group of patients (ADD adults) included a series of 22 who were described in a paper published in 1985 (Gualtieri et al., 1985). The second group of 31 (TBI adults) included a series of 15 who were described in 1988 (Gualtieri and Evans, 1988). It was the policy of the Neuropsychiatry Clinic to follow these patients very closely on a monthly basis over the years, and we have reviewed their long-term follow-up status.

Of a total of 78, there were no cases of stimulant abuse in any traditional sense. No patient ever evidenced inappropriate drug-seeking behavior, or expressed the need for increasing doses as time went by. There were no cases of social disruption, disorganization, or toxic psychosis. No one went on to other drugs of abuse, such as cocaine. In fact, most patients discontinued treatment after 6 to 18 months, mainly because the drug had seemed to exercise its maximum benefit and further treatment was no longer necessary.

Of the 78, 4 patients were compelled to discontinue stimulant treatment because of psychological difficulties. One fellow took an overdose of methylphenidate during an argument with his wife; 3 women developed mild depressive disorders, in 2 cases related to severe family problems, and they were hospitalized because of suicidal ideation. In one case, there was a severe depression and a suicide attempt. All of these patients had ADD; there were no such problems with TBI patients.

It has become our policy to monitor adults on stimulants very carefully for the development of depressive disorders. It is not surprising that some people with a lifelong history of academic and occupational failure might develop depression at some time during their adult lives, and the prevalence of depression in this sample is not really any higher than it is in the general population (e.g., Blazer et al., 1988). But there is always the risk that chronic stimulant therapy may lead to a depressive state, and patients should be monitored accordingly.

Phencyclidine

Phencyclidine (PCP) has been used clinically as an anesthetic agent, and there has been an epidemic of PCP abuse since the early 1970s. Although it has been classified as an hallucinogen, it has an amphetamine-like activity that can be blocked by chlorpromazine, and it causes barbiturate-like effects (Balster, 1987). It is severely disruptive to learning and memory, and it has a range of very serious psychiatric effects from mild dissociation and amnesia to schizophreniform psychosis to violent aggression (Balster, 1987). After the PCP-induced psychosis clears, the patient may experience a long period of depression. Other clinical signs associated with PCP intoxication include catatonia, agitation, and excitement, gross motor incoordination, catalepsy, aphonia diaphoresis, and hypacusis (Petersen and Stillman, 1978).

PCP has anticonvulsant effects in various animal models, which suggests that withdrawal from prolonged intoxication may be an extremely unstable state. It is also capable of enhancing the action of classical CNS depressants such as barbiturates and alcohol. It is believed that heavy use of PCP may be dementing (Peterson and Stillman, 1978), and there is preclinical evidence that PCP may be neurotoxic to specific populations of brain neurons (Olney et al., 1989). PCP and the other hallucinogens such as LSD and mescaline can cause cerebral vasospasm, hypoxia, and cell death (Altura and Altura, 1981).

The other hallucinogenic drugs, like lysergic acid (LSD), psilocin, 2,5-dimethoxy-4-methylamphetamine (DOM), mescaline, and *N,N*-dimethyltryptamine appear to constitute a distinct drug class based on similar phenomenological effects in humans and the fact that cross-tolerance can be demonstrated among many of them (Jacobs et al., 1982). It is thought that what is common to the hallucinogenic drugs is an effect on serotonin neurotransmission, although their effects on this system are complex, with mixed agonist, antagonist, and modulatory actions (Jacobs et al., 1982).

If one considers the use of cannabis or alcohol to be a reckless act for the TBI patient, the use of drugs like cocaine, PCP, LSD, MDA, or other hallucinogens represents a self-destructive activity too gross to countenance. It is not only the severely disruptive effect such drugs have on behavior and organization of thinking; there is also the risk of further brain damage, whether overt or microscopic.

Opiates

Opiate abuse, especially heroin, is almost an anticlimax after a discussion of drugs like cocaine and PCP that are extremely destructive over the short term and that may be associated with neurotoxicity. The most dangerous elements of opiate addiction are secondary: the adoption of an antisocial lifestyle to support an expensive habit; the abandonment of social ambitions and family ties; and the intravenous route of administration with its attendant risks. In contrast to cocaine and hallucinogenic drugs, however, the opiates are remarkably free of direct neuropsychological effects aside from their general property as CNS depressants. They appear to be free of direct neurotoxic effects, and long-term administration of opiates like methadone appears to be safe, medically and psychologically (Kreek, 1987).

There are even reports of treatment for neuropathic patients with opiate derivatives, such as the use of naltrexone for post-concussional syndrome (Tennant and Wild, 1987) or to promote recovery following spinal cord injury (Faden, 1984), and of propoxyphene and codeine for akathisia (Walters et al., 1986). Naltrexone, however, may be hepatotoxic in some people at high doses (Kreek, 1987).

Drugs Prescribed for Medical Reasons

There are licit drugs, illicit drugs, and drugs that doctors recommend. It is arguable that more harm is done from the last; arguable, but meretricious. After all, physicians recommend drugs that are necessary, and the risks of medical treatment are calculated risks. Sometimes.

We have mentioned metaclopramide (Reglan) in Chapter 3, with the neuroleptics, because it is a neuroleptic although some people contend that it is not. It is sometimes necessary to prevent distension and reflux in TBI patients with gastrostomy or jejunostomy tubes. But it should be used only when the indication is severe and unequivocal, because it is a neuroleptic and does nothing to hasten the course of cortical recovery, to say the least.

Three classes of antihypertensive drugs are also discussed in Chapter 3: the beta blockers, clonidine, an alpha agonist, and the calcium channel blockers. They are mentioned as the sometime treatment for behavior problems in TBI patients, and in this regard they show great promise. They are also extremely important antihypertensive drugs, but it is ironic that although they may be preferred as psychotropics, they are second-choice antihypertensives. Sedation and depression are side effects of the beta blockers and the alpha agonists when they are prescribed for blood pressure, and irritability is a side effect of the calcium channel blockers. These are side effects that may limit their utility in the TBI patient.

Antihypertensives like reserpine and methyldopa may also be depressants, and methyldopa and propanalol have been shown to produce memory impairment (Solomon et al., 1983). The preferred antihypertensive for TBI patients might be a thiazide diuretic or an ACE inhibitor like captopril, drugs that have no negative neuropsychological effects at all (Croog et al., 1986). Captopril may even be an antidepressant (Deicken, 1986).

H2 Receptor Antagonists

The best-selling drugs in the world are the H2 receptor antagonists, cimetidine (Tagamet), ranitidine (Zantac), and famotidine (Pepcid). They act on the gastric parietal cell, to block the binding of histamine to the H2 receptor and thus to inhibit gastric acid secretion. They heal and prevent duodenal and gastric ulcers. The worldwide best-seller once was diazepam. It is a measure of the times that one is now content simply not to be so uptight; 20 years ago, the ambition was to mellow out.

The major psychological problem that arises in patients treated with cimetidine, and, to a lesser degree, ranitidine, is mental confusion or delirium, an effect that may be more common in elderly patients and patients with hepatic or renal dysfunction (Sharpe and Burland, 1980; Hughes et al., 1983; Silverstone, 1984; Epstein, 1984). It is possible that H2-antagonist delirium is more likely in patients who are treated concurrently with benzodiazepines (Goff et al., 1985), which makes sense because the H2 antagonists have a benzodiazepine-like effect on GABA and benzodiazepine receptors in the central nervous system (CNS) (Lakoski et al., 1983).

It is possible that famotidine is less likely to exercise CNS effects than ranitidine or cimetidine, although none of the H2 blockers can be said to be completely free of behavioral toxicity. If it is true, though, that famotidine is also a drug that decreases gastric emptying time, it might be a good alternative not only to ranitidine and cimetidine, but also to metaclopramide; it might be used, for example, for the comatose patient with a gastrostomy feeding tube to prevent reflux esophagitis, stress ulcers, and gastric distension.

Sympathomimetics

Drugs that stimulate alpha- or beta-adrenergic receptors are used widely; alpha adrenergics like phenylpropanolamine, ephedrine, and pseudoephedrine are available as over-the-counter (OTC) nasal decongestants. They work by causing vasoconstriction in the nasal mucosa. They are also sold as anorectics, sometimes in preparations that contain caffeine. Beta adrenergics like theophylline are prescribed as antiasthmatics. You have to expect that something so ubiquitous, popular, useful, and cheap is going to be dangerous.

No one is surprised to learn that sympathomimetics can cause nervousness, irritability, emotional lability, insomnia, and agitation. Or even the odd case of hallucinosis, or frank psychosis, or depression. These are problems that can arise from therapeutic doses, or at least from the doses that are packaged in OTC formulations and purported to be therapeutic. In overdose situations, or when the patient is on a concurrent drug like a monoamine oxidase inhibitor, the alpha adrenergics can lead to hypertensive encephalopathy, tachyarrhythmias, and seizures (Pentel, 1984).

The beta agonists are associated with the same pattern of CNS irritability, especially in vulnerable individuals, and the typical case is a hyperactive child who is out of control so long as he has to take slophyllin for asthma. TBI patients have to be included as a group of patients particularly vulnerable to the behavioral toxicity of sympathomimetics.

But that is behavioral toxicity, and although it is a perennial clinical problem, and although it may be a severe problem, it is nothing to the potential neurotoxicity of the beta agonists. Theophylline, for example, is a potent cerebral vasoconstrictor, and it may cause cerebral infarction, seizures, and hemiplegia (Clancy et al., 1984; Noetzel, 1985). Most of the reports have been of children, but there is no reason to believe that the problem should be restricted to children; severe consequences are more likely in circumstances of overdose, but toxicity to theophylline, for example, may occur across a broad range of doses and blood levels (Bertino and Walker, 1987). Nor does there appear to be one beta agonist that is potentially less neurotoxic than any other.

The fallacy, of course, is to think that a drug that is sometimes neurotoxic is always a dangerous drug. The problem, however, is how to ascribe acute neuropsychiatric decompensation to prior treatment with a drug like theophylline, known to be capable of neurotoxicity, absent other overt signs of drug toxicity.

Antispasticity Drugs

Spasticity is a motor disorder characterized by a velocity-dependent increase in tonic stretch reflexes ("muscle tone") with exaggerated tendon jerks, resulting from hyperexcitability of the stretch reflex, as one component of the upper motor neuron syndrome (Young and Delwaide, 1981). The three usual pharmacological alternatives for the treatment of spasticity are dantrolene, a peripherally acting drug that inhibits the release of calcium ions from the sarcoplasmic reticulum of muscle fibers, thereby preventing activation of the contractile apparatus; baclofen, a lipophilic derivative of gamma-aminobutyric acid (GABA) that binds to $GABA_B$ receptors on brain and spinal cord cell membranes, but whose major action is probably at the spinal cord level; and the benzodiazepines, especially diazepam, which work as GABA mimetics and enhance presynaptic inhibition in the spinal cord (Davidoff, 1985). None of the antispasticity drugs works especially well in the TBI patient, although they may appear to alleviate spasticity over the short term; it is not at all clear that decerebrate rigidity is a model of spasticity. All the existing antispasticity drugs are potentially sedating, however, and baclofen has been associated with acute encephalopathy (Abarbanel et al., 1985). It is not clear, then, that the conventional antispasticity drugs are indicated in most cases of TBI.

The question is, what is? and the answer lies in the realm of clinical investigation and new drug development. There has been interest in the phenothiazines and phenytoin, but not from this quarter; in the alpha-adrenergic blockers; carbamazepine; opiate-receptor antagonists; thyrotropin-releasing hormone; calcium channel antagonists; tetrahydrocannabiol (yes, THC); glycine; and progabide, a GABA-mimetic drug with anticonvulsant properties (Davidoff, 1985; Weintraub and Evans, 1985; Faden, 1987; Whyte and Robinson, in press).

CHAPTER 5

Epilepsy

There are four things to consider in this chapter:

1. Neuropsychiatric problems that arise in people with epilepsy;
2. Neuropsychiatric conditions that are not epilepsy, but that are kin to epilepsy;
3. The neuropsychological and behavioral effects of anticonvulsant drugs; and
4. Psychotropic drugs as convulsants and anticonvulsants.

These issues have been discussed extensively in recent books (e.g., Reynolds and Trimble, 1981; Blumer, 1984; Trimble and Zarifian, 1985; Trimble, 1985; Lishman, 1987), especially the first and the second issues, but it is appropriate to go over old ground. For mentally retarded people, for head injury patients, and for children with severe behavior disorders, epilepsy is a common problem, and it is always high in the differential diagnosis of paroxysmal disorders. The psychotropic anticonvulsants carbamazepine (CBZ), valproate (VPA), and clonazepam (KLON) are among the agents most commonly prescribed for behavior disorders. And the influence psychotropic drugs exercise against the seizure threshold accounts for much that transpires in therapeutics and in behavior toxicity.

Neuropsychiatric Conditions in Epileptic Patients

The problems that arise in epileptic patients may be related directly to the disorder or they may be treatment related. Aberrant behavior or extreme emotional events may be ictal, preictal, or postictal phenomena. There is also an "interictal" syndrome that develops in some epileptic patients; changes in personality, in behavior, in emotional expression, or in thinking that is somehow caused by the evolution of the disease itself.

Treatment-related difficulties may be the consequence of behavior toxicity from anticonvulsant drugs, or they may be the consequence of partial or imperfect treatment. Anticonvulsants may cause impairment in cognition; or, impaired cognition may be the result of epileptic activity that is only partially treated. Anticonvulsant treatment may visit a psychiatric disorder on the patient; phenobarbital causes hyperactivity, ethosuccimide causes depression, phenytoin leads to dementia, and CBZ can *make* patients aggressive. Alternatively, continued behavior problems in an epileptic patient may be the consequence of imperfect anticonvulsant therapy.

It is not always possible to distinguish precisely which element may be operative in a given patient. An antiepileptic drug, for example, may be sufficient to control ictal events, but not paroxysmal outbursts of untoward behavior. The problem, then, arises with the disease itself, but it is prolonged or aggravated by inadequate treatment. Theoretically, a psychiatric syndrome may be "kindled" in a patient with an epileptic focus who is treated with a drug that controls ictus but not kindling; the problem never would have arisen, theoretically at least, if the patient had been treated with an anticonvulsant with antikindling properties. That some patients with epilepsy deteriorate intellectually is clear (Reynolds, 1861). That there is a progressive dementia associated with long-term phenytoin or primidone treatment is also well established (Trimble, 1981; Thompson et al., 1980). Depression is a recognized interictal psychiatric problem in epilepsy (Robertson and Trimble, 1983), but depression is also a side effect of antidepressant drugs like ethosuccimide and phenobarbital.

The third element to complicate one's interpretation of psychological events, as they unfold in an epileptic patient, is the influence of the underlying pathology that yields on the one hand seizures and on the other aberrant behavior. Thinking about epileptics is a little like thinking about schizophrenics; so long as one is dealing only with the behavioral manifestations of a neuropathic process, and so long as the neuropathic process itself is poorly understood, correlations and cause-and-effect relationships will always be ambiguous.

Intelligence

A gradual deterioration of intellectual ability in epileptic patients was described in the era before anticonvulsant drugs (Brown and Reynolds, 1981). The mental competence of an epileptic patient may be compromised by genetic proclivity, neuropathic abnormalities acquired before the onset of seizures, epilepsy itself and the neuropathic sequelae of fits, psychosocial isolation, and, of course, overdose with sedative anticonvulsant drugs (Lennox and Lennox, 1960).

The IQ scores of epileptic patients are skewed to begin with. Mentally retarded patients are overrepresented, and intellectually average patients relatively underrepresented, in populations of epileptic children and, to a lesser degree, in epileptic adults (Tarter, 1972).

Epilepsy that is idiopathic or familial is less likely to be associated with mental handicap or dementia than epilepsy that is associated with overt brain damage or a neuropathic process such as tuberous sclerosis or Parkinson's disease (Tarter, 1972; Ellenberg et al., 1986). "Symptomatic" epileptics are more likely to deteriorate cognitively than idiopathic epileptics (Lennox and Lennox, 1960).

The positive correlates of epilepsy and mental impairment include age of onset, duration of the disorder, number of seizures, higher initial seizure frequency, poor response to anticonvulsant medication, and an excess of focal combined with generalized seizures (Tarter, 1972; Brown and Reynolds, 1981). These same correlates are also associated with prognosis of the seizure disorder.

That there is an "epileptic dementia" associated with cerebral atrophy is clear (Lishman, 1987). It is also clear that seizures can, by themselves, provoke neuropathic and metabolic changes in the brain, especially when they are frequent or prolonged (Meldrum and Brierly, 1973; Wasterlain, 1977; Menini et al., 1979). It is not clear, however, that one can distinguish epileptic dementia from anticonvulsant-induced dementia, or that one can exclude all other possible causes of dementia in an epileptic patient with intellectual decline.

Personality

The list of personality traits attributed to individuals with epilepsy is said to be limited only by one's industry in ferreting out fresh derogations (Stevens, 1975). The idea that there is an "epileptic personality" is quaint, but presumptuous. "Epilepsy" and "personality" are two broad and multifaceted constructs that can hardly be expected to unite in a single strain.

The idea, though, that some epileptic patients might be given to one or another of several nonpathological personality traits is less ambitious. The idea that the list of traits to which they are given is relatively circumscribed is amenable to empirical test. In epileptics with temporal lobe foci, for example, quantitative studies have demonstrated a profile of interictal changes in behavior (obsessiveness, circumstantiality), thought (religious and philosophical preoccupation), and affect (anger, emotionality, and sadness) (Bear and Fedio, 1977; Hermann and Riel, 1981; Brandt et al., 1985). Other traits attributed to the temporal lobe epileptic include interpersonal "stickiness," "viscosity," humorlessness, dependence, passivity, hypermoralism, personalization, and hyposexuality.

Whether these traits are a consequence of the epileptic process, or the underlying temporal lobe focus, or a synergy between the two, is an open question. It is likely that they are not related to the convulsive process in its general sense, but rather to some specific aspect that has to do with the anatomic focus. We have on several occasions noted such traits in head injury patients with temporal lobe lesions who were not overtly epileptic.

Nothing, however, in the literature should prepare the reader to expect an inevitable connection between temporal lobe foci and the personality traits in question, or an absence of association, on occasion, with foci in other regions. It is a curious development that serious discussion of the psychiatric concomitants of temporal lobe epilepsy come at a time when epileptologists have abandoned the term, and refer instead to complex-partial seizures, or partial epilepsy, and then refer to the specific focus, if it is known. It would be a singular event, indeed, if the research literature were unequivocal on behalf of a temporal lobe origin to all the traits attributed to that organ (e.g., Mungas, 1982; Tucker et al., 1987). We know that functions that are normally localized to a cortical region can be designated to another as the consequence of trauma, for example, and we know that the organs of brain are insulated one from another only imperfectly. The effects of displacement of function, activation by contiguity, reciprocal inhibition, encephalization, kindling, and the development of mirror foci militate against any single-minded localization, especially to complex features like personality traits.

Dual personality, multiple personality, and dissociative states have also been described in association with temporal lobe epilepsy (Schenk and Bear, 1981; Mesulam, 1981; Benson et al., 1986)

Depression

Emotions, as part of the epileptic experience, may be preictal, ictal, or postictal events. Fear, depression, pleasure, displeasure, and anger have all been documented as ictal manifestations (Hurwitz et al., 1985). Depression as an *interictal* state, however, is an important issue in neuropsychiatry. Epileptic patients have more depressive characteristics on psychological tests; depression is a common reason for hospitalization, and epileptics have a suicide rate that is five times higher than that of the general population (Mendez et al., 1986).

Depression in epileptics is associated with vegetative features, but there seem to be fewer "neurotic" symptoms like self-pity and brooding. Between major depressive episodes, epileptics are said to manifest a chronic dysthymic state, with more irritability, emotionality, and humorlessness than controls. Their affect is described as detached or distant rather than dysphoric (Mendez et al., 1986). They may be prone to agitated depressive states, with psychotic symptoms; alternatively, they may present as psychotics with strong affective symptoms (Betts, 1981).

It is appropriate to mention that studies of psychiatric patients with major affective disorders, unipolar and bipolar, reveal a high frequency of symptoms suggestive of temporal lobe epilepsy (Silberman et al., 1985; Lewis et al., 1984).

Peculiar Behavior

The epilepsy literature has some good ones, like "giggle incontinence" (Rogers et al., 1982) and self-induced photosensitive absence seizures with orgasmic ictus (Faught et al., 1986). The range of phenomena that occur, especially in association with complex-partial seizures, is staggering. It is not always possible, therefore, to distinguish behavior related to ictus from behavior that is "psychiatric" simply on the basis of topography, or whether it is associated with an identifiable provocation. That would be like differentiating between tardive dyskinesia and Huntington's disease simply on the basis of the topography of the abnormal movements; it cannot be done.

Complex-partial seizures of frontal lobe origin are sometimes associated with bizarre behavior outbursts that may be considered hysterical. Kicking and thrashing, finger-snapping, hand-clapping, shouts, obscenities and raps, singing and humming, pelvic thrusting and genital manipulation, bouncing, groping, picking, chewing, lip-smacking, and bizarre facial expressions have all been described in association with frontal lobe seizures (Waterman et al., 1987; Williamson et al., 1985; Boone et al., 1988).

Sudden attacks of pain that flash from one part of the body to another may be associated with mesodiencephalic discharges (Andy and Jurko, 1985). Painful auras preceding generalized seizures have been described (Penfield and Gage, 1933). Although painful partial seizures are probably rare (Trevathan and Cascino, 1988), central pain may be associated with lesions in thalamus (Dejerine and Roussy, 1906) and in the secondary sensory area (Biemond, 1956).

Fear and panic may be preictal, ictal, or postictal; but a seizure can make your hair stand up even without sensations of fear ("pilomotor seizures") (Brogna et al., 1986).

Patients with complex-partial seizures of left temporal lobe origin may be more "verbose" than other epileptic patients (Hoeppner et al., 1987). Left temporal lobe epileptics may also be given to hypergraphia (like Dostoievsky), but there is a converse form of epilepsy that is induced by writing (Cirignotta et al., 1986) and a contrapositive that is induced by reading (Kartsounis, 1988).

"Forced thinking" as an epileptic phenomenon may be confused with obsession, and the "flood of ideas" of epilepsy may be confused for the flight of ideas in mania. Seizures may be associated with hallucinations that are visual or auditory or vertiginous or olfactory or gustatory or somatosensory or all of the above (Daly, 1975).

Autoscopy is the sense that one can perceive oneself projected onto an external visual space. Macropsia and micropsia are sensations of perception through different ends of a telescope. Deja vu, of course, is the sense that something new has happened before; jamais vu is the sense that something familiar is altogether new.

Psychosis

In light of the extraordinary list just given (and a very incomplete list it is at that), it is little surprise that frank psychosis may also be an accompaniment of seizure disorders. But it is a relatively new idea, and there was once a time when psychiatrists and neurologists felt that epilepsy and schizophrenia were incompatible or antagonistic diseases. That was the rationale for "treating" schizophrenic patients by making them seize.

The relationship between psychosis and epilepsy has several dimensions: the two disorders arising as disparate manifestations of an underlying lesion; psychosis as an ictal phenomenon, like generalized nonconvulsive status epilepticus; psychosis as a late manifestation of temporal lobe epilepsy; and psychosis as the consequence of anticonvulsant toxicity.

It is the psychosis of temporal lobe epilepsy that has received the lion's share of attention, and for two good reasons. The late development of psychosis is consistent with a kindling model that obviously has broad import for the study of psychopathology in general (Waxman and Geschwind, 1975; Stevens and Livermore, 1978). The second compelling idea is that the schizophreniform psychosis of temporal lobe epilepsy is localized, relatively speaking, to the left hemisphere, while the psychosis of right temporal lesions is more likely to be affective (Flor-Henry, 1969).

The psychosis of temporal lobe epilepsy would be better termed temporal lobe psychosis, because it has been observed in patients with temporal lesions and no overt seizures (Barnhill and Gualtieri, 1989). It may also be termed late-onset psychosis because there is a delay, of varying length, between the initial insult, or the first seizure, and the development of psychosis. The psychosis is described as schizophreniform, but there are some key differences between temporal lobe psychosis and schizophrenia. The former is associated with many of the interictal personality traits of temporal lobe disease, especially cosmic preoccupation, hyperreligiousity, and paranoia. Demonic hallucinations are typical, or thoughts that one is hearing the voice of God. Hallucinations may be transient or intermittent; they may occur in "spells," along with diminished mentation or perceptual abnormalities. The episodic nature of the symptoms may be the only clue to an epileptic origin. The patients may be given to sudden and abrupt changes in mood, and the moods may vary from ecstasy to profound depression, from laughter to crying or angry explosions. Suicide attempts are not uncommon (Tucker et al., 1986).

"Primary" or Schneiderian symptoms are usually more common than negative or deficit symptoms. In one's relationship with the patient, there is a sense that he is afflicted with psychotic symptoms, but that the ego is intact, and has not been submerged or subsumed by a pervasive psychotic process. When negative symptoms do arise in a temporal lobe psychotic, one must be alive to the possibility of a concurrent depression, and treatment with antidepressants may be necessary.

The treatment of temporal lobe psychosis requires CBZ or VPA as essential agents. There may only be a partial response, however, with reduction in emotional intensity or outbursts and elimination of spells. Persistent hallucinations, delusions, and paranoia may require the coadministration of low doses of a high-potency neuroleptic, especially fluphenazine or pimozide, which are least likely to lower the seizure threshold. Centrencephalic epilepsy is associated with confusional psychosis (Dongier, 1959; Flor-Henry, 1969) and should to be treated first with VPA.

The localization of temporal lobe psychosis, manic to the right and schizophrenic to the left, was introduced by Flor-Henry in 1969, and has since won great currency. But the literature is not unanimous. There are also reports of depression occurring more frequently in patients with left hemisphere lesions (Robinson et al., 1983a; Robinson and Szetela, 1981; Starkstein et al., 1988b). Be that as it may, it has not assuaged the impulse to explain the laterality of epileptic psychosis in terms of the organization of affect in left temporal and frontal lobe structures, analogous to the organization of language on the left (Ross and Stewart, 1987; Ross, 1981; Ross and Rush, 1981), or in the asymmetry of distribution of neurotransmitter projections (Rosen et al., 1984; Schneider et al., 1982; Jerussi and Glick, 1975; Oke et al., 1978).

Absence

One is trained to associate lapses in attention or daydreaming with petit mal or absence epilepsy, but that is not a particularly helpful approach to the practitioner who tends to developmentally handicapped patients or to head injury patients, because they are even more prone to lapses in attention and what appears to be daydreaming. Nevertheless, the diagnosis of epilepsy must always be entertained in patients with severe disorders of attention.

The diagnosis of absence epilepsy is easier if there is "complex absence"; that is, if the seizures are accompanied by mild clonic movements, like eye-fluttering, mouth-twitching, or movements of the upper extremity; changes in postural tone, especially head drooping or mild slumping; autonomic phenomena or urinary incontinence; or automatisms. It may be impossible to distinguish such cases from complex partial seizures without an EEG (Lockman, 1985). Hyperventilation will evoke an absence seizure but not a complex-partial seizure (Adams and Lueders, 1981).

Nonconvulsive generalized status epilepticus ("petit mal status") is a state lasting for 1 hour or longer, with slowness in behavior and mentation, confusion, and sometimes stupor or coma. There is generalized epileptiform activity on the EEG, continuous or nearly so, with spike waves, polyspike waves, or more complex discharges (Guberman et al., 1986). The duration may range from 12 hours to 4 days; the longest known attack was 31 days. The onset of the disorder may be at any age, and it is not an easy form of the disease to control. Naturally, the presentation may be confused with some of the psychiatric disorders; on the other hand, it is not unusual for patients with nonconvulsive generalized status to have severe psychiatric symptoms, including psychosis (Guberman et al., 1986).

Posttraumatic Epilepsy

This is not a form of epilepsy with any special proclivity to induce psychiatric symptoms, but it has an important bearing on neuropsychiatric practice. This is because seizures frequently enter the differential diagnosis of behavior disorders occurring in head injury patients, and because anticonvulsant "prophylaxis" complicates the long-term management of head injury patients and may even retard the recovery process.

Within 5 years after closed head injury, the incidence of epilepsy is 2%–5%; a considerably higher percentage of patients with penetrating injuries will develop seizures (Epstein et al., 1987). Depressed skull fracture and dural penetration are risk factors for posttraumatic epilepsy. "Early epilepsy," that is, ictus within the first week after injury, does not predict the development of subsequent epilepsy although it raises the percentages, and there is even preclinical evidence to suggest that early seizures may exercise a protective effect on the recovery process (Feeny et al., 1987). Epileptiform EEG abnormalities are not predictive of posttraumatic epilepsy in the first year after injury, but they are more significant later on.

Other factors that increase the risk of posttraumatic epilepsy are intracranial hemorrhage (D'Allessandro et al., 1982), persistent focal deficits like aphasia or hemiparesis, and centroparietal or temporal location of the lesion (Feeny and Walker, 1979). Although the onset of seizures is most often within 5 years of injury, later onset has been reported in a substantial number of patients (Salazar et al., 1985).

In considering the wisdom of anticonvulsant prophylaxis, one is guided by the presence of risk factors and the established value or lack thereof of prophylaxis (McQueen et al., 1983; Young et al., 1983). Clearly, there is no place for anticonvulsant prophylaxis for the patient who has sustained blunt trauma, with no other elements of risk. When such patients are seen in consultation, the beneficial effects of a recommended anticonvulsant withdrawal can be dramatic. It is not really clear that prophylaxis works at all, and it may just suppress seizures in patients with epilepsy and suppress recovery in patients without epilepsy.

Phenytoin is probably used more frequently for "prophylaxis" than any other anticonvulsant, because it is begun in the neurosurgical ICU where it can be given parenterally. If a patient must be on anticonvulsants at all, CBZ and VPA are the recommended agents. Phenytoin does not make sense as a prophylactic drug because it is relatively weak against kindling. And whatever it is about phenytoin that causes dementia, it cannot be a good thing with respect to the cortical recovery process.

Psychiatric Conditions That May Be Related to Epilepsy

These are conditions that are fairly and squarely in the camp of psychiatric disorders, but they bear some relation to epilepsy either in their structure (paroxysmal disorders, kindled disorders), natural history (association with seizures), or treatment response (e.g., to the psychotropic anticonvulsants). These conditions include intermittent explosive disorder, major affective disorder, multiple personality, "borderline" personality, and autism.

Intermittent Explosive Disorder

Intermittent explosive disorder ("episodic dyscontrol") refers to the occurrence of extreme emotional outbursts, with rage and sometimes with violence, in patients who have no clearly defined cause, lesion, or psychiatric diagnosis. The evidence for an association with epilepsy is threefold: the common occurrence of such symptoms in patients with epilepsy, especially complex-partial epilepsy; the common finding of temporal lobe abnormalities on neurodiagnostic testing in nonepileptic patients with intermittent explosions; and the good response of explosive patients to CBZ or to VPA.

The cooccurrence of violence with epilepsy has led, naturally, to controversy over whether to "treat" violent citizens with amygdalotomy (Mark and Ervin, 1970) or whether criminal violence may ever occur as a purely ictal phenomenon. The first idea has little empirical (or even theoretical) support, and the second represents a crucial misunderstanding of the nature of neuropsychiatric disorders such as epilepsy and of the nature of personal responsibility for actions that are precipitated by an underlying cerebral disorder.

The idea that epilepsy is an all-or-none phenomenon is attractive, and consistent with the electrical event that accompanies ictus. It is inconsistent, however, with the fact that epilepsy may be partial, and that complete loss of conscious control is not an invariant feature of the disease. It is not consistent with the surmise that the lesion that gives rise, on occasion, to ictus may, on other occasions, give rise to alternative manifestations, to paroxysms that are not readily identifiable as seizure.

The question of violent behavior as a correlate of epilepsy opens a serious line of reflection concerning personal responsibility for behavior that is potentially criminal in nature. This is the kind of question that is argued by experts in criminal proceedings, where strong convictions are sometimes expressed that do not have unequivocal support in the scientific literature. The arcane opinions of learned experts in such matters makes one grateful for the wisdom of a jury of peers.

It is hard to maintain that an act of ictal violence may occur in a patient who is not clearly given to overt seizures. It is also hard to believe that a complex act of interpersonal violence could be a purely ictal event, because the automatisms of complex-partial epilepsy are by definition fragmented, purposeless, and without definite and identifiable goals (Delgado-Escueta et al., 1977). It is also hard to distinguish between ictal violence and postictal or interictal violence, the latter being a relatively nonspecific aspect of a psychopathological condition (Delgado-Escueta et al., 1981).

Affective Disorder

No one has suggested that affective disorder is a variant of epilepsy, but the idea has been raised that the pathophysiology of kindling might be an analogue for the behavioral sensitization that occurs, for example, in response to chronic stress. The experimental model of behavioral sensitization is seen after chronic treatment with dopaminergic drugs like apomorphine or cocaine, when the animal shows increasing hyperactivity or stereotypy to the same dose. The phenomenon occurs, of course, in the absence of ictus, so it is not simply a variant of the kindling model; it seems to involve different neural systems, and the two processes are affected differentially by pharmacological interventions (Post et al., 1982b). The theory suggests that recurrent affective disorder, cycling more rapidly and precipitated more readily by external events as the years go by, is a function of this behavioral sensitization.

The larger, more cogent paradigm is the process of learning in its broadest terms. Kindling and behavioral sensitization are laboratory events that address the gradual acquisition of pathological behavior through repetition and increments of response. It is as if the process of learning itself can be bent by a neuropathic event to serve an increasingly toxic outcome. It is analogous to the perversion of the immune response that characterizes the autoimmune disorders; to the loss of inhibitory feedback control that governs some of the endocrinopathies. It is the description of neuropathophysiology in terms that are exaggerations or derangements of a normal physiological process.

Multiple Personality

The literature pertaining to this bizarre clinical entity refers to several patients who were epileptics, specifically temporal lobe epileptics (Schenk and Bear, 1981). There is said to be an unexpected frequency of multiple personality in patients with complex-partial seizures (Benson et al., 1986; Schenk and Bear, 1981; Mesulam, 1981). The fact that dissociative symptoms are so common in epileptic patients renders a link between this most extreme dissociation and epilepsy that much more credible. If there is a connection, one must wonder if it is ictus or the lesion itself that is operative.

"Borderline" Personality

The so-called borderline personality is typified by symptoms of interpersonal intensity, emotional instability, impulsive and self-destructive behaviors, episodic psychosis, and dissociative behavior. Such patients, to the degree they can be characterized at all, are relatively refractory to psychotherapeutic and pharmacological intervention. Recently, however, there have been reports of successful treatment with the psychotropic anticonvulsant CBZ (e.g., Cowdry, 1988). These are only tentative reports, of course. But it is not unreasonable to suggest that at least some patients who are identified as borderline may, in fact, have atypical psychoses or interictal traits that stem from an epileptiform limbic focus.

Autism

Patients with developmental language or communication impairments may be presumed to have temporal lobe lesions, and lesions like mesial sclerosis are well known to arise from comparatively minor perinatal hypoxic episodes. It is not surprising, then, to find a high frequency of epilepsy and of epileptiform disorders in these people. The incidence of epilepsy in autistic people may be as high as one in three, and complex-partial seizures are the most common type (see Chapter 9, this volume). When an autistic patient or a language-handicapped patient is seen in consultation for severe behavior problems, the possibility of an epileptiform disorder should always be explored.

Neuropsychological and Behavioral Effects of Anticonvulsant Drugs

Carbamazepine (CBZ, Tegretol)

CBZ was first synthesized in the 1950s. It was introduced as an anticonvulsant in Europe in 1962, and its beneficial effects for trigeminal neuralgia were first noted at that time. In 1968 it was approved in the United States for prescription for neuralgia, and in 1974 it won labeling approval as an anticonvulsant for adults. In

1978 it was okayed as a second-choice anticonvulsant for children 6 years and older (Evans and Gualtieri, 1985).

The earlier literature suggested that CBZ was a second-line treatment for seizure disorders, and this was largely from misunderstanding the effects it had on hematopoiesis. In fact, "serious and fatal hematopoietic disturbances" (e.g., thrombocytopenia, agranulocytosis, aplastic anemia) are actually quite rare (Schain et al., 1977; Schmidt, 1982). The old warning to monitor bloodcounts at weekly intervals was rescinded only 2 years ago. Now, CBZ is used by pediatricians as a first-line treatment, even for uncomplicated familial epilepsy. They have learned that the catastrophic side effects of CBZ have been wildly exaggerated, and they are increasingly aware of the neurotoxicity of old-line, sedating anticonvulsants.

The pediatricians have also learned that CBZ, prescribed as an anticonvulsant, will often lead to improvement in behavior problems such as aggression or hyperactivity that may also occur in epileptic children. In fact, the beneficial behavioral effects of CBZ were first apparent long ago. From 1970 to 1978, there were no fewer than 40 published reports of beneficial CBZ effects on mood and behavior in epileptic patients (Dalby, 1971; Ballenger and Post, 1978).

The first report of CBZ effect in bipolar affective disorder (manic-depressive illness, MDI) was published in Japan (Takezaki and Hanaoka, 1971), and the subsequent development of CBZ as treatment for MDI was pursued in Japan by Okuma (Okuma et al., 1973; Okuma et al., 1975; Okuma et al., 1979). (The Japanese were interested in CBZ because of *their* exaggerated fears of lithium toxicity.) The development of CBZ as a psychotropic drug in the United States began in 1978 with Ballenger and Post. Within 10 years, it has become an established treatment for neuropsychiatric disorders ranging from depression to schizophrenia.

CBZ is an iminostilbene derivative, a tricyclic compound with a steric structure that resembles that of imipramine, chlorpromazine, and maprotiline (Post et al., 1982a; Rodin, 1983). It also shares structural features with the anticonvulsants phenytoin, clonazepam, and phenobarbital (Dalby, 1975). In structure and in function, then, it is a psychotrope and an anticonvulsant.

CBZ is highly lipophilic and it is almost completely absorbed from the gastrointestinal tract (slowly at first, more rapidly with long-term treatment). The half-life is 20 to 25 hours, and clinical dosing is usually bid or tid. Some patients, however, require a qid schedule (Dalby, 1971; Morselli and Bossi, 1982; Levy et al., 1975). Although the pharmacokinetics of CBZ are not necessarily linear, and serum levels may not correlate with oral dose, serum levels do seem to be correlated with therapeutic efficacy, at least for seizure disorders. The therapeutic range is usually given as 4 to 12 ng/ml. The most reliable time to draw a serum level, in light of the problem of intraindividual variability, is first thing in the morning, after an evening dose but before the first morning dose.

There is also interindividual variation in CBZ serum levels, and no correlation has been established between serum levels and therapeutic response in psychiatric conditions (Evans and Gualtieri, 1985). Therefore, the 4–12 guideline is only an approximation, and some patients do well at 3 to 4 ng/ml, while others require serum levels as high as 16. The importance of serum level monitoring, therefore, is really a question at the beginning of guaranteeing that the full range of therapeutic opportunity has been explored. Over the long term, it is a question of following the individual patient over time. Serum levels, relative to a fixed maintenance dose, may change: if the patient's metabolism changes with age, from childhood to adolescence when it slows down considerably, and slows down again in the elderly patient; if the patient begins a drug or is withdrawn from a drug that interacts with CBZ metabolism; or if the patient is inadvertently switched from the CIBA-Geigy preparation to Brand X.

CBZ induces the enzymes of its own metabolism, but serum levels should stabilize within a week after treatment has begun. Begin with a test dose, for example, 200 mg bid for an adult, or 100 mg bid for a small child (less than 40 kg). After 3 days, increase to a tid schedule, and then change doses and monitor blood levels at weekly intervals.

The reason for the test-dose interval is that some people simply cannot take CBZ. About 5% of patients treated with CBZ have to discontinue treatment because of toxic reactions (Schmidt, 1982). Skin reactions, nausea and vomiting, irritability, dyskinesia, and agitation may be early side effects that one can detect during a test-dose interval.

We have reviewed the side effects of CBZ on two earlier occasions (Evans and Gualtieri, 1985; Evans et al., 1987a). The important things to reiterate concern behavioral toxicity, epileptogenesis, and dyskinesia.

In terms of behavior toxicity, CBZ compares favorably to the old-line anticonvulsants, but that does *not* mean it is free of adverse behavioral effects. In fact, a substantial proportion of patients will have serious behavioral problems from CBZ. These are not, as a rule, in the direction of blunting, like phenytoin, or disinhibition, like the barbiturates, or depression, like ethosuccimide. Sometimes the behavior toxicity of CBZ is like the tricyclic antidepressants: disorganization, agitation, delirium, hallucinations, psychosis (Silverstein et al., 1982). More commonly, however, the side effects are stimulant like: irritability, aggressiveness, dysphoria, restlessness, and emotional lability (Evans and Gualtieri, 1985).

If a patient develops behavioral toxicity to the first few doses of CBZ, it is usually futile to raise the dose in search of a therapeutic window. Such action is likely only to make the problem worse.

The following dyskinetic movements have been described in connection with CBZ: tics, dystonia, orofacial dyskinesia, myoclonic jerks, ballismus, asterixis, and choreoathetosis (Evans and Gualtieri, 1985). CBZ usually aggravates tardive dyskinesia and akathisia. It is not helpful in the treatment of tics or Tourette's syndrome.

CBZ can cause seizures, or can aggravate a seizure disorder, especially at high serum levels (i.e., greater than 8 ng/ml). Patients who are given to *absences,* or who have a spike-and-wave pattern on EEG, are likelier to seize on CBZ (Snead and Hosey, 1985).

The toxicity of CBZ is overt and easy to recognize when one knows what to look for, and the problems we have listed will remit when the dose is lowered or after the drug is discontinued. Side effects are not necessarily related to high blood levels, with the exception of seizures, as we have mentioned; leukopenia is also more likely to arise at very high levels.

The only side effect of CBZ that hardly anyone looks for is memory impairment. Much is made of the relative safety of CBZ in terms of memory, especially when it is compared to anticonvulsants like phenytoin, and in a small study we conducted with CBZ in hyperactive children, there was an actual increment in memory performance with increasing doses of CBZ (from 1 to 2 to 3 mg/kg/day) (Gualtieri, 1990). Nevertheless, in the susceptible individual one can see memory impairment with CBZ. It is not at all frequent, but it can occur. CBZ is also, unfortunately, a teratogenic drug. Not as teratogenic as phenytoin, but perhaps, more so than VPA.

It is clinical lore among epileptologists that the "psychotropic effects of CBZ may appear after months of treatment, but it may also be evident after only a few days" (Dalby, 1975). The psychiatric literature, however, supports a CBZ effect within a few days (Hooshmand et al., 1974; Lutz, 1977; De Vogelaer, 1981; Moss and James, 1983; Ballenger and Post, 1978). Initial improvement with CBZ may diminish within the first 2 weeks of treatment with enzyme autoinduction and lowered serum levels.

CBZ is known to have a depressant effect on neurotransmission, a putative affinity for specific limbic structures, an antikindling effect, and specific neurochemical and neuroendocrine effects. CBZ may have a neuronal "stabilizing" effect, similar to that of lithium, decreasing sodium and potassium conductance and membrane leakage (Schauf et al., 1974). It selectively depresses neurotransmission in polysynaptic pathways (Theobald and Kunz, 1963), and it depresses synaptic transmission in the nucleus of the trigeminal nerve (Hernandez-Peon, 1965). Its known effects in depressing posttetanic potentiation may be related to its ability to control the spread of seizure discharge (Krupp, 1969). CBZ can inhibit activity in thalamic nuclei, in reticulothalamic and thalamocortical projections (Holm et al., 1970) and in projections from amygdala and hippocampus to thalamus (Sillanpaa, 1981).

CBZ appears to have a special affinity for limbic structures; it is the most effective anticonvulsant, for example, in suppressing amygdaloid focal seizures (Albright and Burnham, 1980). In a variety of experimental preparations creating epileptogenic foci in hippocampus, CBZ was successful in suppressing not only the spread of electrical activity but also the focus itself (Julien and Hollister, 1975). It is particularly effective in preventing the development of sustained afterdischarge in the amygdaloid-kindling cat, as well as the development of motor seizure manifestations (Wada et al., 1976).

It has been suggested that the antikindling effect of CBZ is responsible for its antidepressant rather than its anticonvulsant properties, because it behaves so differently from other anticonvulsants in the kindling model and because the antidepressant effect in epileptic patients can be dissociated from improvement in seizure status (Babington, 1967). The blockade of limbic afterdischarges in the kindling preparation is an effect that CBZ seems to share with the other antidepressants (Rodin, 1983; Schmitt 1966).

The phenomenon of kindling itself, although it is used mainly as a model for studies of neuranatomic relationships, epilepsy, and anticonvulsant drugs, has also been advanced as a model for certain forms of learning (Goddard and Douglas, 1975) and of psychopathology (Wada, 1977; Stevens and Livermore, 1978). The fact that CBZ is the prototypic antikindling drug represents an extraordinary clinical challenge, because the question is posed whether it might be applied prophylactically to prevent the progression of certain neuropsychiatric conditions aside from epilepsy. Of course, because it is not clear that any neuropsychiatric condition is progressive by virtue of kindling, the question is moot. One is inhibited from advancing a potential treatment, it seems, by virtue of a weakness in theory. If the theory of kindling were better understood, one would expect the therapeutic potential of CBZ to be advanced accordingly.

CBZ is a norepinephrine reuptake blocker, approximately 25% as potent as imipramine (Purdy et al., 1977). It is not clear that this noradrenergic effect is related to its anticonvulsant properties, because DPH, with anticonvulsant properties that are not dissimilar to those of CBZ, has no known effects of catecholamine systems (Rudzick and Mennear, 1965). It has been suggested, however, that "brain catecholamines may also, at least partially, mediate the anticonvulsant activity of CBZ" (Quattrone and Samanin, 1977). Because this information derives from a 6-hydroxydopamine-treated animal preparation, however, it is conceivable that the anticonvulsant effect is a secondary consequence of a CBZ effect on cortical recovery. That is what may be mediated by its noradrenergic mechanism.

CBZ inhibits the action of enzymes that metabolize the putative neurotransmitter GABA and decrease GABA turnover; the net effect of increasing effective levels of GABA may mediate the anticonvulsant effects (Sillanpaa, 1981). It is known to increase brain levels of the amino acid neurotransmitter taurine, to decrease levels of glutamate, and to increase striatal levels of acetylcholine (Sillanpaa, 1981). It has direct or indirect vasopressin-like effects, which accounts for its success in treating diabetes insipidus (Post et al., 1982b).

The first issue to consider is the importance of comparison. When the neuropsychological effects of CBZ are compared to the neuropsychological effects of phenytoin, the barbiturates, and the benzodiazepines, one may expect a favorable comparison. Phenytoin, for example, has been reported to influence, in a negative way, attention (Stores et al., 1978), memory (Delaney et al., 1980), and overall test intelligence (Smith and Lowrey, 1972). The barbiturates and the benzodiazepines are also known to exercise negative cognitive effects (Livingston, 1966). In controlled studies, investigators have established that the sedating anticonvulsants influence performance on tasks requiring attention, memory, and motor concentration in a negative way, and there is a trend for increasing serum levels to be associated with decrements in performance (Thompson et al., 1980; Matthews and Hurley, 1975). So, if CBZ is compared to phenytoin, mysoline, or clonazepam, it will naturally appear to improve the patient's neuropsychological test profile. There is no question but that it is less toxic than *those* drugs.

How it compares to VPA or to DMX one cannot say, because the comparison has never been made, and it may be an irrelevant comparison anyway because they are probably not equivalent anticonvulsants. On the other hand, they may be equivalent psychotropes, for example, for rapid-cycling MDI.

The second issue is the population under study. When one considers the cognitive and motor effects of an anticonvulsant, it is essential to consider the type of persons using it. A group of high-level children with benign familial epilepsy, for example, may have sufficient psychological "reserve" to render the negative cognitive effects of phenytoin or phenobarbital imperceptible. Such patients will do well, even in spite of a drug that hinders performance, just as they do well in the face of adversity like a parental divorce, or a poor teacher, or a school year with a number of absences to go to Europe with their family on a business trip.

The negative cognitive and motor effects of a drug are best studied in a population with compromised function to begin with, with limited psychological reserve. It is they who are most likely to feel the negative effects of a drug like phenytoin, and who are most likely to benefit from the substitution of a drug like CBZ.

The third problem is that epilepsy by itself may be associated with blunting of motor performance, cognitive ability, or other aspects of personality. It may be difficult to dissociate drug effects in epileptic patients from the psychological effects of the disease for which the drugs were originally prescribed. The assessment measures that are used in such studies have neither been designed for nor have they been standardized on epileptic patients, who represent a clinically diverse and heterogeneous population. The measures of attention, memory, motor performance, and processing speed that are most commonly used are also known to be negatively affected in epileptic populations not receiving drugs (Matthews and Harley, 1975; Thompson et al., 1980; Loiseau et al., 1983).

We reviewed the neuropsychological effects of CBZ in children and adults in an earlier publication (Evans and Gualtieri, 1985). CBZ was clearly superior to penytoin and to barbiturate anticonvulsants in measures of attention, alertness, reflectiveness-impulsivity, visual scanning, and cognitive flexibility; in memory for words and pictures, and in immediate and delayed recall; in measures of motor speed, motor accuracy, and constructional praxis. In one study that compared CBZ to VPA, however, no difference was found between the two drugs on memory tasks (Butlin et al., Danta, 1980).

The difference, however, is not always in the direction of one up, two down. In other words, the CBZ effect may simply be one of *less decrement* when compared to phenytoin or to phenobarbital. It is important to appreciate that CBZ is not necessarily a benign drug, from the neuropsychological point of view. It may simply be less toxic than the alternatives.

This element is important, for example, when one is considering the wisdom of anticonvulsant prophylaxis in a head injury patient. For such patients, CBZ is clearly the better choice than DPH. But if anticonvulsant prophylaxis is not clearly indicated, neither CBZ nor DPH is appropriate, and both may exercise negative effects on the recovery process. The fact that one is worse does not make two an innocent choice. At best it is supernumerary; at worst, it may retard the patient's recovery.

Carbamazepine as Psychotrope

It has been observed on repeated occasions that treatment with CBZ has a beneficial effect on epileptic patients beyond the control of epilepsy. There was an increase in "psychic tempo" in patients with the "epileptic personality," with improvement in attention, concentration, and perseverance (Dalby, 1971). Physicians described activation and stabilization, normalization of confused or of paranoid episodes, relief from periodic depressions, increased alertness and initiative, decreased "sluggishness of thought and stickiness of personality," and a decrease in emotional overswings. Affective symptoms, emotional instability, and aggressive outbursts were particularly affected (Evans and Gualtieri, 1985).

The development of CBZ as an alternative to lithium in the treatment of MDI was described earlier. CBZ has a prophylactic effect (Okuma et al., 1979), it has direct effects in acute mania (Okuma et al., 1975), it is effective in patients who fail to respond to lithium (Nolen, 1983), it is synergistic with lithium in patients who fail to respond to either drug alone (Nolen, 1983), it may prevent the reoccurrence of periodic unipolar depressions (Post et al., 1984; Stuppaeck et al., 1990) and it is effective in cases of schizoaffective disorder (Nolen, 1983). This extraordinary pattern of success, broader than any other antidepressant drug, has naturally led to considerations of affective disease in terms of physiological processes like kindling (Post et al., 1982b).

The psychotherapeutic effects of CBZ are not however by any means limited to affective disorder. It is an effective adjunct in the treatment of certain subgroups of schizophrenics (De Vogelaer, 1981; Hakola and Laulumaa, 1982; Neppe, 1981; Luchins, 1983; Klein et al., 1984). It is an essential part of the treatment of late-onset psychosis following brain injury and in the related psychosis that sometimes accompanies temporal lobe epilepsy (Barnhill and Gualtieri, 1989).

CBZ, like VPA and lithium, is effective in the treatment of "episodic dyscontrol syndrome," or intermittent explosive disorder, although the literature on this point is largely anecdotal. Although many of these patients have neurodiagnostic evidence of temporal lobe lesions, such as an epileptiform EEG, the presence of such a finding is not necessary to justify a trial of CBZ.

Finally, CBZ appears to be a reasonable choice for treating virtually any severe behavior disorder that occurs in a child, a mentally retarded person, or a brain-injured patient. A global statement like this is not likely to find specific support in the research literature, but it is supported by the weight of clinical experience. One would prefer to say that disorders most likely to respond to CBZ are characterized by extreme emotional variability, behavioral disorganization, or paroxysmal outbursts, but the list of odd patients who seem to do well on CBZ after all else has failed includes a number who defy any such neat attempt at prediction or classification.

Among neuropsychiatrists, CBZ has become a favorite drug. It has achieved a degree of importance that could never have been predicted 10 years ago, when it was only a second-choice anticonvulsant and fears of catastrophic toxicity left it in the hands only of the intrepid or the reckless. The only limitation to its wider use, among an extraordinarily wide swath of neuropsychiatric disorders, is its troubling side effects—irritability and agitation—in a substantial number of patients, and its proclivity to induce or to aggravate the occurrence of centerencephalic seizures. The other limitation is external: the development of an alternative psychotropic anticonvulsant, valproic acid, with an equally broad spectrum of effects and an even more favorable toxicity profile.

Valproic Acid (VPA, Depakene, Depakote)

The pattern for VPA is uncanny for its parallel to CBZ: anticonvulsant properties discovered in 1963 (Meunier et al., 1963); release in the United States in 1978; widespread fears of catastrophic toxicity soon thereafter; and then an explosion of prescription, 10 years later, as an anticonvulsant and as a psychotropic.

It was promoted first as a drug that was more effective in controlling generalized rather than focal seizures (Lewis, 1978), and this has led to the unfortunate surmise that it is never effective for focal or for complex-partial seizure disorders; nothing could be further from the truth (Turnbull et al., 1985). It was first used as an alternative to ethosuccimide, tridione, and other drugs for absence seizures, but now it is considered to be a worthy alternative to CBZ, especially for refractory seizures of many types (Barnes and Bower, 1975). As a beginning point for treatment, however, most epileptologists hold to the idea that VPA is the first choice for patients with absence fits, or a spike-and-wave pattern on the EEG; CBZ is preferred for complex-partial seizures, and fits that arise from a temporal lobe focus.

VPA is a simple structure. The compound, a carboxylic acid, was first synthesized in 1881. It is structurally unrelated to currently available anticonvulsant drugs, but it is similar to the major inhibitory neurotransmitter in the mammalian cortex, gamma-aminobutyric acid (GABA) (Buchhalter and Dichter, 1986). It is rapidly absorbed from the gastrointestinal tract; peak levels occur 1 to 4 hours after an oral dose, and the half-life of the parent compound is 8 to 12 hours.

The anticonvulsant effects of VPA are sometimes presumed to be related to its interaction with GABA neurotransmission. VPA inhibits GABA-metabolizing enzymes such as GABA transaminase, and raises whole-brain GABA concentration. It potentiates GABA-mediated inhibition. It also is known to effect brain levels of glutamic acid and aspartic acid, two amino acid neurotransmitters that are believed to play a role in epileptogenesis (Slevin and Ferrara, 1985). However, it is not clear that these effects are sufficient to explain the anticonvulsant action of VPA, because it is also capable of inhibiting spike generation independent of the GABAergic system (Buchhalter and Dichter, 1986).

The major concern over VPA administration has been the hepatotoxicity, which may be catastrophic. Fatal hepatotoxicity occurs in the first 6 months of therapy, but it appears to be concentrated in children, especially young children (less than 2 years old), and when VPA is used in conjunction with other antiepileptic drugs.

The other serious side effects of VPA are thrombocytopenia, which may occur even after years of treatment, and inhibition of platelet aggregation. The most common side effects are gastrointestinal: nausea, vomiting, and indigestion. Anorexia may be a troublesome effect. VPA can also cause alopecia.

The CNS side effects are usually in the direction of stimulation: insomnia, agitation, excitement, hyperactivity, and disorganization. Occasionally, however, a patient will be sedated on VPA. VPA has been reported to have negative effects on psychological measures like tapping and reaction time but no effect on memory and attention (Sommerbeck et al., 1977).

Like CBZ, VPA was noted to improve some of the psychiatric problems of epileptic patients. In 1966, Lambert and his colleagues discovered antimanic properties for the anticonvulsant dipropylacetamide, which is metabolized rapidly to valproate (Lambert et al., 1966), and in 1980 Emrich et al., described the successful treatment, with VPA of manic patients who had failed to respond to lithium. The development of VPA as an antimanic drug has been summarized by McElroy et al. (1987).

It appears that lithium, CBZ, and VPA represent three points on a triangle of potential agents for the treatment of bipolar affective disorder and schizoaffective disorder, and, by extension, organic affective disorders. Sovner has reported the successful treatment of four mentally retarded patients with what appears to be an organic affective disorder with VPA (Sovner, 1989). Either drug may be effective by itself, although the two anticonvulsants may be more effective in rapid cyclers. Any combination of two of the three drugs may be effective in patients who are refractory to treatment with one by itself.

Although clinical experience and research with VPA as a psychotrope is much less extensive than experience and research with CBZ, the initial experiences of clinicians seems to indicate that the two drugs may be entirely interchangeable, and that only the patient's indiosyncratic reaction will decide which is the better choice. The major advantage of VPA seems to be its lower likelihood to induce irritability, a major difficulty with CBZ in many neuropathic cases.

Clonazepam

Clonazepam (Klonapin, KLON) was originally approved in 1976 as an anticonvulsant for absence attacks, infantile spasms, petit mal variant, myoclonic seizures, and akinetic seizures. It is one of two benzodiazepines (nitrazepam is the other) that is effective orally as an anticonvulsant. Clonazepam suppresses seizure activity in many animal models, and it suppresses many types of paroxysmal activity on the EEG; generalized EEG abnormalities are more readily suppressed than focal abnormalities. Clonazepam often limits the spread of discharge from a focal lesion while not suppressing the primary focus. These observations may be explained by the ability of benzodiazepines to enhance polysynaptic inhibitory processes at all levels of the CNS (Browne, 1978).

Clonazepam does not have any special toxicity beyond that which the benzodiazepines have as a class. In fact, it has been said to be the "safest drug alternative" for the treatment of mania (Chouinard, 1985; see following). What is special about the side effects of clonazepam is largely a function of the patient population for whom it is prescribed. Behavioral and emotional disturbances are especially common, especially in children, and the rate of behavioral toxicity has ranged from 2% to 52% of the subjects in various studies (Browne, 1978). Patients on clonazepam may become irritable, dysphoric, aggressive, violent, noncompliant, and hyperactive. This is the typical manifestation of behavioral disinhibition that has always limited the use of benzodiazepines, for example, in the treatment of TBI patients; people with serious epilepsy do not seem to be much different.

The frequency of this behavioral toxicity, coupled with the problem of tolerance to the anticonvulsant effects of the drug in about one-third of patients (Browne, 1978), has limited the use of clonazepam as an anticonvulsant to only the particular patients, and the particular seizure disorders, where it is uniquely effective. In contrast to carbamazepine and valproate, clonazepam has never been an anticonvulsant to impress the neurologist with its favorable psychological profile.

In fact, it was Chouinard, when examining the effects of treating mania with serotonergic drugs such as tryptophan combined with lithium, who selected clonazepam by virtue of its ability to stimulate serotonin synthesis. His group described acute antimanic effects with clonazepam, and then a wider range of clinical effects, for example in nonspecific agitation, steroid psychosis, tricyclic-induced mania, neuroleptic-induced somnambulism, atypical psychosis, and the schizophrenia-like psychosis of epilepsy (Chouinard, 1985). The presentation is clonazepam as an acute antipsychotic, the first legitimate alternative to the neuroleptics for acute management of the severely disturbed patient. Chouinard's work has been replicated (Victor et al., 1984; Freinhar and Alvarez, 1985a; Freinhar, 1985; Freinhar and Alvarez, 1985b; Chouinard et al., 1983; Aronson et al., 1989).

These investigators found that clonazepam was an effective drug for panic disorder by virtue of comparison with alprazolam, a high-potency benzopiazepine with a short half-life; clonazepam was a high-potency benzodiazepine with a longer half-life, so the problem of rebound was not likely to be so much a problem. Its subsequent efficacy for panic disorder was reported by Fontaine (1985), Beaudry et al., Annable (1986), and Pollack et al. (1986). Tolerance does not seem to develop to the antipanic effects of the drug, and the effective dose is very low (0.25–6.0 mg/day) (Pollack et al., 1986).

Not only is clonazepam a reasonable substitute for the class of drugs that appear to cause tardive dyskinesia CTD, but it also seems to be an occasional treatment for TD (Bobruff et al., 1981). It appears to provide some symptomatic relief for selected patients, perhaps until the problem cools down of its own accord. But whether it is better than other benzodiazepines in this regard, one cannot say. It is also prescribed as one of the only effective treatments for tardive akathisia, but that is not to say it is especially effective in this regard (Kutcher et al., 1989). It has been effective, too, for Meige's syndrome, a form of idiopathic tardive dyskinesia, if you will (Goldstein et al., 1986). The idea is that the benzodiazepines, as GABAmimetic drugs, inhibit striatal dopaminergic hyperactivity, which they may do at times.

Acetazolamide

Acetazolamide is an inhibitor of carbonic anhydrase, an enzyme that catalyzes the hydration of carbon dioxide and the dehydration of carbonic acid. It is a diuretic that promotes the renal loss of carbonate ion. In the eye, it reduces the secretion of aqueous humor and cause a drop in intraocular pressure, which accounts for its use in the treatment of glaucoma. It is also prescribed to prevent altitude sickness, and it can prevent the neuropsychological decompensation that often accompanies this syndrome (White, 1984).

Acetazolamide was used as an epileptic in the 1960s, but it fell from favor because rapid tolerance is developed to its diuretic and anticonvulsant effects. Its major use in epilepsy now is as an intermittent treatment in the prevention of catamenial seizures. Prescribing the drug for 2 weeks on and 2 weeks off seems to prevent the development of tolerance. Its use as an adjunct to other anticonvulsants, like CBZ, may be a function of its effect in raising brain levels of the CBZ.

There is an interesting report from Hiroshi et al., (1984) that describes a number of patients with "atypical psychosis" who responded to acetazolamide treatment. The rationale for the study was that the acetazolamide had effects of ion flux across the neuronal membrane similar to that of lithium. The best results were observed in patients who had periodic psychosis that coincided with the menstrual cycle, which is consistent, of course, with its use in catamenial epilepsy.

Acetazolamide has an extremely favorable toxicity profile, and the dose range is narrow—500 to 1000 mg/day. It may be added to CBZ or to VPA in the event of a partial response to the primary drug, as is done by epileptologists. Whether this strategy is also useful for the treatment of certain psychiatric disorders remains to be demonstrated, but it is not an outlandish idea to pursue.

One of our most difficult cases was a prepubertal girl with complex-partial seizures and severe aggressive and self-injurious behavior. The seizures were only partially controlled with phenobarbital and phenytoin, but the behavior was severe. Changing to CBZ led to a substantial improvement in behavior, but seizure control was still given to frequent failure.

After years of relative failure, she entered menarche, and her seizure pattern and the pattern of misbehavior changed dramatically. Seizures and aggression tended to cluster around her menstrual periods, and before each period she would become bloated and dysphoric. Cotreatment with acetazolamide led to a dramatic improvement in seizure control and in behavior control, and this effect was sustained over prolonged follow-up.

Such a case is particularly given to a trial of acetazolamide for its diuretic effects, its action to enhance brain levels of CBZ, and its known effects on catamenial seizures. Perhaps the drug has a wider application; we shall see.

Psychotropic Drugs as Convulsants and as Anticonvulsants

This subject has been discussed at a number of points in this volume, especially in Chapter 3 where the various drugs are discussed individually. Nevertheless, it is appropriate to review some of the principles involved.

Virtually all the psychoactive drugs are capable of exercising an effect on the seizure threshold if the dose is sufficiently high or if the change in dose is sufficiently abrupt. The effect is the usually easier to detect if it is in the direction of lowering the seizure threshold, and that is because a drug-induced seizure is a notable event. The effect of the drug, however, is probably less important than the individual's particular sensitivity. One should never be surprised, therefore, if the introduction of a psychoactive drug is associated with a change in the clinical status of an epileptic patient. One should never be surprised in any neuropathic patient if a sudden change in dose, especially a big change, provokes a seizure.

Psychoactive drugs may change the seizure threshold by (1) altering the metabolism or protein binding of an anticonvulsant; (2) stabilizing the patient's psychological condition and thus improving the general stability of other systems; and (3) exercising a direct effect on the mechanisms of epileptogenesis. Most of the known effects of psychotropics on the seizure threshold fall into the latter category.

Dopaminergic drugs like the psychostimulants and amantadine have a biphasic effect. In low doses, they are known to raise the seizure threshold and to improve seizure control. Amphetamine and amantadine have even been used as anticonvulsants (Livingston et al., 1948). Higher doses, however, may have the opposite effect. A TBI patient taking amantadine should be advised against alcohol ingestion, because that combination may lead to seizures.

Dopaminergic drugs like cocaine may cause seizures. Of all the "recreational" drugs, cocaine is probably the likeliest to induce seizures. Seizures from amphetamine abuse are more likely in association with intravenous administration. Seizures may also occur with phencyclidine intoxication, but not with heroin abuse (Alldredge et al., 1989).

The antidepressants and the neuroleptics are the psychoactive drugs most commonly associated with a lower seizure threshold (Messing et al., 1984). There is hardly any disagreement on that point. The incidence of seizures in people on tricyclic antidepressants is about 1% and in patients on neuroleptics about 1% to 2% (Messing et al., 1984). The important question is whether any particular drug in the class is more or less likely to carry the effect.

Maprotiline is probably the likeliest antidepressant to induce a seizure (Schwartz and Swaminathan, 1982). It may be that amitriptyline is the least likely, although this information is based on a preclinical study (Clifford et al., 1985). It is a counterintuitive finding in light of the sedative and anticholinergic properties of amitriptyline, as well as the results of clinical surveys (Trimble, 1978). Bupropion has an unfortunate reputation in this regard, an unearned reputation in the author's opinion; the likelihood of a seizure with bupropion is only about 0.5% (Davidson, 1989).

Among the neuroleptics, there is some disagreement; the old saw is that thioridazine and mesoridazine are the least likely drugs to lower the seizure threshold (Itil and Soldatos, 1980). In fact, a more modern technique suggests that molindone and fluphenazine and pimozide should be the preferred neuroleptics in patients who are prone to epilepsy (Oliver et al., 1982). This would be more in accord with the author's clinical experience.

Lithium was supposed to be a drug that lowered the seizure threshold (e.g., Brumback et al., 1975), but it probably has a beneficial effect, at least for some patients (Jus et al., 1973). The beta blockers seem to have a membrane-stabilizing effect and so are useful adjuncts to anticonvulsants in the treatment of epilepsy. Buspirone does not seem to effect the seizure threshold one way or the other; in contrast to benzodiazepines, there is no risk of seizures if buspirone is abruptly withdrawn.

CHAPTER 6

Neuropsychiatric Disorders in Mentally Retarded People

The utility of psychiatric diagnosis may be overstated, or it may be disparaged, depending on one's point of view. So, it is appropriate to consider what a psychiatric diagnosis really is. It is a fallacy to think that all the so-called psychiatric disorders are meaningful entities, from a classical medical, that is, an etiopathogenic, point of view. It fact, none of them are. Whatever validity they have is based on no more than natural history, genetic associations, or response to specific treatments.

There has been so much criticism of the DSM-3s that it is almost mendacious to assert that there may be some intelligence behind the thing, tool that it is to advance the hegemony of psychiatrists and to fatten the coffers of their professional association. The DSM-3 and its baby sister, the DSM-3r, are composed of nothing more than systematized descriptors that borrow heavily from the research traditions of the past few years. The diagnostic entities contained therein are nothing more than phenomenological constructs, and their purpose is as much to improve communication and understanding among researchers as it is to systematize clinical practice. It says nothing about etiopathogenesis, which is what most people suppose medical diagnosis is really about. It says nothing about pathophysiological mechanisms that may be manifest in different ways among people with different levels of cognitive ability.

The legitimate question, of course, is not how mentally retarded people may be stretched or shrunk into a Procrustean bed of DSM categories, but to what degree, if any, those categories have any useful relevance to understanding and managing certain individuals who also happen to be mentally retarded. Or to what degree it is a useful intellectual exercise, something that advances medical science. And to what degree it is a useful clinical endeavor, something that will advance the understanding and the treatment of some individuals and not simply justify, post hoc, the administration of psychotropic drugs.

And, finally, to what degree it is irrelevant. For the fact is that there are a great many behavioral problems that occur in mentally retarded people that are not contained in the DSM, unless they are fit into wastebasket categories like "organic personality disorder" or "atypical psychosis." The only mental retardation categories that the DSM contains are the old American Association for Mental Deficiency (AAMD) ratings, "mild," "moderate," "severe," and "profound," a slender offering, to be sure.

The Psychiatric Treatment Manual (PTM), the companion to the DSM, recognizes the limitations of established psychiatric categories in retarded people (Gualtieri, 1989a). As far as treatment is concerned, the PTM has taken this approach: there is a role for the traditional psychiatric categories, albeit a small one. There is also a role for an alternative diagnostic schema.

The alternative schema for diagnosis includes a body of neurobehavioral disorders that are classified as specific mental retardation syndromes, like Lesch–Nyhan and Down's. These are referred to as "pathobehavioral syndromes" because they are associated with a predictable constellation of pathological behaviors (Lesch–Nyhan and self-injurious behavior), or with the development of a specific neuropsychiatric disorder (Down's syndrome and Alzheimer's disease).

The alternative schema also includes a group of disorders that do not fit into either the traditional psychiatric or the pathobehavioral categories. These disorders, defined in purely behavioral terms such as aggression, pica, self-injurious behavior, and stereotypy, are referred to as "behavioral disorders," which is not a very imaginative term.

The alternative schema also includes a group of disorders like phenylketonuria (PKU) and the Prader–Willi syndrome that might be considered "pathobehavioral syndromes," but which are joined under the hypothetical construct "disorders of serotonin regulation." This is a purely theoretical construction that is presented for the sake of argument. There may prove to be many alternative approaches to neuropsychiatric diagnosis like this one as our knowledge of the chemistry of behavior advances.

The organization of this chapter, then, is around four categories of neuropsychiatric disorders: traditional psychiatric disorders, behavioral disorders, pathobehavioral syndromes, and hypothetical constructs based on the neurochemistry of behavior. The system has a certain organizational simplicity, at least for the purpose of composing a chapter. It also has a certain utility, in clinical terms, because it reflects the current state of neuropsychiatric practice in the field of mental retardation. It also reflects the interests of researchers in the field, who write, for example, about "The Diagnosis of Major Affective Disorder," or "The Treatment of Self-Injurious Behavior," or "The Neurobehavioral Correlates of William's Syndrome," and who will one day be writing about "Behavioral Manifestations of Serotonin Dysregulation."

It is, however, a purely arbitrary division. It is simple, but it is by no means pure. There is substantial overlap among the categories. The syndrome of Cornelia de Lange (CDLS), for example, is a pathobehavioral syndrome. But the prevailing problems of CDLS patients are best expressed in behavioral terms: self-injurious behavior, aggression, hyperactivity. And the most interesting question to raise about CDLS is whether there is an association to the major affective disorders, especially that class of the affective disorders that is linked to an abnormality of serotonin metabolism.

So, we do not propose a theory of how the abnormal behaviors of mentally retarded people may be classified. We only propose the simple idea that alternative models, or scheme, are necessary to embrace the full range of abnormal behaviors.

And that no existing system, not even the DSM, is sufficient to capture that full range.

Traditional Psychiatric Disorders

Affective Disorders

A literature spanning more than 60 years agrees that the full range of affective disorders occur in people who are mentally retarded (Sovner and Hurley, 1981). That information comes from clinicians, who have reported individual cases. On the other hand, the survey data are less conclusive. In the Camberwell study, for example, when ICD-8 criteria were used, only 22 of 402 subjects were found to have had current or prior episodes of unipolar or bipolar depression (Corbett, 1979). In the Nebraska study, using DSM-3 criteria, the diagnosis of affective disorder was nil of 114 subjects (Eaton and Menolascino, 1982). These are almost certainly spurious findings, however, the result of applying screening criteria that are not appropriate. Reiss (1982), for example, applied a "broader" diagnostic basis to a sample of 66 mentally retarded outpatients, and found that 13.6% of the patients were in fact depressed. That is a more credible number, although it is higher than survey results in the general population (Blazer et al., 1988). On the other hand, it is also much lower than the rates of depression after stroke or head injury (see Chapter 2, this volume).

One may make the diagnosis of major affective disorder in a mildly retarded person, or in a moderately retarded person who is suitably verbal, by applying traditional DSM-3r criteria. In the severely to profoundly retarded person, however, self-report of mood is not an appropriate criterion, and the diagnosis can only be inferred. It is risky to try to infer someone else's mood state from overt behaviors, but it is the only alternative, and because the treatments of affective disorder are so effective, it is important that we have a low threshold for the diagnosis.

We have suggested, therefore, that the diagnosis of major affective disorder may be made in retarded people on the basis of the following clinical elements (Gualtieri, 1989b):

1. A change is observed in the patient's emotional state, in a negative direction and from an established baseline.
2. This change persists for at least 2 months.
3. The emotional state of the depressed patient may be described consistently as sad, melancholy, or prone to tears; or as irritable, prone to angry outbursts or to tantrums; emotional lability; anhedonia, lack of interest in things that were formerly agreeable; anxiety, fearfulness, panic, agitation; somatic complaints or hypochondriasis or somatic delusions; morbid thoughts, memories, or preoccupations; suicidal thoughts or gestures.
4. The patient's emotional state may be inferred from behavioral changes, like social isolation, withdrawal, anergia, hypoactivity, psychomotor retardation, or agitation.

5. It may be inferred from the development of vegetative symptoms like anorexia or hyperphagia, weight loss or gain, constipation, insomnia, or hypersomnolence.
6. It may be inferred on the basis of developmental regression or a falloff in performance in school or in the workshop.
7. Manic behavior and hypomania are given to a similarly wide range of symptoms: emotional, like euphoria or agitation or irritability; behavioral, like distractibility, off-task, out-of-seat, hyperactivity, aggressiveness, destructiveness, disorganization; vegetative, like insomnia, anorexia, or hyperphagia. One may observe a dramatic increase in whatever "target behavior" the patient was usually given to, and, naturally, a deterioration in social interactions and workshop performance.

The diagnosis of a depressive episode or a manic episode is easy when it hinges on a clearly observed change in the patient's mental state, or when the changes follow a well-defined up-and-down pattern suggestive of cycling or of rapid cycling. There are two problems, though. One is that some depressive episodes may have persisted for such a long time that no one will have remembered a discrete change. Thus, evidence for a change in mental state is not always available to the consultant, and the diagnosis is therefore less secure. The other problem is the problem with cycles. As we should know from reading Vico, everything cycles. The very universe is organized around the continual reoccurrence of cycles. And, since Vico, no one seems to be more adept at detecting subtle but ineluctable cycles in human misbehavior than the psychiatrist with a low lithium threshold. The very mention of an on–off or up–down pattern may be sufficient; we all have met the type. And it certainly does not take a great deal of imagination to read a circular pattern into the day-to-day variability that characterizes the behavior of neuropathic patients.

Nevertheless, with a suitable degree of rigor, one may achieve at least a degree of success in identifying severely retarded people with major affective disorders and treating them accordingly. It really is not that difficult.

If that were all there was to say about affective disorders in retarded people, it would not be very much. It is never a challenge to fit retarded people into a mold that was made for someone else; they are congenial to it and people do it all the time. There is a more interesting aspect to the problem. Is it possible to take what we know about affective disorders in retarded people, and in other groups of neuropathic patients such as stroke and traumatic brain injury (TBI), and in children and the elderly, for that matter, and to construct with it a more embracing and a more useful idea of what exactly "affective disorder" is? Is the study of affective disorder in special populations simply a curious variant, or is there something more important to glean from it?

Let us begin with an alternative construction. This is the premise: that the occurrence of major affective episodes are not, in fact, the essence of affective disorder. Permit us to argue that a specific episode of affective illness is only a breakthrough, an extreme manifestation of an underlying pathophysiological trait.

In patients with normal cortical function, the occurrence of an affective episode is the only way to infer the existence of the trait. But in people whose cortical organization has been disrupted by a severe neuropathic process, the trait may be evidenced in other ways.

What one encounters most frequently in patients with head injury, developmental disorders, epilepsy, stroke, and other neuropathic disorders is the occurrence of affective symptoms that may be extremely debilitating and which may require intensive pharmacological treatment, but which only occasionally meet diagnostic criteria for a discrete major affective episode. This is a problem that crops up again and again in the extensive stroke literature on antidepressant treatment. Stroke patients have severe affective disorders but their occurrence is not characterized by the onset of a discrete affective episode. Their affective symptoms tend to be more variable, more changeable from day to day, more given to extremes of emotional expression.

The same is true of mentally retarded people, among whom symptoms of affective instability are indeed common; in all probability more common than the occurrence of discrete affective episodes. The same is probably also true of children, of the elderly and of closed head injury patients.

The characteristic of affective disorder in special populations, then, is the comparative rarity of discrete affective episodes, in contrast to the extreme frequency of negative mood states that may be chronic but not invariant; and the comparative rarity of prolonged extremes of mood, in contrast to the extreme frequency of emotional instability or of lability.

It is possible that this observation may be open to theoretical expansion. One may propose, by way of theory, that the essence of affective disease is a proclivity to affective instability. This may be an inherited weakness, an inborn familial tendency; a function of receptor dynamics, for example, in the ascending monoamine pathways. Or it may be an acquired tendency, the result of neuropathic damage or of a failure of development. In such cases, receptor dysregulation could be the consequence of a paucity of receptors or of a weakness in neural systems that modulate receptor dynamics.

In normal patients, that is, patients who are not neuropathic cases, there is an intact cortical regulatory system to control the extreme fluctuations of ascending monoaminergic pathways. One should expect to see, therefore, the occurrence of affective breakthroughs only in response to severely stressful circumstances, when cortical regulation is distracted and weakened. Alternatively, there may be spontaneous affective breakthroughs, when midbrain or brainstem structures become so unbalanced that they are able to overwhelm cortical protection. And when subcortical influences in either event grow so strong that they overwhelm the capacity of cortical regulation, it should come as no surprise that the episodes are sustained.

In patients with extensive destruction of white and gray matter, such as stroke patients and head injury patients and mentally retarded patients, one may expect to see a substantial diminution in cortical regulation of affective instability. One should see, rather, the frequent breakthrough of affective instability, even in trivial circumstances. The extreme example is emotional incontinence in patients with extensive cortical disease, like Alzheimer's.

So, one may propose that the clinical manifestations of an affective instability syndrome in retarded people, in neuropathic patients, and even in children emerge as frequent but unsustained expressions. And that sustained affective events, like bipolar disease or melancholia, are much more likely to occur in patients who are cortically intact.

A two-stage model of affective disease is therefore proposed: impulsion, the impulse to emote, which comes from below; and regulation, which resides in the cortex, and which moderates the impulse to emotional expression.

It is a Jacksonian formulation. The expression of emotion is a "primitive" method of communication that is deeply embedded in the phylogenetic past. It is hard-wired in midbrain and brainstem structures. Recognizable emotions are observed in rodents, who hardly have a cerebral cortex at all. In higher mammals, diseases of the gray and white matter lead to the release of affective expressions, even to trivial stimuli. The most dramatic display of emotion one will ever observe is the extreme lability that afflicts patients with extensive cortical destruction.

The regulation of emotion is clearly a learned process, a skill that is acquired with many years of maturation, and a trait that varies widely from one culture to another. It is a power that is lost in the face of overwhelming stress, or when the gray matter is destroyed.

The two-stage model alleviates the burden of trying to fit retarded people, stroke patients, head injury patients, or young children into a nosological system that was devised for people whose physiology is really quite different. The issue should never be, "How do we fit these special groups into the existing nosology?" The proper question is how we can reconcile the affective instability syndromes that occur in neuropathic patients into a wider conception of affective disease.

There is room, then, in the study of retarded patients, stroke patients, children, demented patients, and head injury patients, to speak of affective disease without recourse to the refinements of categorization that are salient to people who are cortically intact. One should eschew such an impulse because it gains little, and it costs a good deal of confusion.

One notes, for example, vain attempts to define affective events in brain injury patients in terms of "mania" (Bakchine et al., 1989), or "panic" in autistic people (Grandin and Scariano, 1986). In fact, there may be a functional neuro-anatomic construction to their behavior in terms of the syndrome of hypervigilance-hyperreactivity (see Chapters 1 and 2 on Traumatic Brain Injury and Chapter 9 on Autism). We have addressed the issue of treatment of this affective syndrome with adrenergic antagonists and beta blockers.

The psychiatric condition that clinicians refer to as "chronic depression" or "depressive personality" includes a large group of people whose energy level is somewhat low and whose outlook is perennially dim. When such a patient is encountered in a brain injury clinic, the appropriate diagnosis is "abulia," and the syndrome is usually attributable to a frontal lobe lesion in the convexity. Alternatively, damage to ascending monoamine pathways may lead to a chronic state of cortical depression; the chronic depression and negativism one observes, for example, in head injury patients with diffuse axonal degeneration. Treatment here is better with dopamine agonists like the psychostimulants amantadine and bromocriptine.

There are "rapid cyclers," and "emotionally unstable characters" who are given to extremes of up and down, and who may bounce frequently from one extreme to another. They may be said to be "atypical bipolar" patients, but they may also be patients with disease of the deep temporal lobe structures, in which case treatment is probably more rational with a psychotropic anticonvulsant.

These are all conditions that are affective, and they are major, but they are not major affective disorders in DSM terms. They are affective diseases, a term that we prefer because they are clearly neuropathic in origin. The DSM term is organic affective disorder, and you can take your pick. Whatever you call them, they respond inconsistently to conventional antidepressant treatments, and most of the time they require a different kind of treatment.

One might prefer, then, to speak, not in terms of the diagnosis of affective disorders, but rather in terms of the differential diagnosis. One may describe the event in terms of the general descriptors in the DSM if that is appropriate, but usually it is not. If the presentation is "atypical," it is not sufficient simply to add that adjective to the label. There should be an attempt to understand the disorder in terms of its etiology and the pathophysiology that is operative for that individual patient. If the patient is abulic, one should hypothesize a lesion, or a functional weakness in the frontal convexity; if the patient is explosive, in the deep temporal lobe; if the patient is hypervigilant-hyperreactive, in the thalamofrontal circuitry. In a right temporal, the depression might be turgid and dense; in a left temporal, manicky or garrulous. In a brainstem case, there should be a global slowdown, or global activation.

Anxiety Disorders

It may be appropriate to include the anxiety disorders and panic in the broad family of affective disorders, for the following reasons.

It is rare to find an anxious patient who has no symptoms of depression, or a panic disorder patient who is not anxious and depressed (Kendler et al., 1987).

There is substantial overlap among the drugs. The antidepressants are equally efficacious for anxiety, and anxiolytics like alprazolam are effective antidepressants (the other benzodiazepines are depressants, however) (Rickels and Schweitzer, 1987).

Within families, people may have slightly different manifestations of what appears to be a genetic proclivity to affective dysregulation: one member of the family may be depressive, another more anxiety prone, and a third given to panic attacks. A fourth might drink to excess, but that is probably from having to live with one, two, and three.

If the anxiety disorders do not breed true, if their margins are blurry, and if they respond in a nonspecific way to pharmacotherapy, is there anything left to say? Very well, then, one should subdivide. If the overarching whole is an untenable position, perhaps the smaller pieces will endure.

So, one may speak of psychic anxiety and somatic anxiety.

The former refers to subjective feelings of nervousness, worry, and fear, and the latter to the experience of autonomic hyperarousal, with rapid breathing and shortness of breath, diaphoresis, palpitations, distal paraesthesias, and the urge to micturate (Fahs, 1989). There are also the discrete anxiety conditions, like performance anxiety and panic anxiety, or agoraphobia, hypochondriasis, and the various phobias. The pharmacotherapy of anxiety is germane to this informal distinction. Tricyclic antidepressants are better than benzodiazepines for panic anxiety, and the two classes are probably equal for generalized anxiety disorder. Beta blockers are better for performance anxiety, and they are also good when symptoms of somatic anxiety predominate the clinical picture. Buspirone is an anxiolytic that has yet to find itself, but it may be dramatically effective for some severely anxious patients with hypochondriasis or elements of the so-called borderline personality.

Symptoms of anxiety and panic are not uncommon in developmentally handicapped people. In some cases, they will fit neatly into DSM categories and respond to the conventional treatments. In other cases, alternative constructions may be appropriate. The concepts of somatic anxiety or of performance anxiety may be more relevant. Irrational fear and panic may be ictal or periictal, related especially to lesions in the temporal lobe. What appears to be panic may be an expression of hypervigilance-hyperreactivity.

The principle is to embrace the formulation that is heuristic; to choose the hypothesis that is not only the most reasonable, but also that lends itself best to empirical proof.

Schizophrenia

There are two forms of schizophrenia, one from Bleuler and one from Kraeplin. Much of the difficulty in understanding the nature of schizophrenia comes from assuming there is only one disease, when in fact there are two.

The Bleulerian form of schizophrenia is a late-onset form. It is distributed equally between males and females, and it has an intermittent, relapsing course, with discrete episodes characterized by "positive" or "Schneiderian" symptoms. Paranoia is an element peculiar to this form of schizophrenia. Its structure is that of the major affective disorders in its course, in its genetic associations, and in its response to drug treatment.

The other form of schizophrenia, what Kraeplin called dementia praecox, is an adolescent-onset variant of mental retardation. It occurs predominantly in males, and is anteceded by premorbid deficits that have been described as "neurointegrative," but which are, in fact, developmental disabilities. It tends to have a deteriorating course and to respond poorly to treatment. Its structure is that of a static encephalopathy.

The variant of schizophrenia that is characterized by positive symptoms, like paranoia, is a relatively specific disorder, and like affective disorder it may be accurately diagnosed only in people who are mildly or moderately retarded. Reviewing our clinical experience and the literature, it is difficult to make a case for this variant of schizophrenia in people who are severely or profoundly retarded.

In cases of Bleulerian schizophrenia, it is appropriate to use the established psychiatric diagnostic criteria, but only in retarded people who are only mildly to moderately impaired, and who express psychiatric symptoms in ways that are similar to the rest of the population. The administration of long-term neuroleptics to such patients is entirely appropriate, and may be justified by the psychiatric diagnosis.

The diagnosis of dementia praecox can be made, in adult patients, not on the basis of their current "symptoms" but on the basis of their clinical history. Such patients have a near-normal developmental sequence into late childhood or adolescence, and then develop a chronic psychosis. There is a global deterioration in personality, socialization, and intellectual capacity, and they finally come to function at a mentally retarded level. They are usually not in the severely to profoundly retarded range, however.

For this group, one may say that functional mental retardation is, in fact, the consequence of an adolescent-onset encephalopathy, and that cognitive impairment is the inevitable result of a dementia praecox. We are beginning to see more and more of these people in mental retardation facilities. They arrive, like refugees, after a long hopeless sojourn through the mental health system. To the psychiatrist, they are schizophrenics with predominantly "negative" symptoms. To people in the mental retardation system, they are clients with functional deficits that require habilitation, and some behavioral peculiarities that require structure and tolerance. Antipsychotic medications are appropriate, and long-term treatment may be necessary, but drug treatment may only be required during periods of decompensation.

Although both forms of schizophrenia occur in mentally retarded people, the major epidemiologic studies have demonstrated that it is primarily a problem of mildly and moderately retarded people, and that schizophrenia "cannot be diagnosed on clinical grounds in the more severe and profound ranges of retardation" (Reid, 1989). The DSM and ICD criteria are entirely appropriate for the diagnosis of schizophrenia in mildly and moderately retarded people.

The importance of the dichotomy between Bleulerian and Krapelinian schizophrenia is for the direction of research. For the former, one would expect that the research strategies that are useful in the study of affective disorders would also be productive. The mandate for research in dementia praecox is different. Not something that psychiatrists are usually interested in, but a strategy that is very familiar to students of mental retardation: to discover an etiology for the deteriorating course. We know it is an encephalopathy of some kind, because it begins early in life and occurs predominantly in males, and because the patients deteriorate in many different dimensions. It is not, however, a congenital encephalopathy. Perhaps it is an autoimmune response to viral infection, which would explain its onset in youth, its high frequency, and its worldwide distribution among all races. If that were the case, then the genetics of such forms of schizophrenia would be the individual's vulnerability to such an extreme reaction to a viral insult—the genetics of vulnerability, like the vulnerability of a PKU patient to the toxic effects of phenylalanine.

There is another view of schizophrenia in retarded people that is different from the schema presented here. There are physicians who understand schizophrenia to be a unitary disorder, simply a complex of symptoms like disorganization, agitation, interpersonal alienation, and bizarre perceptions. They maintain that the disorder is common, if not ubiquitous, among people with severe encephalopathies, and particularly in people who are severely to profoundly mentally retarded. People who take this view are prone to diagnose the disorder in retarded people at every level. They may also make exaggerated claims for the use of antipsychotic drugs.

That approach is almost certainly overly inclusive. After all, what they are talking about is not a complex of symptoms that are unique to a particular lesion or to a particular psychopathological process, but rather the kind of global dysfunction that characterizes a diffuse encephalopathy. There is no advantage to calling any degree of disorganized or bizarre behavior "schizophrenia." It is like adding pigments to black; the color that results is still black.

In severe and profoundly retarded people, who may happen to show an exaggerated complex of symptoms including disorganization, alienation, and agitation, one can only speculate that the encephalopathy that gave rise to their retardation has been so extensive, especially to subcortical structures, that the clinical picture merges with the wider range of specific dysfunctions, like autism, schizophrenia, and affective disorder. In terms of diagnosis, it is better to concentrate on functional deficits, target behaviors, and the neuropathic substrate. In terms of treatment, it is better to justify medication in terms of behavioral response, rather than psychiatric diagnosis. If one is absolutely compelled to concoct a diagnosis for such people, for example, if HCFA requires it, there are always cop-outs like "organic psychosis" or "atypical psychosis." As diagnostic labels, they are so vague and ambiguous that they achieve a certain integrity.

Behavioral Disorders

These are disorders that are described entirely in terms of the particular behaviors at issue. Although they may be seen in association with traditional psychiatric disorders, or with the pathobehavioral mental retardation syndromes, they are more commonly observed to stand alone, with no other diagnostic hallmark save the behavior itself.

Hyperactivity

In the chapter on childhood hyperactivity (Chapter 11), we present the hypothesis that "temperamental" hyperactivity is a dysmaturation syndrome of frontal lobe regulatory systems. In the Autism chapter (Chapter 9), we describe the nature of "pathological" hyperactivity as a form of exploratory behavior. In the section on amantadine in Traumatic Brain Injury (Chapter 2), we presented the idea that presynaptic dopamine agonists are preferable in the first instance and postsynaptic dopamine agonists in the second. All these concepts bear on the issue of hyperactivity in mentally retarded people.

Noncompliance

Child psychiatrists use the term "oppositional." Clinicians who work with schizophrenic patients call it "negativism." In mental retardation, the "target behavior" is usually "noncompliance." The idea is met frequently, in its different forms, but there is virtually no literature on it. Stubbornness and nay-saying are not events that excite scientific interest. They do excite literary interest, though, like *Oblomov* and *Bartleby the Scrivener* and *The Loneliness of the Long Distance Runner*. But that is another story.

Writers have understood noncompliance or oppositional behavior as a fundamental right of individual expression, albeit a negative expression. Oblomov was a lazy aristocrat, a slob; the polite expression is *ennui du siecle*. The long distance runner, in Alan Sillitoe's story, was expressing the outrage of an oppressed class, if you will, or alternatively a sense of despair over his father's meaningless life and death. (Bartleby will always be a mystery. His negativism is a pure type. It looks like simple schizophrenia, but he probably just had a bad case of industrial disease.)

Writers understand negativism and oppositional behavior. If you have ever tried to convince a writer to abandon his Underwood and buy a word processor, you have probably encountered a good case of oppositional behavior. But scientific writers have been reluctant to take the problem on; that is probably a function of their own ineluctable positivism. Have you ever heard a scientist say, "No more research is needed"? Probably not. Anyway, literary allusions aside, it may be that no one writes about oppositional disorder because no one has found an interesting context to frame the problem.

In fact, there is.

I had never had any interest in the problem of oppositional behavior when I worked in a child psychiatry clinic. When I consulted at mental retardation facilities, I would peruse, politely, behavioral graphs of "noncompliant behavior," and then carry on to the next patient. The prescription was to look for specific areas of cognitive weakness or emotional trauma that would be a "setting event" for the negativistic behavior, and to deal with that; to structure the patient's experiences in a developmentally appropriate way; and to handle transitions in a gentle and a creative way. That was all.

It was not until I began to work with patients with closed head injuries that the problem of oppositional behavior got interesting, because it finally began to make sense. The paradigm is the frontal lobe patient, especially the right frontal, who can be as stubborn as a mule. Adult patients with frontal lobe lesions of the convexity can be as intractable and truculent as the most oppositional child. They are inflexible and they have difficulty "changing sets."

The idea of cognitive flexibility refers to the capacity to change behavioral or cognitive sets in response to changing circumstances. It is an idea that arose in neuropsychology, and it is demonstrated in tests like the Wisconsin Card Sort and in a number of Luria tasks. The extreme of cognitive inflexibility is perseveration, which can be demonstrated on these tests. In the Stroop test, the frontal patient is found to have great difficulty operating out of two simultaneous cognitive sets, suppressing one while the other is active.

The function of the frontal lobes is to execute complex programs of activity, to form the orienting basis for action, and to organize its strategy (Luria, 1973). Lesions of the frontal convexity lead to a motor stereotype and to a derangement in the complex forms of organization of behavior, against the background of absolutely intact consciousness. Patients with such lesions have an inertia to maintain the present set. They are inflexible in the face of changing external demands because they cannot dissociate their responses or pull their attention away from what is in their present field (Lezak, 1983). They eschew novel circumstances because they have difficulty maintaining organization in the face of insufficient redundancy (Pribram, 1973); once they get going in a new set, and when redundancy or at least familiarity is established, they can continue in a perfectly suitable way.

Frontal patients, like primates with dorsolateral lesions, are "sluggish" in response to reinforcers; the feedback to actions from their outcomes is impaired, so reinforcers become relatively ineffective (Pribram, 1973). So, it is no easy matter to induce them to be more accommodating by rewarding or punishing selected behaviors.

The pathophysiology of noncompliance, therefore, has to do with the physiology of frontal lobe function, in distributing attention and organized behavior in response to appropriate external requirements, in registering novelty so that habituation or assimilation can take place.

It should not be surprising that similar difficulties should exist in the troubled child, who in the first decade of life has little in the way of frontal lobe resources; or in severely retarded people, who have a diffuse encephalopathy and little in the way of cortical executive function at all.

Understanding the physiology should direct treatment. The principles of treatment for oppositional behavior, based on this understanding, are to look for specific areas of cognitive weakness or emotional trauma that would be a "setting event" for the negativistic behavior, and to contend with that; to structure the patient's experiences in a developmentally appropriate way; and to handle transitions in a gentle and a creative way.

Rituals, Preoccupation with Sameness, and Tyrannical Behavior

The motor stereotypes that characterize frontal lobe patients may have several clinical manifestations in people with severe developmental handicaps. Rituals are extremely complex stereotypes that may grow with accretion over the years. The bedtime rituals of autistic people are classical. If the same pattern of activity is not pursued, in the same order and with the same emphasis, night after night, sleep is impossible, and a horrible scene may take its place. One of our patients heard a doorbell ring during a nighttime ritual that lasted about an hour; thereafter, doorbell ringing at precisely that time was incorporated into the ritual.

The other symptom that is classical for autistic people is preoccupation with sameness: the same arrangement of furniture around the house; going to school by exactly the same route; the same teachers every day; the same, invariant task at work, every day.

Tyrannical behavior refers to the development of stereotyped activities over the years, especially when a severely handicapped person lives at home. As parents grow elderly, they learn that the course of least resistance is to accommodate the rituals and "sameness" behavior of the handicapped child. This only serves to expand the repertoire of stereotyped activity, so the whole day may be spent in gratifying ritual preoccupations. Extricating a family from this deadend can be a major operation.

Stereotypy

"Stereotypies" are repetitious, topographically invariant motor behaviors or action sequences in which reinforcement is noncontingent (Schroeder, 1989a). They are a normal behavioral variant in infancy and early childhood (Sallustro and Atwell, 1978), but they are far more dramatic when they occur in retarded and autistic people and in the congenitally deaf and the blind ("blindisms"). Stereotypies occur in about two-thirds of these populations (O'Brien, 1981).

The most common stereotypies are whole body movements or postures (rocking, twirling); other repetitive movements (head-rolling, head-banging); nonrepetitive movements (posturing, sucking); complex hand movements; manipulation of objects; and meaningless utterances (Berkson, 1967).

"For the most part, the stimuli which initiate, guide and reward stereotyped behavior have their origin within the organism performing the act" (Berkson, 1983). This feature renders stereotypies relatively resistant to behavioral treatment.

Stereotypies arise from two different contexts. They are more likely to occur in people with severe sensory impairments, the congenitally blind and deaf (Guess and Rutherford, 1967; Kaufman and Levitt, 1965). They occur in circumstances of confinement (Warren and Burns, 1970) or restriction (Berkson et al., 1963) or sensory deprivation (Higgenbottam and Chow, 1975; Tizard, 1968). This suggests a functional end in the service of self-stimulation.

"Zoo behavior" or stereotypy in animals (especially foraging animals, like bears) occurs when they are confined or frustrated or isolated. The motor patterns include scratching, hair pulling, masturbation, and endless pacing (Insel, 1988).

The second variant are stereotypies that seem to have an end in the service of tension reduction. They are likely to occur in response to intense environmental stimuli (Forehand and Baumeister, 1970b), frustration (Baumeister and Forehand, 1971), or novel situations (Berkson et al., 1963).

The animal equivalent is "displacement behavior," stereotyped motor acts (or "fixed motor patterns") that are excessive and inappropriate. The particular behaviors, like pecking, grooming, digging, or head-turning are typical within a species but vary greatly between species. They are invariably triggered by an emotionally laden situation, like sexual or territorial conflicts, and it is believed that their service is to reduce tension associated with conflict (Insel, 1988).

Stereotyped motor activity has a well-known neuropharmacological basis, because it can be evoked quite reliably in laboratory rats by lesions or chemical agents that induce a state of hypersensitivity in the postsynaptic striatal dopamine receptor (Lewis and Baumeister, 1983). Apormorphine-induced stereotypy after a 6-hydroxydopamine-induced lesion is a classical preparation. It is reversed by D_2 dopamine receptor antagonists like haloperidol. In clinical circumstances, neuroleptics are very effective in reducing stereotypies; dopamine agonists, like L-dopa and the psychostimulants, may evoke stereotyped behavior, especially in high doses.

Noncompliance, rituals, preoccupation with sameness, tyrannical behavior, and stereotypies are all cuts of the same cloth, manifestations of frontal lobe dysfunction. They are all elements one grows accustomed to when working on a service for head injury patients. They represent, in all probability, a release from descending cortical control of motor programs embedded in the basal ganglia. They are much more complex than the simple dyskinesias we attribute to diseases of the basal ganglia, like Huntington's chorea. But they respond, like chorea, to low doses of dopamine antagonists and they are aggravated, like chorea, by low doses of dopamine agonists.

The pharmacological treatment of stereotyped behavior should therefore be with neuroleptics, to mitigate the influence of striatal hyperreactivity. That is not a good idea, however, because neuroleptics also shut down dopaminergic tonus to frontal structures, and that produces a state of blunting or lethargy that is only rarely a desirable therapeutic outcome. Neuroleptics are also in the long run toxic to the dopamine receptor, and they actually produce severe dyskinesia. Some of the clinical manifestations of tardive dyskinesia, in fact, resemble stereotyped mannerisms.

An alternative treatment strategy is to activate frontal modulation, as one does in the treatment of abulic states, with a stimulant or a dopamine agonist like amantadine. However, it seems to be impossible to stimulate dopaminergic projections to frontal structures without also increasing dopaminergic neurotransmission to the striatum, and that, of course, is only going to make the stereotypies worse.

The pharmacological strategies appear to be contradictory, although it should never be a surprise when opposite stimuli evoke the identical behavioral response. Stereotypies may be evoked by high doses of amphetamine (Iversen, 1977), or they can be suppressed by amphetamine (Insel, 1988). And as we have also seen, stereotypies can be elicited, clinically, in circumstances of sensory deprivation or alternatively of intense sensory activation.

There is a solution to this paradox, in considering the mutual and interrelated roles of frontal cortex and corpus striatum in ritual and stereotyped behavior. Some light may be shed by considering the example of obsessive-compulsive disorder (OCD), and this may also be pertinent clinically. One has often wondered whether the rituals and stereotyped behavior of autistic and retarded people are a variant of OCD. One has also wondered whether the new, successful treatments for OCD may be helpful in treating the former conditions, the serotonin reuptake inhibitors fluoxetine and clomipramine, for example.

The similarity between rituals and stereotyped motor behaviors in developmentally handicapped people and people with OCD does not mean that the former is a brain-damaged variant of OCD. That would be a naive construction. A better way to frame the idea is to propose that the neural substrate for ritual behavior is the same in both disorders. The occurrence of stereotypies ("zoo behavior" and displacement behavior) in lower animals suggests that the neural substrate is subcortical. Thus, one's interest in the functional anatomy of stereotyped behavior, which begins with the consideration of the consequence of frontal lobe lesions, extends caudally along frontal projections to the corpus striatum. This is a natural progression (retrogression) of thought, because the basal ganglia subserve what are usually considered to be frontal lobe functions in immature primates and in lower mammals, like the rat, which hardly possesses a frontal cortex at all (Divac, 1968).

The role of the basal ganglia is probably central to the ritual behavior of patients with OCD, and there is clinical evidence for lesions in the basal ganglia associated with OCD (Rapoport and Wise, 1988; Weilburg et al., 1989). The function of the basal ganglia is presumably to release species-specific motor patterns (Stahl, 1988). Its function is also to respond to levels of motivation, either to persist in motor patterns that are internally driven or to respond to external stimuli (Cools and van den Bercken, 1977). It may be considered as a gate, or a filter between the incentive system, which is input to the caudate, and the motor system, which is output (Broekkamp et al., 1977). The incentives come from above; the appropriate response patterns are delivered to effector systems below.

The release of repetitive, meaningless stereotypes, for example in OCD, are probably the result of something like an aberrant feedback loop around the frontal lobes, limbic cortex, basal ganglia, and thalamus (Stevens, 1977; Rapoport and Wise, 1988; Moddell et al., 1989). One may conceptualize the disorder as a dissociation of the motivational from the motoric, with all of the doubt, dismay, and confusion that will necessarily ensue. A reverberating circuit, if you will, and one that is badly out of balance.

The release of repetitive, meaningless stereotypes in developmentally handicapped individuals probably has a more diffuse origin, but it almost certainly involves a deficit in cortical modulation of striatal activity. It is not a dissociation between the motivational and the motoric. It is a lapse in the capacity of frontal structures to respond to new external stimuli and to generate the motivation for adaptional motor patterns in the striatum. This is the model of a caged animal who is unable to forage, and who finds nothing external that is sufficient to motivate a motor pattern. So it relies on repetitive, internal motor patterns. There is no incentive to anything else.

This is the kind of stereotypy that occurs in severely handicapped people in circumstances of sensory deprivation. It is also the type of stereotypy that should be expected to respond favorably to a dopamine agonist, and it does (Insel, 1988; Chandler et al., in press), or to an antagonist (Stevens, 1977), and it does.

For the second variant of clinical stereotypy, the mechanism is different, although the output is the same. The release of repetitive meaningless stereotypes in the face of intense novel stimuli occurs when frontal structures that are sluggish to respond to novel external stimuli are overwhelmed. New stimuli overflow the circuitry, paralyzing the system, as it were. This leaves the striatal generator once again at the mercy of a much lower, intrinsic order of motivation.

One might expect to have a degree of success against ritualized behavior in handicapped people by manipulating the serotonin system, because it works in OCD. Although the test has never been made, it may not work. The effects of sertonergic drugs on movement disorders, another manifestation of striatal dysfunction, are weak and unpredictable; we discuss that issue in the serotonin chapter (see below). It is a compelling idea, and it merits empirical trials, although preliminary experiments in our clinics have not supported the treatment of ritual behavior in autistic people with serotonergic drugs.

Aggression

There is not a simple way to address the subject of aggression, because its origins plumb the depths of human motivation and its manifestations reflect the breadth of human endeavor. There is certainly no unitary way to code it. There is no single perspective that is inclusive of all forms of aggression.

There is the history of human aggression, its politics and sociology; there is a genetic approach, and a phylogenetic approach; there is a neuropharmacology of aggression, and a psychopharmacology. There are as many psychologies of human aggression as there are schools of psychology.

Fortunately, the clinical approach to the problem of aggressive behavior is not as complicated as the overarching philosophy of aggressive behavior, but it makes more sense if one has a philosophy. The philosophy that I prefer eschews the dichotomy of aggression is innate versus aggression is pathological. There is no choice to make between the alternatives, because both are correct; they are simply different models or paradigms. The two paradigms support a framework for the differential diagnosis of aggression. They support, as well, a philosophy of aggression, and an approach to treatment and to prevention.

The models are temperamental aggression and pathological aggression—aggression as an extreme variant of normal human assertiveness, and aggression as a dramatic manifestation of brain disease.

Aggressive behavior is only one of the many neuropsychiatric entities that can be defined in terms of a "two-stage" model, an idea which is developed more extensively in the discussion of Childhood Hyperactivity (see Chapter 11). In simple terms, the model posits two fundamental kinds of aggressive behavior: temperamental and pathological. The former is an expression of the normal variation of human personality traits. If polygenes for a trait one may call "assertiveness" are assumed to be normally distributed in the human population, one may expect to find a group of people who are "loaded" with such genes and who are assertive to an extreme degree. This is not a radical idea. No one is a stranger to the observation that some individuals are forceful, dynamic, competitive, energetic, and single minded of purpose, even to the callous disregard of the feelings and interests of their fellow humans. And no one can argue that these traits are always bad, or maladaptive or destructive. They may serve a useful purpose; the success of the individual is not always at the expense of the group. Genes to support the phenotype of assertive behavior exist in the genome because they have at least some adaptive utility.

The point at which extreme assertive behavior is defined as aggression is arbitrary, and it is different from one society to another, and from one age to another. It represents a social value, and a mutative value at that.

The value of the polygenic model is that it introduces the concept of a threshold of expression; the expression of the phenotype is variable, and may be influenced by external elements, for example social values. The heroes of one era, even the historical figures we continue to admire, would be hopeless misfits, even criminals, if they were set down today in a suburban mall or an office of CPAs. Assertiveness is admired if it occurs in a socially approved context. If it is inappropriate to the context, it is labeled aggression, and it is bad.

What is "pathological," then, about temperamental aggression is its inappropriateness to the social context. The assertive individual is aggressive if he cannot conform his behavior to the external demands of the situation. The failure is one of social judgment.

The aggressive behavior of such individuals occurs in the context of normal human exploratory or acquisitory behavior; that is, aggression in the service of a specific, understandable end. The behavior may be inappropriate, or the end may be excessive, but it is understandable. There is a rationale for it.

So, the normal genome regulates the intensity with which behavior is directed, but it cannot speak to the context in which behavior occurs, or the threshold that separates appropriate from inappropriate aggression. The genome may regulate one's capacity to read social cues, or to learn from past experience, or to adapt one's behavior in light of past experience. But it cannot influence the view of other people, and it is their opinion that determines the threshold. The genome hardly distinguishes between the robbing of a bank and the founding of a bank.

If one were to seek a neuropathic paradigm for temperamental aggression, one would select the frontal lobe patient who has difficulties conforming to social expectations, and who may lash out violently when he is confronted by external requirements that he can neither read nor understand. The temperamental aggressive has a genotype that expresses assertive behavior; if he has a weakness in genetic endowment that renders his assertions inappropriate, it is in a failure to read social cues or to learn from social experience. That would represent a variant of the frontal lobe syndrome we have postulated in the chapter on hyperactivity (see Chapter 11.)

"Pathological" aggression, on the other hand, represents a behavioral variant that is not encoded in the genome, but that is expressed as a consequence of some extraordinary derangement of the behavioral apparatus. Such aggression occurs in extraordinary manifestations, quite out of proportion to any reasonable provocation or end. The paradigm here is the paroxysmal, explosively aggressive behavior that occurs in patients with deep temporal lobe lesions, or in patients who are in the disoriented, agitated stage of coma recovery. Or the compulsive aggression and self-mutilative behavior that occurs in extraordinary disorders like the Lesch–Nyhan syndrome.

Dichotomies invariably fail, because there is always a grey area in between, and in clinical practice most cases fall into the gray area. But that is the advantage of a model over a theory. A theory can be discredited by the discovery of a single exception. A model can be kept alive so long as there are a few examples that fit.

This dichotomy is supported by a mass of evidence, however. If one examines the most common neuropsychiatric disorders among common criminals, people who are confined for comparatively minor transgressions like burglary or drug-running, one finds nothing more than the common developmental disorders like mild retardation, hyperactivity, dyslexia, and developmental dysphasia. If, on the other hand, one examines the status of the much smaller number of violent criminals who are confined on Death Row, one sees a very high incidence of severe psychiatric disorders, such as schizophrenia, and of brain lesions, which may be congenital or traumatic (Lewis et al., 1985; Lewis et al., 1986).

If the model were correct, one would expect to see this: among mentally retarded people, there should be a higher frequency of operant aggression among the mildly and moderately retarded, aggression in the service of specific aims, petty criminality, sexual transgressions, competitiveness, argumentativeness, and fighting. In people who are severely and profoundly retarded, one would expect to see compulsive aggression (and self-injurious behavior), aggression that has no understandable aim, or that is not specific, or that has no operant properties at all. The study, of course, has yet to be done. But the dichotomy seems to conform to one's clinical observations.

Clinical experience may also guide the differential diagnosis of aggressive behavior in mentally retarded people. The principles are familiar: among higher level patients, the traditional psychiatric categories may be relevant, especially the categories that refer to impulsive behavior and poor social judgment—sociopathy, for example. In lower level patients, one takes recourse to such categories only with a degree of skepticism, and one usually refers to more simple, behavioral definitions. As is the case for self-injurious behavior, a peculiar variant of human aggression, one may utilize a wider differential of etiological, neurological, psychiatric, psychological, and neurochemical constructs.

The two-stage model of aggressive behavior lends itself to a philosophy of treatment. The treatment of temperamental aggression is simply this: teaching the patient to direct his energies in appropriate directions, and rewarding him for doing so; teaching the patient to read external cues more accurately; and structuring the patient's environment to guarantee the success of the lessons one has taught. The treatment of temperamental aggression, therefore, is largely behavioral, educational, and environmental. If psychopharmaceuticals are useful, they are drugs like the stimulants, which tend to reduce impulsive behavior and increase reflective behavior. As in the treatment of hyperactivity, stimulants are intended to increase cortical regulation of impulsive and excitable behavior.

The treatment of pathological aggression on the other hand, like the treatment of self-injurious behavior which we shall discuss later on, is aimed at the underlying neuropathic process. It is not specific to aggression. It is specific to the hypothesized lesion. That is why it is probably an idle endeavor to try to develop a class of "antiaggression" drugs. Because aggression itself is not a unitary construct, it is unlikely that there could be a unitary treatment. In fact, the psychopharmacology of aggression is quite diverse.

The psychotropic anticonvulsant carbamazepine appears to have a tropism for temporal lobe structures like the amygdala, which is also an organ that is linked to a particular manifestation of intense aggressive behavior. But carbamazepine is not effective for all pathological aggressives, or all explosive aggressives, although it is a very good drug. Valproate is an anticonvulsant with a preference for centrencephalic epilepsies, but it is sometimes effective when carbamazepine fails. To what degree the success of these two drugs as antiaggressives is related to their anticonvulsant effects is a perennial source of argument.

There is no unitary mechanism to account for the success of other antiaggressive agents like lithium, the beta blockers, the alpha agonists, and the serotonergics for cases of pathological aggression. Lithium probably acts as a serotonergic drug or as a drug that reduces abnormal neuronal excitability by virtue of its effect on second-messenger systems (see Chapter 3, this volume). The beta blockers and the alpha agonists probably reduce noradrenergic overdrive to cortical inhibitory systems (Chapter 3), thus allowing them to function more efficiently. The serotonergic drugs act in similar fashion, possibly by enhancing the modulation of dopaminergic and noradrenergic systems. Caffeine, a drug that increases irritability, aggression, and self-injurious behavior, does so by antagonizing the inhibitory neurotransmitter adenosine (see Chapter 4).

It is ironic that the drugs most commonly prescribed to aggressive patients are probably, in the long run, the least effective. The neuroleptics are dramatically effective in reducing aggressive behavior in acute or emergency situations, and they are irreplaceable for the treatment of aggressive schizophrenic patients. But their long-term usefulness for the control of aggression in most retarded patients is really quite marginal. In fact, because they may cause a prolonged state of akathisia even after they are withdrawn, they may actually aggravate the problem over the long term.

Pica

Pica is the Latin word for magpie, a bird that is said to eat inedible things. That is also the definition of the behavioral syndrome, although it also pertains to scavenging for inedibles or mouthing them (Kruck, 1989). Pica is a developmental variant in normal-IQ children. It is seen in about half of all 1-year-olds and 10% of 4-year-olds (Barltrop, 1966; Lourie et al., 1963). The most frequently ingested items are paper, clothing, dirt, matches, toilet items, plaster, writing materials, and tobacco.

Pica has been observed in 26% of a population of 991 institutionalized retarded people (Danford and Huber, 1982). The occurrence of pica was more likely in younger patients and in patients who were more severely handicapped intellectually. Its cooccurrence with low levels of iron suggests a nutritional context, and with low levels of zinc, a disgeusic influence. If pica is oriented to cigarette butts, one may consider Nicorette as a substitute.

Zinc deficiency in children has been associated with hypogeusia, dysgeusia, and pica (Hambidge, 1981). Supplemental zinc has also been reported to eliminate pica in children (Hambidge and Silverman, 1973) and in a mentally retarded adult (Lofts, 1986). In severe zinc deficiency, plasma levels are less than 6 μmol/liter (normal range, 10-17) (Hambidge, 1981).

A small number of patients with habitual pica can develop serious medical consequences, such as lead poisoning or intestinal obstruction. In such patients, treatment or prevention is a high priority; there is no current psychopharmacological treatment. The proper treatment strategy is to investigate the possibility of a nutritional deficiency, like low zinc, or an addiction, like tobacco; then to determine whether pica is a function of boredom, frustration, unhappiness, or idleness, or some other emotional state that might be corrected programmatically. The behavioral alternatives are contingent restraint (Singh and Bakker, 1984) and overcorrection (Mulick et al., 1980a).

Copraxia

This term refers to rectal digging, feces smearing, and coprophagia, three repugnant behaviors that are rarely seen outside of large public institutions (Frieden, 1977). It is usually a function of idleness or disorganization. It sometimes occurs in a chain, from scavenging to pica to digging to smearing to coprophagia, although this pattern is by no means invariant; rectal digging, for example, may be masturbatory, or it may be a response to parasites, pruritus ani, or hemorrhoids (Schroeder, 1989b). The treatment is usually behavioral (Frieden and Johnson, 1979).

Rumination

Rumination, or ruminative vomiting, consists of repeated vomiting, chewing, and reingestion of the vomitus. Rumination is not hard to distinguish from vomiting as an acute response to illness or toxic ingestion, or as a manifestation of altered taste sensitivity from burns, cancer, renal failure, zinc or lead toxicity, medication, or hypothalamic disease, or as a symptom of anorexia or bulimia nervosa (Schroeder, 1989c). In contrast, rumination is said to have a significant learned component that is maintained by sensory reinforcement; it is a complex, chronic problem that is highly resistant to therapeutic intervention. Like pica and copraxia, it may occur in normal children as a developmental variant (Richmond and Eddy, 1957; Kanner, 1959).

Rumination may occur in 5% to 10% of the institutionalized retarded population (Ross, 1972; Singh and Dawson, 1980), especially in the severe and profoundly retarded and in autistic individuals. The onset is usually after years of institutionalization, and because it is often accompanied by stereotypies, it appears to be a form of self-stimulation. It is only rarely associated to an overt anatomic or a physiological abnormality (e.g., hiatal hernia), although it may be caused by poor positioning or, conceivably by oral-motor dyspraxia. It is not life-threatening, as a rule, but it may lead to weight loss, dehydration, respiratory infections, periodontitis, halitosis, and caries, as well as social isolation, as you can imagine (Schroeder, 1989c). The behavioral treatment is multiple small feeding to satiety, with active involvement in activities that are stimulating and diverting (Mulick et al., 1980b).

There is no established pharmacotherapy for rumination, or for copraxia or for pica. It is possible that some of the pharmacological investigations currently applied in the treatment of hyperphagia in the Prader–Willi syndrome (see following discussion) or in anorexia and bulimia nervosa may be applicable to some individuals with these disorders.

Compulsive Water Drinking (CWD)

Disturbances in water and thirst regulation are not uncommon in the chronically mentally ill, and also in head injury patients and in the mentally retarded. Virtually all the research has been done in psychiatric patients, but the principles are the same for all three groups. Polydipsia may be, first, the manifestation of a disease like diabetes mellitus or diabetes insipidus; second, it may be a drug effect; third, the result of hypothalamic injury or of neuropathic change in that area; or, last, a compulsion or an acquired habit, a peculiar form of addiction or of self-stimulation.

It is a serious problem, whatever the patient group. Uncontrolled drinking can cause water intoxication, a potentially fatal event. The differential diagnosis is very important, because management based on misdiagnosis can be disastrous. And the drugs we use quite frequently in retarded people and in patients with head injuries, especially carbamazepine (CBZ) and lithium, can affect the regulation of salt and water balance.

Primary polydipsia refers to "the ingestion of water in excess of that required to maintain normal water balance" (Stevko et al., 1968). Compulsive water drinking (CWD) refers to continuous or habitual drinking of excessive amounts of water, and psychogenic polydipsia refers to the consumption of extraordinary quantities over a short period of time (Singh et al., 1985).

Polydipsia is a common behavior, but it does not necessarily lead to intoxication, because the kidneys can compensate by excreting large amounts of dilute urine. Compulsive drinkers may have low urinary specific gravity, but most of them do not develop severe hyponatremia. It is estimated, however, that one-quarter to one-half of the patients with psychogenic polydypsia do go on to develop water intoxication at one time or another (Illowsky and Kirch, 1988).

Excessive drinking occurs in 3.3% to 17.5% of chronic mental patients (Jose et al., 1979; Blum et al., 1983), but it is not specific to any particular diagnostic group. Most of the cases, though, are psychotic, and there may be an association between the encephalopathy that gives rise to schizophrenia and the inappropriate secretion of antidiuretic hormone (ADH, vasopressin or arginine vasopressin, AVP) (Hobson and English, 1963; Khamnei, 1984). It has also been suggested that polydypsia is a hypothalamic manifestation of an underlying hyperdopaminergic state in psychotic patients (Singh et al., 1985). For example, adipsia can be induced in rats after chemical lesions to ascending dopaminergic pathways (Ungerstedt, 1971).

When compulsive drinking leads to water intoxication, the symptoms include headache, blurred vision, vomiting, diaphoresis, incoordination, irritability, and excitability; in severe intoxication, when water intake overwhelms renal output, hyponatremia develops; there is sudden dilution of body solutes, and the patient may exhibit muscle cramps, twitching, delirium, stupor, coma, and convulsions (Singh et al., 1985).

Excessive fluid intake may also be a symptom of diabetes insipidus (DI), a disorder characterized by polyuria and secondary polydypsia. It is important to distinguish between CWD and DI, because the management is really quite different. Administration of ADH to a patient with CWD can lead to hyponatremia and signs of water intoxication; restriction of water to a patient with DI may lead to hypernatremia and serious dehydration (Lishman, 1987).

Diabetes insipidus may be neurogenic, by virtue of reduction of ADH production in the hypothalamus; or nephrogenic (NDI), a circumstance that arises when the distal tubule of the glomerulus is unresponsive to physiological levels of ADH. Polydipsia in diabetes insipidus is a normal physiological response to the primary metabolic derangement, so if the diagnosis is missed and if fluid intake is restricted, the patient may develop a serious fluid and electrolyte imbalance (Lishman, 1987).

Diabetes insipidus is similar to CWD in that water consumption and urine output are excessively high, and the concentration of the urine is low. In DI, however, serum sodium, blood urea nitrogen (BUN), and serum osmolality tend to be high in contrast to CWD (Singh et al., 1985).

Symptoms of NDI may arise in patients who are treated with lithium, a drug that blocks the ADH receptor in the distal tubule. Lithium causes an NDI-type syndrome, with thirst and polydypsia and polyuria, in a substantial number of patients who have blood levels in the therapeutic range. Fluid restriction is not appropriate in lithium-induced NDI.

Chlorpromazine, thioridazine, and other neuroleptics may also cause polydipsia through a direct hypothalamic effect, perhaps on dopaminergic neurons that govern thirst, drinking behavior, and ADH secretion (Smith and Clark, 1980).

DI may be caused by destructive events such as tumors or cerebral infection. DI has been described after traumatic brain injury (TBI), in association with symptoms of rage, hyperphagia, and dementia, and in association with lesions in the posterior hypothalamus (Reeves and Blum 1969).

The polar opposite of DI is the syndrome of inappropriate ADH secretion (SIADH), caused by ectopic production (e.g., oat cell carcinoma of the lung), Guillain–Barre, acute intermittent porphyria, central nervous system (CNS) insults like tumors, stroke, or TBI, or by drugs. SIADH is associated with elevated levels of ADH, increased urinary osmolality, and decreased serum osmolality and hyponatremia (Illowsky and Kirch, 1988), whereas compulsive water drinkers tend to have dilute urine with low urine osmolality (Singh et al., 1985).

Inappropriate ADH secretion may, however, be seen in association with or as a consequence of CWD (Ferrier, 1985); for example, there is evidence of supersensitivity in the ADH receptor in psychiatric patients with CWD (Goldman et al., 1988). This may be a reset secondary to a prolonged period of low ADH secretion to accommodate the chronic water load (Hariprasad et al., 1980).

SIADH may be induced by treatment with anticonvulsants like phenobarbital, phenytoin, or CBZ, or by neuroleptics (e.g., thiothixene, chlorpromazine, fluphenazine), or tricyclic antidepressants (e.g., amitriptyline) (Ferrier, 1985).

The effect of CBZ is not only to enhance the release of ADH from the neurohypophysis (Smith et al., 1977; Thomas et al., 1977), but also to increase the sensitivity of adenyl cyclase in the distal tubule. Therefore, CBZ is an effective treatment for DI, although it has variable effects against lithium-induced NDI (Henry et al., 1977; Braunhofer and Zicha, 1989; Brooks and Lessin, 1983). On the other hand, it is not an effective treatment for primary NDI, because its renal effect is relatively weak, and it is not effective for DI in patients with a total failure of ADH secretion (Bonnici, 1973).

The mechanism of direct CBZ effect on the posterior pituitary may lead to hyponatremia in patients on CBZ for epilepsy or for disorders of behavior (Yassa et al., 1988). The effect is dose related (Henry et al., 1977). Hyponatremia may be the reason that some patients become irritable and aggressive on high doses of CBZ (Yassa et al., 1988), or even why some patients lose seizure control at high doses (Snead and Hosey, 1985).

Treatment with thiazide diuretics has been associated with impaired free-water clearance and water intoxication in psychiatric patients with CWD (Day, 1977). Thiazides are potentially lethal when they are used in patients who consume excessive amounts of water.

The treatment of compulsive water intoxication is restriction of fluid intake and attention to intrinsic or extrinsic factors that may be aggravating the situation. There are reports in the literature to support direct treatment either with propanalol (Shevitz et al., 1980) or demeclocycline, an antibiotic that induces a reversible NDI (Nixon et al., 1982). Captopril, an inhibitor of the angiotensin I converting enzyme, blocks the formation of angiotensin II, a potent dipsogen; captopril has been reported to reduce polydipsia in at least some psychiatric patients with CWD (Lawson et al., 1988).

CBZ, a drug that may cause SIADH, may be used to treat DI. CBZ may also reverse the effects of lithium-induced NDI (Brooks and Lessin, 1983). Lithium, on the other hand, may be used to treat SIADH. That would seem to make lithium and carbamazepine a natural combination. In fact, the combination can be neurotoxic. A delirious patient who has been on CBZ and lithium together probably does not have water intoxication, but he may well be neurotoxic from the drugs themselves (Shukla et al., 1984; Chaudry and Waters, 1983).

Pathobehavioral Mental Retardation Syndromes

These are eponymic syndromes with behavioral stereotypes and a well-defined genetic origin (Lesch–Nyhan syndrome), or syndromes with a clear genetic basis but a variable behavioral phenotype (PKU, Down's syndrome), and syndromes with a consistent behavioral stereotype but only the suspicion of a genetic/metabolic basis (Cornelia de Lange syndrome, Prader–Willi, Rett's).

The Lesch–Nyhan syndrome (LNS) is discussed in the following chapter on rational pharmacotherapy of self-injurious behavior (SIB) (Chapter 7). Neuropharmacological models of LNS were the foundation of our initial studies of the dopamine D1 receptor antagonist, fluphenazine.

The Cornelia de Lange syndrome (CDLS), another SIB syndrome, is described in Chapter 8 where the results of a large-scale behavioral survey are presented.

The Prader–Willi syndrome (PWS) is described in a succeeding section, because it is, arguably, a prototype for the serotonergic disorders. The discussion of PKU is also to be found, rightly or wrongly, in that section.

Autism is really in a category by itself, because it is already listed in the DSM, and it is also discussed in a separate chapter (Chapter 9). It is not a mental retardation syndrome in the sense of having a unitary genetic or biochemical basis, or a relatively invariant behavioral stereotype, although some people think it has. If there is a behavioral stereotype to autism, though, in the author's opinion it is most likely to be in autistic people who are not mentally retarded. If you work with severe and profoundly retarded people, you begin to believe that every patient is autistic, or, alternatively, that no one is.

The phakomatoses, like tuberous schlerosis and Von Recklinghausen's disease, are often associated with mental retardation, seizure disorders, and severe behavior problems. There is not an extensive psychiatric literature, however, on these disorders, and the author's experience is usually to treat the seizure disorder vigorously and intelligently, and to allow the behavior to follow along.

Down's Syndrome

Down's syndrome (DS, Trisomy 21) is the prototypical mental retardation syndrome, with a phenotype that is familiar to people who take no interest whatever in dysmorphology; it is the commonest known genetic cause of mental retardation, unless the fragile X syndrome is more frequent. Considering the efforts that are made to prevent the birth of DS children to older mothers, and the relative ignorance concerning prevention of fragile X, it is only a matter of time. The incidence of DS is about 1 per 1000 live births (1.2/1000), and DS people comprise no fewer than 16% of the mentally retarded population (Fryns et al., 1984b).

It is hardly necessary to reiterate the characteristic dysmorphic features of DS, or its association with disorders of the immune system, the endocrine system, and the cardiovascular system. DS people are mentally retarded, of course, although not every DS person is retarded, and many are only mildly or moderately retarded.

As people, they tend to be sociable, positive in outlook, and affectionate, if sometimes bullheaded. Nevertheless, they may be prone to any of the psychopathological conditions that afflict other people (Gath and Gumley, 1986), and I have consulted on cases of DS patients who were hyperactive, aggressive, or self-injurious. The striking pathopsychological association, however, is with Alzheimer's disease.

DS people are prone to signs of early senescence, with thin hair, dry, wrinkled skin, and cataracts, as well as neuropathic changes, as early as the third decade (Gualtieri, 1989a). In fact, virtually all DS patients develop neuropathic changes in brain tissue characteristic of Alzheimer's disease by the age of 40, although they may not show behavioral or cognitive signs of decline until much later (Lott, 1982; Thase et al., 1984). The diagnosis of dementia in patients with DS may be made on the basis of personality changes or developmental regression on standardized tests. Seizures may be a manifestation of dementia, gait deterioration, sphincteric incontinence, frontal release signs, or serial computer tomography (CT) scans (Lott and Lai, 1982). On the other hand, there may be reversible causes of dementia, like hypothyroidism (Thase, 1982), and depression may mimic the symptoms of dementia or accelerate their onset.

The prevalence of dementia in one prospective study of institutionalized retarded people is 8% at 35 to 49 years, 55% at 50 to 59 years, and 75% at 60 or older. Seizures developed in 84% of the DS patients with dementia, and 20% had parkinsonian features. Brain tissue loss on CT scan was most pronounced in the temporal lobes (Lai and Williams, 1989).

The psychopharmacological treatment of dementia is too broad a subject to discuss in any depth here, but the author prefers aggressive treatment early in the course of the disorder and a relaxed approach when it is far advanced. There is a developing literature of the use of cholinergic treatments, but nothing that can be translated into specific recommendations at this point. There is often something to be gained from a trial of stimulants or amantadine (Erkulwater and Pillai, 1989), or of an antidepressant (Reifler et al., 1989), or of vitamin B_{12} (Lindenbaum et al., 1988), or thiamine (Gibson et al., 1988; Blass et al., 1988). There will probably be some interest in L-deprenyl, nimodipine, and tetrahydroaminoacridine, too. Most of these issues are discussed in the chapter on the Psychopharmacology of Traumatic Brain Injury (Chapter 3).

Rett's Syndrome

Rett's syndrome occurs only in girls, and is characterized by autistic behavior, dementia, apraxia of gait, loss of facial expression, and stereotyped use of the hands. Based on studies in Sweden and Scotland, the prevalence of Rett's syndrome has been estimated to be 1.0 to 1.2 per 15,000 girls (Brase et al., 1989).

The onset is toward the end of the first year of life or early in the second year, after a period of normal development; thereafter it follows a progressive, deteriorating course (Rett, 1966; Hagber et al., 1983). The patient may then stabilize in a severely retarded state that may last for decades. Additional features of the syndrome include loss of functional use of the upper extremities, jerky truncal ataxia, acquired microcephaly, spastic parapareses, vasomotor disturbances of the lower limbs, intermittent hyperventilation, and epilepsy (Hagber et al., 1983).

The pathophysiology of Rett's syndrome has not been worked out. Pathological alterations, depigmentation in the substantia nigra for example, have been found (Hillig, 1985). The only biochemical abnormalities have been reduced levels of metabolites of the biogenic amines norepinephrine, dopamine, and serotonin in cerebrospinal fluid (CSF), and elevated levels of biopterin (Zoghbi et al., 1989).

Some of the clinical elements of Rett's syndrome have been compared to the effects, in laboratory animals, of exogenously administered opiate compounds. In rodents, exogenous opiates lead to a deceleration of brain growth and development; stereotypies, for example, excessive grooming behavior; respiratory depression and apnea; myoclonic jerks and seizures; indifference to pain; nystagmus; decreased REM sleep; and motor incoordination. The CSF of Rett's syndrome patients indicate a significant elevation of beta-endorphin-like immunoreactivity, and improvements in sleep, apnea, and seizure control have been described in Rett's syndrome patients treated with the opiate antagonist Naltrexone (Brase et al., 1989).

If it is true that endorphinergic hyperactivity has a role to play in the pathophysiology of Rett's syndrome, one might hope that early treatment with opiate antagonists might attenuate the development of microcephaly and some of the other characteristics of physical and mental retardation (Brase et al., 1989).

The genetics are not understood either, but the exclusive affliction of females, correlated with findings from pedigree analysis, has suggested a dominant mutation on the X chromosome that results in affected girls and nonviable male hemizygous conceptui (Hagber et al., 1983; Hillig, 1985). However, a hereditary link to the X chromosome has not been established.

Rett's syndrome has been particularly interesting to students of autism, not only because the girls are autistic, but also because the pattern of developmental regression after a period of normal development is often seen in autistic children who do not have Rett's. The stereotyped hand-washing movements of Rett's patients are also familiar to parents of autistic children. It is likely that there is are several degenerative diseases involving brain-stem and subcortical tissues that may cause autism and mental retardation when they arise early in development, or dementia praecox when they develop later, in adolescence.

Williams' Syndrome

This syndrome is a disorder of unknown etiology with characteristic elfin-like facies, vascular disease (e.g., supravalvular aortic stenosis), and infantile hypercalcemia. There is also a distinct neurodevelopmental profile, including mild-to-moderate mental retardation with relative verbal strengths, marked motor and perceptual deficits, and an outgoing personality (Pagon et al., 1987). Hyperactivity and short attention span are the most common behavioral features. The social demeanor of these patients is friendly, loquacious, and socially disinhibited, and their language is described as "cocktail chatter" (MacDonald and Roy, 1988).

The neuropsychological profile is striking, with fluency in language and facility in reading, in contrast to a substantial deficit in visual–motor–perceptual performance. The patients are overly talkative and have no obvious problems with vocabulary or syntax. People may overestimate their intellectual abilities, impressed as they are by their fluency. But they also tend to overuse cliches, and there may be a tangential quality to their language. They may say much more than they mean—their capacity to express may be far in excess of what they are capable of processing.

What all this represents is a developmental variant of fluent aphasia. It is characteristic of Williams' syndrome patients, although it is by no means limited to that group. "Cocktail chatter" is also described in hydrocephalic children.

If the phenomenon were not observed in prepubertal children, one would be inclined to attribute the neuropsychological profile of Williams' syndrome to a relative strength in left hemisphere linguistic processing and a relative weakness in communicative pragmatics in the right hemisphere. Such a formulation would predict a relative weakness in other right-hemisphere-mediated abilities such as visual–motor performance, which is, of course, exactly what is observed in these patients. But there is no evidence beyond the functional to support the idea of a hemispheric deficit in Williams' syndrome. The pragmatics of language are the rules that govern its appropriate use, depending on the situational context (Blumstein, 1981). It is exactly this component of language that is impaired in patients with right hemisphere lesions.

Although Williams' syndrome patients are usually friendly, sociable, and affectionate, there have been cases of autistics with this syndrome (Reiss et al., 1985). It is possible that such cases represent an extreme variant of the dissociation between language processing and pragmatics.

Fragile X Syndrome

Most of us have known people whose chromosomes were fragile, likely to break at the drop of a social slight or an untoward remark. It is reassuring, then, to discover that popular wisdom has been affirmed by genetic science. There is, in fact, a class of people who have a chromosome with a nonstaining gap; it is a hereditable feature (Mendelian codominant) and "fragility" is defined, at least in terms of chromosomes, by the production under certain circumstances of acentric fragments, deleted chromosomes, and multiradial figures (Michels, 1985). The author himself can vouch for a few multiradial figures in his past, and just about everyone has left an acentric fragment behind, somewhere; so the topic is something that anyone should be interested in.

Everyone should, because the discovery a new class of X-linked disorders is no small event. People have always known that there were many more handicapped males than females, and that males are vulnerable to just about everything compared to females. There is nothing like finding a rationale on the X chromosome. It explains so much. But it is tantalizing to think that it may, one day, explain some things that today we have not even thought of as needing an explanation. The march of science is not only to answer the open questions we have not answered; it is also to ask some questions we have not thought to ask.

The fragile X is like that. More than just a poetic name, it is something that has emerged, without sensation, into a world that knew something must be brooding in the realm of selective male affliction (Gualtieri and Hicks, 1985c), but never really knew exactly what that something might be. People were content to think that Down's syndrome was the most common genetic diagnosis in mental retardation. But that never accounted for more than a fraction of cases, and it is usually cited that one-half or two-thirds of mental handicap is undiagnosable. That was not a biological given, or an immutable law; it was simply a recognition of the state of callow ignorance we found ourselves in.

In 1969, Lubs described a "fragile site" on the long arm of the X chromosome in a retarded male (Lubs, 1969). A short time later, the association of a fragile X with severe retardation and marcoorchidism was described by Escalante et al. (1971). The fragile X syndrome was soon established to be by far the most common X-linked cause of mental retardation (Opitz and Sutherland, 1984). With current technology, which may not be as sensitive as some newer techniques, the fragile X syndrome has been found to account for no fewer than 10% of all cases of mental retardation (Rogers and Simensen, 1987). This is one of the most dramatic developments of the generation in medical genetics and neuropsychiatry. It is so important that its full impact has yet to be measured. Its impact will certainly grow as we learn more about the psychological concomitants of the carrier state, and when the test for the fragile site is improved (i.e., linkage analysis) and its price comes down.

The diagnosis of fragile X is established by a special karyotyping technique that will reveal the unstained or fragile sites. The diagnosis should be suspected in males with mild to profound mental retardation who have a family history suggestive of familial retardation, especially with an X-linked pattern and characteristic dysmorphic features, including a long face with a prominent forehead, broad-based large nose, prognathism, and large, abnormally structured ears. Marcoorchidism is probably the most important dysmorphic feature, but it may not be apparent until after puberty. The dysmorphic features are variable, however, so only about 60% of adults males have the classic triad (mental retardation, long face, megalotestes) (Fryns, 1984). Thus, male, mental retardation, and familial neuropsychiatric history is probably sufficient information to warrant a karyotype. The issue of preventive screening is all important (Turner et al., 1986).

Not every male with fragile X is retarded (Daker et al., 1981; Howard-Peebles and Friedman, 1985), although nonretarded males may be hyperactive and learning-disabled (Hagerman et al., 1985). Conversely, not every female carrier is asymptomatic. About 30% of the female carriers have been found to be borderline or mildly retarded, with a high frequency of psychiatric disturbance, especially psychosis and affective disorder (Knoll et al., 1984; Fryns, 1986; Reiss et al., 1986). Fragile X patients may have seizures (41%), dyskinesias (35%), or motor incoordination (59%) (Finelli et al., 1985), but the neuropsychiatric manifestations are more impressive; The males are often hyperactive and they may also be aggressive; autism and self-injurious behavior are not uncommon, and stereotypies are frequent concomitants (Finelli et al., 1985; Fryns et al., 1984a; Gillberg et al., 1985). There is evidence for decline in intellectual performance from childhood to adult life (Lachiewicz et al.,1987), but no mention of dementia or psychological deterioration later on. There were early reports of successful behavioral treatment with folic acid, which made some sense because the fragile marker at the q27 site is demonstrated in a folic-acid-depleted environment, but the encouraging early reports have not been replicated (Gillberg et al., 1986; Hagerman et al., 1986; Rosenblatt et al., 1985).

It remains to be seen to what extent the fragile X Syndrome will influence the diagnosis of children and adults who present, not with mental retardation, but with learning disabilities, hyperactivity, and behavioral and psychiatric disorders. The abnormality is not frequent in the normal population, but it remains to be seen whether it is frequent in neuropsychiatric populations. One wonders how many things like fragile X are out there—etiologies, causes, origins, things that can explain clinical entities in ways that we have never thought to find an explanation.

Disorders of Serotonin Regulation

It is possible to consider neuropsychiatric disorders in terms of their hypothetical neurochemical basis. This is an alternative to the purely phenomenological approach taken by the psychiatrists and the behaviorists. For example, one might think in terms of specific disorders of serotonin regulation.

Serotonergic neurons project from brainstem nuclei in the dorsal raphe to innervate cortical structures in the frontal lobes and subcortical structures in the striatum, hippocampus, and septum (Molliver, 1987). Like the other monoamine neurotransmitters, serotonin seems to exercise a neuromodulatory or a neuroactivating effect on higher systems. Serotonin effects seem to be specifically devoted to the modulation of appetitive or vegetative functions like regulation of the sleep and waking cycle, the expression of mood, and the intake of water and sustenance (Meltzer and Lowy, 1987).

The clinical meaning of such associations to serotonin metabolism has been developed, with some success, in the study of affective disorders (e.g., Van Praag, 1978; Meltzer and Lowy, 1987). On a theoretical level, there seems to be a subcategory of affective illness that is primarily mediated by serotonin systems, and there is a practical benefit to be gained from the administration of a cascade of serotonergic antidepressants, including lithium and L-tryptophan, to some patients with refractory depression (Hale et al., 1987; Blier et al., 1987).

There is also an association, replicated on numerous occasions, between low levels of the serotonin metabolite 5-HIAA, in the CSF of patients who attempt suicide (Virkkunen et al., 1989; Arora and Meltzer, 1989). The connection, however, appears in patients from virtually every diagnostic group, and it does not seem to be a function of a depressive state so much as a tendency to impulsive, aggressive behavior. There is also a well-founded association between low levels of serotonin metabolism and aggressive behavior, exclusive of suicide (Eichelman, 1977; O'Neal et al., 1986).

Serotonin neurotransmission must have a role to play in the genesis or at least the maintenance of obsessive-compulsive disorder (OCD), because the effective treatment usually involves a serotonergic antidepressant like clomipramine or fluoxetine and because augmentation with L-tryptophan and/or lithium may be successful in refractory patients (Insel and Murphy, 1981; Rasmussen, 1984; Zohar et al., 1987). The association is reinforced by studies of serotonin metabolites in OCD patients (Zohar et al., 1987).

Anorexia and bulimia nervosa are two other disorders that have also been linked to serotonin and that may be treated successfully with the serotonergic antidepressants (Herzog and Copeland, 1985; Goldbloom et al., 1989).

All these clinical examples are the encouraging results of thinking that is based on the established physiology and anatomy of serotonin neurotransmission pathways. One develops hypotheses on the basis of serotonergic lesions in laboratory preparations. These are tested by examining markers of serotonin metabolism in patient groups, and then by evaluating the effects of serotonergic drugs. The value of the approach can be measured in the dramatic improvement in pharmacological treatment of refractory affective disorders, OCD, disorders of aggression, and sleep disorders. Serotonergic drugs like clomipramine, fluoxetine, trazodone, L-tryptophan, propanalol (Jefferson, 1974; Yudofsky et al., 1981) and lithium (Craft et al., 1987) have become the mainstays of modern psychopharmacology.

In fact, the only relative failure in this rich field of investigation has been the study of serotonin metabolism in autism (e.g., Hanley et al., 1977; Minderaa et al., 1989), which seems to have led nowhere. But that is the exception that proves the rule. The rationale for the study of serotonin metabolism in depression, aggression, suicide, and eating disorders is based on an understanding of what serotonin systems do, and a credible connection between that function and the disorder in question; for example, the modulation of affective expression, or the modulation of appetitive function, or the promotion of sleep. In autism, there has never been such a rationale. So, it is not surprising that the work has not been fruitful, that the results of metabolic studies have not been consistent, and that the results of treatment with antiserotonergic drugs has been a relative failure.

Self-Injurious Behavior

There are, however, developmental disorders that may well be linked to abnormalities of serotonin neurotransmission. The role of serotonin in modulating aggressive behavior leads one, naturally, to the consideration of developmental syndromes that are characterized by high rates of self-injurious behavior. We shall discuss the serotonergic hypothesis of Cornelia de Lange syndrome, for example, in an ensuing chapter (Chapter 8). In the Lesch–Nyhan syndrome, also, there is evidence for decreased serotonin turnover in the CNS (Castells et al., 1979; Silverstein et al., 1985; see Chapter 7, this volume). What is common to patients with these disorders, in addition to the self-injurious behavior (SIB), is a degree of affective instability that is manifest clinically as dysphoria, irritability, emotional lability, and hyper-reactivity to environmental stimuli.

The rationale for serotonergic treatment of developmentally handicapped people with SIB is sound, but untested. There is one obscure report of an individual with Cornelia de Lange syndrome and SIB who had low levels of whole blood Serotonin and responded well to the combination of L-tryptophan and trazodone (O'Neal et al., 1986). We have studied another individual with severe SIB whose problems were eliminated with combined treatment with L-tryptophan and fluoxetine.

One of our SIB patients, and one of the most difficult, was a profoundly retarded 4-year-old white boy with Pierre-Robin syndrome who had a 3-year history of sleep disturbance, up all night, with progressive SIB, head-banging, and head- slapping. He lived at home, and although he had good programming during school hours, his parents were required to spend the rest of the waking hours, and most of the (non)sleeping hours attending to the child, restraining him to prevent severe self-injury. They were prepared to institutionalize the child, even though that likely meant a lifetime of physical restraint and neuroleptic drugs. In fact, he had previously been treated with neuroleptics to no good effect.

We tracked his disorder with the SIBQ, as well as by counting the number of self-directed slaps and the number of times he had to be put into physical restraints. Over 3 weeks of baseline, he was put in restraints 71 times a week. After treatment was begun with L-tryptophan (2 g/day) and fluoxetine (20 mg/day), and for the next 90 days, restraints were applied only 17 times a week, and over the next period of 132 days, he was not in restraints at all. When an attempt was made to reverse the protocol, and the L-tryptophan was discontinued, the child became increasingly irritable and dysphoric, and the number of restraints increased to 14 per week. When the L-tryptophan was again added to the fluoxetine, the number went back down to 6 per week during 60 days of follow-up. For ratings of SIB on the SIBQ, he scored 8.5 on drug-free baseline, 4.4 after treatment was initiated, 1.8 during the 132-day optimal period, up to 2.1 when the L-tryptophan was withdrawn, and back down to 1.6 after it was begun again.

The combination of L-tryptophan and fluoxetine seemed to exert the same beneficial effect that O'Neal et al. (1986) noted in a retarded, aggressive, and self-injurious individual on L-tryptophan and trazodone. It would appear that serotonergic treatment may hold a degree of promise for self-injurious patients.

Phenylketonuria

Phenylketonuria (PKU) is a genetic deficiency of the phenylalanine hydroxylase, and the major metabolic consequence is hyperphenylalaninemia. There are several phenotypes, defined in terms of different components of the phenylalanine hydroxylating system, and at least one of the phenotypes is associated with a malignant neurological course, even in the face of dietary restriction of phenylalanine-containing foods. However, dietary restriction has been largely successful in reducing the occurrence of mental retardation as a consequence of PKU, and admission of PKU patients to mental retardation facilities has declined dramatically since the introduction, more than 20 years ago, of dietary treatment (Scriver and Clow, 1980).

Although it is clear that hyperphenylalaninemia is a central event, it is by no means clear precisely what the biochemical basis is for the mental retardation and behavioral abnormalities of PKU patients. The possibilities include perturbation of energy metabolism, amino acid transport, and cellular amino acid pools, synthesis of macromolecules, and synthesis of neurotransmitters (Scriver and Clow, 1980). Plasma serotonin, norepinephrine, and epinephrine concentrations are reduced in PKU, and there are reduced concentrations of dopamine, norepinephrine, epinephrine, serotonin, and their metabolites in the brain (Lasala and Coscia, 1979). In "malignant" PKU, caused by a deficiency in tetrahydrobiopterin, there is impairment of the tyrosine and tryptophan hydroxylases, and the condition is characterized by deficiency of catecholamines and serotonin in the central and peripheral nervous systems (Kapatos and Kaufman, 1981). In PKU, there may be alterations in serotonin metabolism by virtue of competition between phenylalanine and tryptophan for uptake into neurons (Wortman and Fernstrom, 1975). Even in treated PKU with good metabolic control, there may be a chronic inhibition of 5-hydroxy tryptophol synthesis (Giovannini et al., 1988).

It may be inaccurate to define PKU as a primary disorder of serotonin metabolism, but that is an important component of the neurochemistry of the disorder, and it may have a bearing on some of its behavioral manifestations. Laboratory animals with PKU have been compared to low-serotonin preparations; they are anxious, "in a state of general preparedness" (Chamoye, 1984). Chronic dietary administration of phenylalanine to monkeys produces lethargy, irritability, and diminished reactivity in a normal environment, but abnormally heightened levels of activity in response to novelty or to stress (Chamoye, 1984).

The major controversy over treatment of PKU has centered around the wisdom of terminating the phenylalanine-free diet at some point in adult life. The results of studies on dietary termination have been conflicting, especially with respect to deterioration of intellectual function, and no uniform policy has come of this research. Workers who have identified decrements in cognitive performance after termination have suggested a chronic metabolic encephalopathy, possibly related to phenylalanine interference with neurotransmitter synthesis (Seashore et al., 1985).

Behavioral and emotional disturbance and overt psychiatric disorders are known to be associated with PKU, even when the disorder is treated successfully and mental retardation does not occur (Graham and Rutter, 1968). PKU children have been described as impulsive, irritable, immature, and aggressive, and studies have documented poor interpersonal relations, and mood and behavior problems (Realmuto et al., 1986). The diverse and nonspecific nature of these difficulties may speak to the broad band of neurotransmitter abnormalities that have been associated with hyperphenylalaninemia.

There have been conflicting results, too, from clinical trials that have attempted to alleviate these behavioral symptoms by restricting dietary phenylalanine. This also must be expected, given the several phenotypes of PKU. Nevertheless, it is not inappropriate to attempt a trial of dietary treatment for selected cases, or even to consider a trial of L-tryptophan, L-dopa, and a dopa decarboxylase inhibitor.

Prader–Willi Syndrome

Because serotonergic neurons are known to modulate appetitive behavior, there has been interest in applying treatment with drugs that enhance serotonin neurotransmission to the treatment of eating disorders like anorexia and bulimia nervosa (Mitchell and Groat, 1984; Pope et al., 1988). The Prader–Willi syndrome (PWS) is an extraordinary disorder of appetitive instability that may also be amenable to a serotonin solution.

The PWS was described in 1956 by Prader et al. as a syndrome of mental retardation, short stature, obesity, hypogonadism, and muscular hypotonia. More than 200 cases have been reported since; the estimated incidence is between 1 in 5,000 and 1 in 10,000 (Crnic et al., 1980) or alternatively 1 in 25,000 (Bray et al., 1983). It is one of the five most common syndromes seen in birth defect clinics, but is only one-fifth to one-tenth as common as Down's syndrome (Holm and Pipes, 1976).

Several specific chromosomal abnormalities have been described in association with PWS (Goh et al., 1984), although no genetic defect that is central to the disorder, or unique or pathognomonic to PWS, has been identified. Etiology and pathophysiology are unknown, although virtually all the abnormalities observed in PWS point to a disturbance in the development and function of the midline structures of the brain, including the thalamus and the hypothalamus (Gualtieri, 1989a).

Although most PWS people are mentally retarded (IQs about 40 or 50), it appears that about 40% are not retarded at all. They have typical facies: a narrow bifrontal diameter, almond-shaped eyes, and a triangular mouth, features that may be lost after they gain weight. It has been observed that there is a decrement in cognitive development at about the same time that PWS begin to engage in hyperphagia. It has even been suggested that PWS children whose hyperphagia is controlled at an early age may continue to develop intellectually (Crnic et al., 1980).

These children begin to gain weight during the preschool years, after an infant period with failure to thrive; thereafter there is a rapid increase to morbid obesity if it is not controlled. In fact, hyperphagia is the most compelling behavioral symptom of the PWS, and it may be severe, bizarre, and life-threatening. Eating behaviors include an insatiable appetite, stealing, foraging, and gorging. PWS sufferers try to consume enormous amounts of food with no concern for taste or quality: garbage, dog food, frozen bread, and other unappetizing things. They may be devious to the level of minor genius in their attempts to get at food, and they may be aggressive or prone to tantrums when their attempts are thwarted. They are not bulimic, because they do not eat in binges, and there is no induced vomiting.

In fact, it may be that PWS people cannot vomit. Nor is what they do pica, because they confine their intake to recognized if unappetizing foodstuffs.

The driving force behind the obesity of people with PWS is hyperphagia and increased caloric intake. Measures of fat mobilization have been found to be normal (Bier et al., 1977). Glucose tolerance is normal and so is the growth hormone response to insulin-induced hypoglycemia (compared to obese controls). The thyrotropin-releasing hormone (TRH) response to thyroid-stimulating hormone (TSH) is elevated, and because hypogonadism is a defining characteristic of PWS it should be no surprise that the response to luteinizing hormone-releasing hormone (LHRH) is absent (Bray et al., 1983). The activity level of PWS children is not invariably reduced (Nardella et al., 1983). In the absence, then, of any peripheral mechanism, or any clearly defined endocrinopathy aside from luteinizing hormone, one may surmise that a hypothalamic mechanism is responsible for the hyperphagia and its attendant morbidity.

The neuropharmacology of eating behavior is complex, and all the monoamine neurotransmitters appear to be implicated, although which, or which complex of neurochemical effects, is most salient to PWS remains to be seen. Through alpha-adrenergic receptors in the paraventricular nucleus of the hypothalamus, norepinephrine can be a powerful inducer of eating behavior in rats (Herzog and Copeland, 1985; Leibowitz, 1984). Lesions of ascending dopaminergic pathways have been associated with aphagia in laboratory animals (Ljungberg and Ungerstedt, 1976); dopamine agonists are known to produce anorexia (Evans and Eikelbloom, 1987), and dopamine antagonist drugs, like the neuroleptics, are known to lead to obesity, especially in mentally retarded people. Manipulations that increase serotonin synthesis are known to reduce appetite (Herzog and Copeland, 1985), and the serotonergic antidepressant fluoxetine has impressive effects in reducing appetite and weight (Fuller and Wong, 1989).

The serotonin antagonist fenfluramine has been noted to reduce hyperphagia in one PWS patient, but L-tryptophan, in doses as high as 15 g/day, had no effect on eating behavior in a larger group (Bray et al., 1983). We have actually had success with one mildly retarded gentleman with PWS whose weight and hyperphagia had been stabilized behaviorally, but who still was given to episodes of angry aggression. He improved, behaviorally, on L-tryptophan at 4 g/day.

It would seem natural to explore the possibility that hyperphagia in PWS would respond to treatment with serotonergic drugs, perhaps with L-tryptophan or fluoxetine or perhaps with the cascade of serotonergic drugs that is described in the SIB chapter of this volume (Chapter 7), and that has already been used successfully for the treatment of refractory affective disorder (Hale et al., 1987) and obsessive-compulsive disorder (Rasmussen, 1984).

The only systematic trials of pharmacotherapy for PWS are attempts to explore the opiate hypothesis of hyperphagia. The endogenous system is known to exercise a stimulatory effect on eating behavior in lower animals (Morley, 1980), and naloxone, an opiate antagonist, is known to suppress eating behavior induced in animals by stress or by benzodiazepines (Morley and Levine, 1980; Stapleton et al., 1979). Naloxone has also been found to reduce daylong caloric intake in obese subjects (Wolkowitz et al., 1985). Unfortunately, trials of opiate antagonists in PWS subjects have not been especially convincing (Kyriakides et al., 1980). The current treatment for PWS is entirely behavioral (Gualtieri, 1989a).

Movement Disorders

Neuropsychiatric approaches to the movement disorders have traditionally concentrated on dopamine and acetylcholine neurotransmission, and most therapeutic interventions are oriented toward drugs that affect those systems. There are indications that serotonergic compounds may be pertinent.

It is known that hindbrain serotonin systems project to the caudate nucleus and to the substantia nigra, and that serotonin neurotransmission may modulate dopamine activity (Bunney and DeReimer, 1982). Serotonin neurons are known to control or to modulate brainstem and spinal motor neurons (Jacobs et al., 1982). Stress-induced stereotypies in the rat may be reduced by drugs that increase serotonin release (Knott and Hutson, 1982). It appears that serotonergic systems may mitigate the activity of dopaminergic systems.

There also seems to be a reciprocal interaction between serotonin cell bodies in the midbrain raphe and norepinephrine cell bodies in the locus coeruleus of the pons. Serotonin axons appear to regulate beta-adrenergic receptors in brain (Stockmeier et al., 1985).

This reciprocal relationship with dopaminergic and noradrenergic neurotransmission systems is probably responsible for some of the clinical effects of serotonergic drugs on the expression of abnormal movements. For example, L-tryptophan has been reported successful in the clinical management of restless legs syndrome (Sandyk, 1985). It has also been reported to suppress motor and phonic tics induced by stimulants (Chandler et al., 1989). On the other hand, L-tryptophan has not been notably effective in the treatment of tardive dyskinesia (Prange et al., 1973).

The serotonergic antidepressant fluoxetine has been reported to aggravate extrapyramidal symptoms in psychiatric patients, and other serotonin reuptake inhibitors have led to motor decompensation in parkinsonian patients (Bouchard et al., 1989; Tate, 1989; Brod, 1989).

Myoclonic jerks, especially nocturnal myoclonus, may be side effects of tricyclic antidepressant therapy, especially with serotonergic antidepressants; myoclonus may occur with L-tryptophan alone or in combination with an monoamine oxidase (MAO) inhibitor (Levy et al., 1985). In experimental preparations, application of serotonin may initiate myoclonic seizures after serotonergic neurons are lesioned (Stewart et al., 1976).

But in neuropharmacology, one must grow accustomed to conflicting results and seemingly contradictory drug actions (Munsat, 1977). The combination of serotonin and carbidopa has been shown to reduce myoclonus in patients with anoxic or other brain damage (Van Woert et al., 1977) and the anticonvulsant effects of trimethadione have been attributed to increased brain levels of serotonin (Diaz, 1974).

CHAPTER 7

Self-Injurious Behavior

Self-injurious behavior (SIB) is an extraordinary affliction of human behavior. SIB refers to repetitive acts of physical violence directed against oneself. It occurs most commonly in mentally retarded people, about 8% to 14% of those who reside in institutions (Schroeder et al., 1980), and probably an equal number of retarded people who live in community-based facilities (Phillips, 1988).

Although most cases of SIB occur in people who are mentally retarded, especially the severely retarded, it is not by any means restricted to retarded people. It occurs, in the form of head-banging, as a developmental variant in normal infants, but it is rarely so severe that it leads to tissue damage (Hoder and Cohen, 1983). It is not uncommon in the chronically mentally ill, especially schizophrenics and people with the "borderline" personality disorder, although it is more likely to be paroxysmal and self-mutilatory in those patients (Favazza, 1987). It may also have occurred as a ritual experience in certain primitive peoples (Favazza, 1987), and it has been said to occur on occasion in present-day torture victims.

Caged animals will sometimes engage in self-mutilation; for example, psittacine birds will pluck their chest feathers and even gouge their pectoral muscles if they are isolated and unhappy. Rhinos will grind their noses against a wall, repetitively, compulsively, even to the point of grinding their horn down to a mere nub.

So, SIB is not a rare occurrence, by any means, but it is an extraordinary event, whenever it occurs. It is one of those behaviors that affects caregivers as much as patients, or even more. It is not only the pain, the disfigurement, and the horror it conveys; it is the vexing question, why should such a thing happen at all? What psychology can possibly explain it?

It was not that question that brought the author to his clinical interest in SIB. His introduction to the problem was with a group of behaviorists, led by Steve Schroeder, who cared less for the underlying psychology of the phenomenon, and more for its ecology and for devising treatment strategies to correct the problem. This was the SIB Project at the Murdoch Center, a mental retardation center in North Carolina. It was a very important program, and Schroeder, Mulick, and

Parts of this chapter appeared in substantially modified form in *Psychopharmacology Bulletin* 25: 358-363 and 25: 364-371, 1989.

Rojahn were amazingly effective at reducing, even eliminating, the problem of SIB, at least for a while.

After the special SIB program was terminated, most of the clients did well, at least for a period of time, but over the years many of them reverted to their old bad habits. The purely behavioral interventions designed to correct the problem were so expensive that they could not be sustained. So the clients spent their days in restraints or on massive doses of sedating drugs.

Many of the patients who had participated in the SIB Project came to the author's attention again during a series of tardive dyskinesia (TD) studies at the Murdoch Center when they were systematically withdrawn from neuroleptic drugs. Some patients relapsed after the drugs were taken away; it was not a good idea to return to neuroleptics, however, because the incidence of TD was so high, and the drugs had never worked very well. The reader is aware, of course, that SIB is the frequent occasion of pharmacotherapy in retarded people, but the efficacy of drug treatment has never been established. There are only anecdotal data and single case studies to support treatment with neuroleptic drugs, lithium, or opiate antagonists, antidepressants, or anything else (Singh and Millichamp, 1985).

In fact, SIB has not been the focus of extensive pharmacological research in humans. The only established treatments have been the various behavioral interventions, like contingent restraint, differential reinforcement, and overcorrection (Singh, 1981). These require an extraordinary investment in time and professional effort, and good behaviorists who can mount such efforts are few in number. Such intensive treatments are available only to a minority of people with SIB. Restraint with helmets, handcuffs, or leather straps represents the usual "treatment" for most people with SIB.

In 1984, we set about the task of developing a rational pharmacotherapy for SIB. It began with the assumption that SIB was a unitary disorder; that although there might be a wide range of different origins to the problem in any particular individual, there must be a common final pathway for all self-injurious patients, a neurochemical endpoint, a single channel that mediated the behavioral stereotype. In retrospect, it was an idea that was hopelessly naive. But like most wrong ideas, it had a perfectly reasonable argument behind it, and it seemed like a good idea at the time.

The origin of the idea lay with a singular anomaly of human behavior, the Lesch–Nyhan syndrome (LNS), an SIB syndrome that is associated with a grotesque form of compulsive mutilation (self-mutilatory behavior, SMB). The fact that the LNS has been associated with a very specific biochemical derangement suggested that pharmacological correction of an underlying deficit was not an unreasonable hope (Lloyd, et al., 1981). The fact, too, that certain drugs are known to cause SMB in experimental animals, and the fact that the pattern of drug effects to evoke SIB is consistent with the neurochemical basis of the LNS, also spoke to a neuropharmacological basis to the behavior that could be reversed or at least attenuated. If there were a neuropharmacological basis to SIB in the LNS, there might be a pharmacological treatment. If the treatment were effective for one SIB syndrome, perhaps it would work for others.

LNS is a prototype of SIB. LNS children engage in severe self-mutilation—they bite themselves—and they begin doing so in the first or second year of life (Lesch and Nyhan, 1964). They also have choreoathetoid movements and dystonia, and most of them, but by no means all, are mentally retarded. LNS is an inborn error of purine metabolism, and the specific biochemical defect is an inherited deficiency of the purine salvage enzyme, hypoxanthine-guanine-phosphoribosyl transferase (HGPRT), resulting in massive overproduction of uric acid (Lesch and Nyhan, 1964; Wilson, 1983).

In normal human beings, HGPRT activity is highest in brain tissue and it is particularly high in the basal ganglia. In brain tissue from LNS patients, the activity of this enzyme is markedly reduced or absent (Seegmiller et al., 1967). No specific neuropathological changes have been identified in postmortem tissue, and the nature of neuropathic "lesion" in LNS is unknown. However, a variety of neurotransmitter abnormalities have been reported in Lesch–Nyhan patients. These include abnormal adrenergic function peripherally and decreased serotonin turnover in the central nervous system (CNS). Castells et al. (1979) reported a decrease in dopamine and serotonin metabolites in cerebrospinal fluid (CSF) in a single patient. Lloyd et al. (1981) reported significant regional decreases in dopamine metabolites in three postmortem Lesch–Nyhan brains. Decreased levels of CSF homovanillic acid (HVA) and 5-HIAA were reported in four LNS patients, with a rapid decline in the first 3 years of life (Silverstein et al., 1985).

The amazing thing about the LNS is the predictable association of SMB with a specific biochemical deficit. This naturally led to research in experimental animals (rats and mice) to reproduce elements of the LNS and thus to clarify the neurochemical substrate of the behavior abnormality. SMB has been induced in experimental animals by administration of pharmacological compounds that influence monoaminergic systems, especially dopamine. These include caffeine (Minana et al., 1984), amphetamine (Mueller 1982), pemoline (Mueller and Nyhan, 1982), and clonidine (Mueller and Nyhan, 1983).

In 1984, Breese and his associates developed a model of SMB (Breese et al., 1984) that seemed especially promising. Neonatal treatment with 6-OHDA is known to selectively destroy dopamine-containing fibers in the rat. When these animals are treated as adults with L-dopa, severe SMB is observed. The effect is dose dependent, and is blocked by the D1-dopamine blocker *cis*-flupenthixol but not by the D2-dopamine antagonist haloperidol. This suggested to Breese that a D1-dopamine receptor supersensitivity state could be the pharmacological basis of SMB in the neonatal 6-OHDA-treated rat (Breese et al., 1984).

Monkeys with ventromedial tegmental lesions of the brain stem applied when they were very young (2–3 years) have also been observed to develop SMB when they are challenged, as adults, with dopamine-agonist drugs (Goldstein et al., 1985b). This, too, has been attributed to sensitivity at the D1-dopamine receptor. For example, when the monkeys with tegmental lesions were treated with D1-dopamine blockers (fluphenazine, SCH 23390), the SMB was eliminated (Goldstein et al., l985a).

The same group also reported success in controlling SIB in a 20-month-old LNS patient with the D1 blocker fluphenazine (FPZ). They hypothesized a relationship between the specific enzyme deficit in LNS and dopamine receptor supersensitivity, and this was related to the modulating effect of guanosine triphosphate on the activity state of dopaminergic receptors (Goldstein et al., 1985b).

The D1-dopamine hypothesis conveyed the potential of a rational pharmacotherapy for SIB. In fact, it was one of the only credible theories of SIB. The major competing theory—the opiate hypothesis, which we shall discuss further on—was being examined quite vigorously by Barbara Hermann's research group in Washington. It made sense, then, to examine the D1-dopamine hypothesis in North Carolina.

The first effort was a small pilot study of the mixed D1/D2-dopamine blocker FPZ in six of the most severely self-injurious patients, who had been refractory to previous treatments. The second effort was a placebo-controlled trial of FPZ in nine more SIB patients. The results of these two preliminary studies have been described in Gualtieri and Schroeder (1989), Gualtieri (1989b), and Gualtieri (in press).

The Pharmacotherapy of SIB

LNS is a rare disorder, and the vast majority of SIB patients are not LNS. Nevertheless, the D1-dopamine model of SMB in LNS is interesting to clinicians, not because they see many LNS patients—even specialists see very few—but because the D1-dopamine supersensitivity model could represent a common final pathway.

The neuroleptic FPZ antagonizes both D1- and D2-dopamine receptors (Seeman, 1981), but is the most potent D1-dopamine blocker that is commercially available in the United States. In fact, there is no pure D1-dopamine blocker available for human use anywhere in the world at this time. Cis-flupenthixol and clozapine may be stronger D1-dopamine blockers than FPZ, but they were not available in this country (Titeler, 1983; Anderson and Nielsen, 1976) at the time.

Fluphenazine, then, is added to a long list of neurotropic drugs that have been tried in patients with SIB. The pharmacotherapy of SIB has been reviewed (Singh and Millichamp, 1985; Farber, 1986). In fact, there are probably more review papers on the subject than papers describing successful treatment trials. Specific medications attempted in reasonably well-conducted trials include:

> Naloxone and naltrexone (Beckwith et al., 1986; Richardson and Zaleski, 1983)
> Neuroleptics (D2 blockers) (Mesulam, 1986; Mikkelson, 1986)
> Neuroleptics (D1/D2 blockers) (Gualtieri et al., 1989)
> Lithium (Sovner and Hurley, 1981)
> Tricyclic antidepressants (Hardy 1983)
> 5-Hydroxytryptamine (Mizuno and Yugari, 1975)
> Trazodone and Tryptophan (O'Neal et al., 1986)
> Beta blockers (Ratey et al., 1986)
> L-dopa (Nyhan et al., 1980)

The list is not necessarily exhaustive, but it is long enough to make a point: There is no successful pharmacotherapy for SIB. The most recent treatment trials, with opiate antagonists for example, have been only partially successful (Herman et al., 1987). Only some patients appear to respond; many patients respond only to a degree, but are still self-injurious, and none of the reports have described long-term follow-up.

Testing the D1 Model

A decision having been made to pursue clinical trials of FPZ, it was necessary to develop an appropriate method. It was necessary to sidestep many of the conventions that are current in psychopharmacology (e.g., Sprague and Werry, 1971). If the purpose of the research were simply to test the D1 hypothesis, one would design a controlled study to compare the effects of FPZ to the effects of a drug like haloperidol, a relatively pure D2-dopamine receptor antagonist. But there were competing considerations:

One, if the drug had any merit at all, its value should be tested immediately. Because FPZ is not an experimental drug, and because neuroleptic treatment is quite common in self-injurious individuals, there was really no obstacle to immediately examining its effects in the context of clinical treatment.

Two, it was impossible to treat self-injurious people in any drug protocol that would compromise the treatment programs that were already in existence. Considering the enormous investment of staff time to care for such individuals, it would superimpose on the staff additional chores of a controlled study; it was hardly ethical to do so on behalf of a mere hypothesis, and one that had virtually no support from clinical trials in human beings.

Three, the first hypothesis to test was not the D1-dopamine hypothesis, but the more fundamental hypothesis, that SIB is a unitary disorder. After all, if the clinical sample is not sufficiently homogeneous, no amount of experimental rigor can compensate for that inherent weakness.

And four, it was more important to appraise the success of treatment over the long term. Other treatments, like L-hydroxytryptamine, have been found to work well, too, for a short time, but not over the long term. One would be ill advised to recommend treatment with a drug as troublesome as FPZ on the basis of a short-term study. It is possible to blind a longitudinal study, but it is extremely expensive to do so.

Finally, there is the penicillin effect. We were interested in penicillin: that is, a drug that would stop the problem of SIB, when no other drug had previously been effective; a drug that would give more than a statistically significant result (e.g., "episodes of head-banging reduced by 50%, one-tailed test, $p<.05$), but rather, a drug that would eliminate the problem altogether. If FPZ were such a drug, and if the effect were sustained, it should be readily apparent. There are times when one can trust one's eyes.

To begin, therefore, we selected six severely self-injurious patients whom we had followed for a long time at the Caswell Center and at the Neuropsychiatry Clinic. They have been described in greater detail by Gualtieri (in press). They were all drug free, but that was because they had been treated before with a series of psychoactive drugs, including the neuroleptics, with no success at all. These were people whose self-injurious behavior had been sustained over many years. They were in restraints virtually all the time, or they required one-on-one staff attention. Two were blind from head punching or eye-gouging, and all had significant tissue damage.

The initial design was A-B-A-B, which was our usual method for assessing psychoactive drug effects at the Center. Each condition was intended to last for several months.

Five of the six patients responded dramatically to treatment with low doses of FPZ: from 2 to 8 mg/day. Higher doses tended to cause akathisia, with an attendant return of the SIB. One patient, who had been in restraints for no fewer than 32 years, was able to spend more than 90% of his waking hours out of restraints. In the other four, the results were equally impressive (Gualtieri, in press).

The effects were sustained during 16 to 24 (mean, 21.4) months of follow-up, except in one case, an unfortunate young man who had blinded himself from head-punching. He developed tardive akathisia after 16 months on FPZ, and there was no way to recover the original beneficial effects. Now he spends most of his day in restraints, as he did before the medication began.

The success of the treatment, however, led us to abandon the original design. In cases like this, it was impossible to withdraw a medication that was so clearly effective. So, the A-B-A-B design was set aside. (It would not be the last time that the demands of a controlled trial would be rejected in the face of a seemingly effective treatment of a dread disorder. The same has been done now, many times, about the treatment of AIDS.)

There was a second series of nine severely self-injurious, retarded people treated with FPZ with the introduction of at least a degree of control, a placebo baseline of variable length before the drug was introduced under double-blind conditions. In this group, there were six responders. The beneficial effects of the drug were again seen at very low doses, and were sustained over a follow-up period that lasted for 8 to 23 months (mean, 15.3) (Gualtieri and Schroeder, 1989). There was only one dropout for failed response, after 6 months.

From the total group of 15 patients who were evaluated in these clinical trials, therefore, 4 subjects were nonresponders and 11 showed a very favorable response. One of the responders failed after 6 months, and another after 16 months. The others have shown no diminution of response over time. Because the doses were low, sedation was not a problem, and indeed the responders were more alert and attentive when they were on the drug. The only problem with treatment was the occurrence of extrapyramidal side effects ($N = 4$), especially akathisia ($N = 3$). The risk of tardive akathisia, of course, is something that looms over all patients who continue on the drug.

The D1-dopamine receptor antagonist FPZ was effective, then, in at least 9 of

16 retarded people who had severe self-injurious behavior. They had not responded to other neuroleptics. Their baseline rates of SIB had been high for months of drug-free baseline, and there was no indication of positive effect during a placebo-controlled baseline period. The favorable effects of the drug were sustained over a prolonged follow-up.

Higher doses of FPZ were not helpful. In most cases, higher doses were accompanied by symptoms of akathisia that actually made the SIB much worse, after an initial favorable response. In four cases, the patient was classified as a "low-dose responder" because titrating the FPZ dose downward led to significant improvement, compared to baseline, placebo, and high-dose results.

Because FPZ is a dopamine antagonist at both the D1 and the D2 receptors, one cannot really distinguish the actual site of drug action in a clinical trial like this. Therapeutic response to FPZ in SIB may be a D1-dopamine effect, a D2 effect, a combined effect of blocking both receptors, or the result of some other unknown action of the drug. There is no direct measure to address this question, short of positron emission tomography with appropriately labeled ligands, but there are indirect measures of dopamine receptor activity. Extrapyramidal reactions and neuroleptic-induced hyperprolactinemia are believed to be the consequence of D2-dopamine antagonists in the corpus striatum and the hypothalamus, respectively.

Prolactin response to neuroleptics is believed to be mediated by the D2 receptor, and D1-dopamine receptor blockade is reported not to alter prolactin secretion at all (Ioria et al., 1983). We measured prolactin levels while patients were on optimal therapeutic doses of FPZ, and as one might expect, most of the subjects had prolactin levels that were higher than normal baseline. (Assume, for the moment, that the normal baseline prolactin also is "normal" for self-injurious patients.) However, 2 of the eleven responders had morning venous prolactins less than 10; that is, no neuroleptic-induced elevation at all. This suggests that a therapeutic response to FPZ occurred in at least 2 patients at a drug dose that did not yield a significant degree of D2-dopamine receptor blockade. Neither of these patients experienced extrapyramidal side effects to FPZ, another indicator of D2-dopamine receptor antagonism. It appeared, therefore, that D2-dopamine receptor antagonism is not essential to the therapeutic effects of FPZ in SIB. Dopamine receptor blockade at the D1 receptor may therefore be the mechanism behind the therapeutic success of FPZ.

The Differential Diagnosis of SIB

The FPZ trials offered some degree of support to the D1 dopamine hypothesis of self-injurious behavior. But they did not really address the question of whether SIB was, in fact, a unitary disorder.

It is possible that supersensitivity at the D1 receptor is a final common pathway for many cases of SIB. But it is not likely that there is a common neurochemical mediator to all cases of SIB. The SIB that is induced in laboratory animals in the D1 paradigm is compulsive, continuous, and self-mutilatory. Self-biting is a key feature, just as it is in the Lesch–Nyhan syndrome (LNS). It is clear, however, that the manifestations of SIB in retarded people are not always like that. In fact, self-mutilation and compulsive SIB are unusual manifestations of the problem.

The topography of SIB is wide ranging. It includes head-banging, self-hitting, eye-gouging, and self-scratching, -pinching, -rubbing, digging into orifices, pulling hair, throwing oneself down, etc. The occurrence is also diverse. It may be compulsive and continuous, or it may be intermittent, occurring in cycles, in patches, or in isolated explosions. The ambience is like that of stereotypy. It may occur in circumstances of isolation, when it seems to be like a form of self-stimulation, or it may occur in circumstances of stress, when it seems to be a form of tension reduction. There are times when it appears to have operant properties, when it seems to be a way to get attention or to communicate displeasure or pain.

The etiology is also diverse. It may be associated with specific mental retardation syndromes, like the LNS or the Cornelia de Lange syndrome, in which SIB is a typical event, or with mental retardation syndromes like Down's, in which it is an unusual event, or it may be associated with the nonspecific encephalopathies. Its strongest neuropsychiatric correlates are epilepsy on the one hand and aggressive behavior on the other. SIB may occur in very young children, and subside as the years go by, or it may continue into adult life, or it may arise for the first time in adolescence.

Now it is possible that every such case must channel its outcome through the D1 dopamine receptor, but it is not very likely. It is possible that every case of SIB will respond favorably to D1 blockers, especially when some good ones come along. But is does not seem likely, to the author at least, and one must wonder whether any new series will match the extraordinary results of our FPZ trials when two-thirds of the cases did very well indeed.

There is probably a great deal more to the problem of SIB than behavioral definition. One should prefer, instead, to develop a system for the differential diagnosis of SIB. It is possible, for example, to understand at least some cases within the framework of existing neuropsychiatric paradigms and to treat them accordingly. It is also possible to take the 'idiopathic' cases of SIB, who are not diagnosable in any such framework, and to develop alternative neurochemical hypotheses about their origin, their pathophysiology, and their appropriate treatment. The first group should be treated conventionally. The second group should be candidates for experimental treatments that use novel neuropharmacological models to advance experimental treatments.

Now, one may make a strong case for the value of a neuropsychiatric differential diagnosis, but it is important to remember that the method of differential diagnosis cannot be applied to a patient in a confused and unstable system. It is not possible to attribute structure and pattern to a behavioral disorder that arises in the context of isolation, frustration, and dismay. A patient whose life is spent in such circumstances may only show a random and meaningless pattern of behavior, confronted as he is by developmentally inappropriate expectations, by contingencies and consequences administered fitfully and unpredictably. Before one can posit some order to a behavior like SIB, one must be assured that fundamental programmatic rules are addressed.

It is not necessary to elaborate on what comprises a humane environment, a developmentally appropriate program, or an effective behavior management system. It is necessary to iterate, however, that to the degree such elements are absent from a patient's life, to that degree will the process of medical diagnosis and treatment be weak and ineffective. To the degree one can ensure that these elements are operative, then medical diagnosis and treatment can be a cogent force.

The first element of the differential diagnosis, then, is to ensure an appropriate developmental and behavioral program, administered by competent and humane professionals. Within this context one is advised to collect baseline data on the occurrence of SIB and of related behavior problems, using specific targets like the number of self-injurious outbursts, or time in or time out of restraints, as well as a more global measure of the patient's clinical condition, such as the Self Injurious Behavior Questionnaire (SIBQ) (Gualtieri, 1989b). As baseline data accumulate, the diagnostic process may unfold.

After the patient is followed for a period of time in a well-managed, developmentally appropriate program, and once a reliable data system is in place, it is possible to proceed with the differential diagnosis approach. The approach includes three broad categories: medical, neurological and psychiatric.

General Medical

Any chronic painful condition can lead to SIB, as an expression of pain and discomfort or an attempt to communicate the desire for relief. At various times, we have tended patients whose SIB was the consequence of undetected physical disorders: migraine, otitis, peptic ulcer disease, esophagitis, endometriosis, premenstrual distress, menopause, cystitis. When the disorder is brought under control, the SIB usually goes away.

On the other hand, if SIB is the manifestation of a painful condition that is not treated soon enough, it is possible that it will become a habitual behavior sustained by its own dynamic, and in such cases alleviating the root cause may not correct the outcome. This is an old saw from psychosomatic medicine: A psychosomatic symptom may have a psychological origin, but if it continues long enough, it achieves a degree of "autonomy," a life of its own. It is like the process of "encephalization." Phantom pain from an amputated digit will clear up, early on, with local anesthetics. If it persists for a longer while, a brachial root nerve block will be necessary to control the symptom. Longer still, and stereotactic psychosurgery may be the only thing that works.

Medical conditions like reflux esophagitis are the likely origin of SIB in young Cornelia de Lange patients, as I shall describe in the next chapter. One can make a perfectly credible case that repeated self-injurious responses to such conditions are the sensitizing events that ultimately lead to the development of severe SIB when the patients get older.

One should treat painful conditions then in handicapped people because they are painful, and because they should be treated. But it is also important to spare the person pain, to the degree one is able to do so. If they learn pain, it may become a habit.

Some drugs may cause SIB. The most common culprits are the sedative anticonvulsants, phenobarbital, primidone, phenytoin, and ethosuccumide. Other drugs that may cause SIB are the xanthines, theophylline, and caffeine; and the neuroleptics, especially high-potency neuroleptics like haloperidol, which can cause akathisia and dysphoria. As a general rule, any medication that can cause sedation, dysphoria, depression, irritability, or restlessness can cause or aggravate SIB.

Epilepsy

Mentally retarded people are prone to seizures, and many require long-term treatment with anticonvulsants. One can usually improve the quality of treatment for seizure disorders in retarded people by pursuing the goal of anticonvulsant monotherapy; by withdrawing patients from anticonvulsants after their seizures have been under control for several years; or by choosing anticonvulsants that are psychotropes, like carbamazepine (CBZ) or valproic acid (VPA), in preference to anticonvulsants that have behavioral toxicity. Blood levels must be monitored periodically. Blood levels that are sufficient to control overt seizures may not control behavioral accompaniments of epilepsy like aggression, disorganization, or SIB.

It is a prudent first step to seek optimal anticonvulsant therapy for SIB patients with a history of seizures, an active seizure disorder treated with phenytoin or a barbiturate, or, in some cases, with no overt seizure history but a clearly defined record of paroxysmal SIB.

Paroxysmal SIB may be considered a "seizure equivalent" or the manifestation of what psychiatrists label "explosive disorder." In either event, the treatments overlap, and prescription of CBZ or VPA may be indicated.

SIB may also occur in connection with neuropathic conditions like dysautonomia, or after tissues are denervated and the sensation of pain is lost. In such cases, the SIB is not paroxysmal, but compulsive. It may be an example to support the "exploratory" model of SIB, which is discussed further.

Psychiatric Disorders

Retarded people are vulnerable to the full range of psychiatric disorders. This simple fact has been obscured in the past, when virtually any misbehavior that arose in a retarded person was treated with neuroleptics. It was impossible to differentiate among the major psychiatric diagnoses and the nonspecific behavior problems that are peculiar to retarded people. Now more attention is given to the issue of psychiatric diagnosis and treatment, and we are discovering the benefit in conventional psychiatric treatments. Antidepressants and lithium for affective disorders; antidepressants, benzodiazepines, or beta blockers for panic disorder; neuroleptics for schizophrenia; and lithium, beta blockers, and the psychotropic anticonvulsants for explosive disorders and aggression. One wishes that there were more research on the subject of psychiatric diagnosis and treatment in retarded people, but there is not, so one is guided for the present by extrapolations from other patient groups.

The problem, of course, is accurate diagnosis. It is no simple job to diagnose a "thought disorder" in someone whose IQ is 17. But simply because the margins of diagnostic accuracy are less precise in this population does not mean that the conventional diagnostic processes should be abandoned entirely. Like the case of "seizure equivalents," one's confidence is high enough to support a conservative trial of a likely, specific treatment. Not so high, though, that it will support an extraordinary treatment, like electro convulsive therapy for example. (Not that we are so far removed from such extraordinary interventions. It has not been an uncommon event at all, in the author's experience, to meet a mentally retarded person in his thirties or forties who had psychosurgery, *as a child*, for aggressive or for self-injurious behavior.)

In traditional psychiatry, self-injurious behaviors of varying intensity are observed in a wide range of conditions (Pattison and Kahan, 1983): in affective disorders and anxiety states, in major psychoses, in antisocial or borderline personalities, and in posttraumatic stress syndrome. This also seems to be true for retarded people who are self-injurious. In our recent clinical experience, and in an emerging literature, SIB is observed in mentally retarded patients who appear to be schizophrenic, in patients with major affective disorders and panic disorder, in patients with Tourette's syndrome, and in patients with intermittent explosive disorder. In these cases, the appropriate psychiatric treatment is expected to bring about a substantial reduction in SIB, along with the other symptoms of the primary condition. A successful response to the specific treatment affirms the psychiatric diagnosis; not a "scientific" affirmation, by any means, but a practical one. If a systematic attempt at psychiatric treatment is unsuccessful, the patient may go on to join the 'refractory' or 'idiopathic' SIB patients for whom experimental treatments may be indicated.

Among the SIB cases who have been referred to our clinic, only about half can be successfully diagnosed and treated according to the medical and neuropsychiatric paradigms we have discussed. The most severe SIBs—the LNS cases, for example, or young children—do not seem to fit very well at all. They are candidates for a new approach, and it is here that research is necessary, to develop new paradigms and new treatments.

Subgroups Related to the Neurochemical Basis of SIB

The divisions we have suggested thus far are in terms of established neuropsychiatric categories. It is an intelligent approach to the individual patient, but it is not a complete solution to the problem of SIB. The algorithms have some value, but they are not universal. For a substantial number of SIB cases, the algorithms are not helpful; the behavior persists, and a new approach must be developed. It is for these refractory cases that one relies on neuropharmacological models and hypotheses to advance experimental treatments.

The D1-dopamine receptor supersensitivity hypothesis is a neuropharmacological paradigm, based on neuropathic findings in LNS patients and an animal model tested in rats and monkeys. It is conceivable that D1-dopamine receptor supersensitivity is a "common final pathway" for the occurrence of SIB, but it is also possible that the neurochemical substrate of SIB is also diverse, and that alternative models may be pertinent.

The major alternative paradigm is the endorphin model, which is based on the observation that endogenous opiates or endorphins are released in the brain following painful stimulation. The chronic stimulation of endorphin receptors by repeated SIB is hypothesized to 'downregulate' the reactivity of these receptors and underlie an "addiction" to chronic painful stimulation. If pain-reducing behavior is reinforced by the release of endorphins onto opiate receptors, then blocking those receptors may be expected to prevent the reinforcing consequences of the behavior and allow extinction to occur (Richardson and Zaleski, 1983). With this rationale, Richardson and Zaleski (1983) attempted the treatment of severe SIB in a 15-year-old retarded boy with the opiate antagonist naloxone, and the treatment, after a brief "extinction burst," was successful.

It is not really known whether SIB patients experience "pain" as other people do. Because many LNS patients and many other SIB patients seem to ask for restraint, it appears that they may be aggrieved by the painful consequences of their behavior. In other cases, however, the threshold for pain appears to be high. The idea that at least some SIB could be attributable to "blunted nocioception" and maintained by the endorphin system was raised by Sandman et al. (1983). Thus a different hypothesis about endogenous opiates led to a treatment study with low dose naloxone, which is known to induce hypalgesia or lowered pain threshold. Intravenous naloxone reduced SIB in one subject and eliminated the behavior in a second (Sandman et al., 1983). Success with naloxone in SIB was replicated in one patient by Sandyk (1985), but not by Davidson et al. (1983) (one patient) or by Beckwith et al. (1984) (two patients).

Because naloxone is a short-acting drug that can only be administered parenterally, these studies could report only very short-term results. The recent availability of naltrexone, an opiate antagonist that is long acting and that can be administered orally, means that more definitive clinical studies of this phenomenon may finally be undertaken. Preliminary results from studies of naltrexone in SIB appear to be encouraging (Thompson, 1985; Herman et al., 1987). On the other hand, only small numbers of patients have participated in naloxone or naltrexone trials, and there are, to the author's knowledge, no long-term studies at all. The limited success of opiate antagonist treatment may be a function of the heterogeneity of the opiate receptor system; the existing antagonists may not block the appropriate opiate receptor.

The serotonin hypothesis of SIB is based on the observation that low levels of serotonin in the CNS may be associated with impulsive and aggressive behavior (Eichelman, 1977); that certain conditions disposed to SIB like Down's syndrome, autism, and Cornelia de Lange syndrome are sometimes associated with low levels of serotonin (Coleman, 1973). One study reported that Cornelia de Lange (CDL) patients with low serotonin levels were likelier to have severe behavior problems (Greenberg and Coleman, 1973). O'Neal et al. (1986) reported one CDL patient with SIB who had low levels of whole blood serotonin. Treatment with the serotonin reuptake blocker trazodone and the serotonin percussor L-tryptophan led to resolution of SIB, and elevation of whole blood serotonin to normal levels (O'Neal et al., 1986).

The adenosine hypothesis of SIB has evolved from an appreciation of the role of CNS purines, elevated in LNS, as neurotransmitters, neuromodulators, and regulators of receptor sensitivity, especially in relationship to adenosine (Kopin, 1981). Caffeine and theophylline can increase SIB in experimental animals (Mueller et al., 1982; Nyhan, 1973); behavioral potency is related to the ability of these agents to block the adenosine receptor (Daly et al., 1981). Clonidine-induced self-mutilation in mice has been attributed to adenosine-A1 receptor blockade and may be inhibited by adenosine or by the adenosine agonist dipyridamole (Katsuragi et al., 1984). Adenosine inhibits self-mutilation in Breese's D1-dopamine receptor supersensitive rats (Criswell et al., 1986).

It is possible that some of the sedative properties of neuroleptic drugs are mediated by adenosine agonist effects (Phillis, 1984). CBZ, on the other hand, seems to be an adenosine antagonist (Phillis, 1984). Dipyridamole is a commercially available drug with few side effects that is an adenosine agonist (Harker and Kadatz, 1983), but clinical trials of dipyridamole in SIB patients, in our program, have not been impressive.

The GABA (gamma-aminobutyric acid) hypothesis has been woven out of similar cloth. Muscimol, a GABA agonist, evokes intense stereotyped behavior, including self-biting, in laboratory animals (Frye et al., 1986), and the rat model of dopamine deficiency in LNS is more sensitive to the SIB produced by muscimol (Breese et al., 1987). Caffeine inhibits the binding of diazepam to receptors, and diazepam also potentiates the adenosine effect in inhibiting the firing rates of neurons (Kopin, 1981). GABA antagonists do not necessarily suppress SIB, however (Sawynok, 1983). Most of our SIB patients have at one time or another been treated with benzodiazepines, with no benefit at all.

The various neurochemical hypothesis have an intrinsic advantage because they lend themselves to empirical evaluation in clinical drug trials. They are compromised by the inability to measure neurotransmitter/neuromodulator function directly, and by the fact that neurochemical systems are inordinately complex and interactive. Because most neuroactive compounds influence several neurotransmitters, there probably is no "clean" drug that is centrally active.

Can treatment response be used to define meaningful subgroups? That is an issue that is central to the clinical approach to SIB, as one accumulates patients who have responded well to different treatments, and whose response is maintained over follow-up. Suppose one were to demonstrate a group of SIB patients who responded well to D1-dopamine receptor blockers, another group of lithium responders, and so on, for CBZ, VPA, beta blockers, serotoninergic drugs, opiate antagonists, etc. It would be tempting to reconstruct a nosology of SIB, especially if certain clinical characteristics typified the individual groups. However, there is so much ambiguity and overlap in the neurochemical effects of neuroactive drugs that behavioral specificity to drug response is more the ideal than reality.

Once I asked a patient of mine why she bit herself. She was a retarded woman who was quite verbal and engaging in spite of her handicap, but she was given to awful tantrums, and when she had one, she would bite her arm furiously. Her wrists were terribly calloused. When I asked her why she did that, why she bit herself, she said she did it because she was hungry.

Her answer affirmed something I had always suspected about the psychology of SIB. There is a reason why some people hurt themselves; it is just not a very good reason.

CHAPTER 8

Behavior in the
Cornelia de Lange Syndrome

The Cornelia de Lange Syndrome (CDLS) is a mental retardation syndrome characterized by short stature, hirsutism, and facial and skeletal anomalies (de Lange, 1933, 1938; Hawley et al., 1985). It is interesting by virtue of association with a unique constellation of behavioral and temperamental attributes. One thinks first of self-injurious behavior (SIB), of course, and CDLS has been compared, in this regard, to the Lesch–Nyhan syndrome.

I have had the opportunity to get acquainted with a large number of CDLS patients and their families as the result of a larger interest in the problem of SIB and its pharmacological treatment. We had developed an approach to the differential diagnosis of SIB (Gualtieri, 1989), and the natural question was where CDLS would fit. As it turned out, CDLS was not at all similar to the Lesch–Nyhan syndrome, in terms of SIB, and neither did it fit any of the other categories. The problem of SIB in association with CDLS was not what one had been led to believe on the basis of the existing medical literature. It turned out to be a much more interesting problem.

CDLS patients are small and hirsute, with a characteristic facies and typical skeletal anomalies (de Lange, 1933; Smith, 1982; Joubin et al., 1980). The phenotype is not invariant; it may change with age, and it may vary in relation to elements such as birth weight (Greenberg and Robinson, 1989). There are associated cardiac, gastrointestinal, and genital anomalies, like ventricular septal defect, gastric reflux, peptic ulcer disease, cryptorchism, hypospadias, etc. (Lachman et al., 1981; Smith, 1982). Almost all the identified cases are mentally retarded, but not all of them, by any means (Gadoth et al., 1982). About 20% have seizures at one time or another (Smith, 1982).

CDLS is probably a genetic disorder, although the genetics have not been worked out. The risk of recurrence within a sibship is said to be 2% to 5% (Pashayan et al., 1969). There are reports of monozygotic concordance (Choo and Bianchi, 1965; Kroth, 1965; Opitz, 1965) and of familial occurrence (Kumar et al., 1985; Leavitt et al., 1985; Bankier et al., 1986), and partial elements of the full syndrome have been identified in family members (Opitz, 1985). It has been proposed that the disorder is an expression of an autosomal dominant gene (Robinson et al., 1985; Leavitt et al., 1985; Bankier et al., 1986), perhaps with incomplete penetrance, or as an "iceberg" dominant (Opitz, 1985). The similarities between CDLS and the phenotype of the duplication 3q [dup (3q)] Syndrome are entirely superficial (Wilson et al., 1985).

The diagnosis is clinical, based on morphological features, and no genetic, biochemical, neurodiagnostic, or psychological measure can affirm the diagnosis. The incidence is 1 in 10,000 live births (Opitz, 1985) or 1 in 50,000 (Beck, 1976). The Cornelia de Lange Syndrome Foundation, in Collinsville, Connecticut, has, at present, more than 700 identified propositi, mostly in the United States and in the other English-speaking countries. (The CDLS Newsletter is published in English.)

The behavioral phenotype of CDLS has usually been described in terms of SIB or self-mutilatory behavior (Shear et al., 1971; Johnson et al., 1976; Bryson et al., 1971; Mueller and Hsiao, 1980), aggression (Andrasik et al., 1979), hyperactivity (Greenberg and Coleman, 1973), and autistic features (Johnson et al., 1976b). In fact, this commentary has been based on relatively small samples, people in institutions, for example, or people who have taken neuroleptics or sedative anticonvulsants. There is the possibility, then, that it may not be an entirely accurate representation.

Although all the behavioral features described in the literature are also represented in the present sample, it is our opinion that they are only one side of the real clinical picture. The whole picture is much more interesting, and it may shed some light, in its contrast to the Lesch–Nyhan group, on the nature and origins of SIB.

The CDLS Survey

A questionnaire was designed with queries about medical background, family history, drug treatment, and abnormal behaviors. The questionnaire also contained two copies of the Self-Injurious Behavior Questionnaire (SIBQ), a rating scale that had previously been developed for pharmacological and epidemiologic studies of SIB (Gualtieri and Schroeder, 1989). Because the SIBQ emphasizes negative behaviors, parents were instructed to fill it out on the basis of how the child behaved over the previous week, and how the child behaved at any point in the past when he or she was at his very worst.

The questionnaire was distributed to the entire membership of the CDLS Foundation via the newsletter, which reaches more than 700 families of CDL people; 111 questionnaires were returned. Twenty-seven questionnaires were also filled out by parents of CDL patients who had consulted with the author directly, either by telephone or at the annual CDL convention in Chicago (in 1988). The data from 138 CDL probands are presented herein.

Because these are survey results from only a small proportion of the known population of CDL, and because they are a sample of young patients living at home with their families, the data are not presented as definitive. Nor has an extensive statistical analysis of the data been undertaken, because the survey was not constructed around an hypothesis. Its purpose was to survey the nature of behaviors exhibited by CDL children, the context in which they arose, and the success of pharmacological treatments.

There were large gaps of missing information, since the informants did not always respond to every query.

Demographics

The respondent probands were mostly white (126 white, 1 black, 1 Hispanic surname) and female (78 female, 60 male). They ranged in age from 1 to 39 years (mean, 10.4; SD, 7.4), so they were in fact a very young group. They were mainly from the United States (118); 18 were from other English-speaking nations. Ninety-nine (of 124) were described as ambulatory but only 44 (of 115) were verbal. Fifty-nine of the respondents had IQ or SQ scores available; they ranged from 8 (sic) to 88 (mean, 48.9; SD, 18.2.).

Medical

Respondents were queried about the coexistence of specific handicaps. The responses are in accord with the results of other such surveys of medical conditions and handicaps in CDLS (Hawley et al., 1985). Among handicaps, the extremities (21) and hearing (21) are listed first; then visual defects (17), cleft lip and palate (8), skeletal abnormalities such as scoliosis (5), and difficulties with gait and coordination (4). Among medical conditions, gastrointestinal difficulties were listed first (56), then head and neck problems such as otitis, bruxism, sinusitis, cataracts, and retinal detachment (45); then respiratory problems like asthma or frequent infections (25), cardiac anomalies (21), and genitourinary problems (hypospadias, cryptorchism, frequent UTIs) (11).

Paroxysmal Events

Myoclonus, the sudden and abrupt stimulation of a large group of coordinated muscles, is well known to occur in CDLS patients. In response to a question about its occurrence, 43 were positive, and 36 said myoclonus was never observed. The most frequent manifestation of myoclonus was arching of the back (25).

Current or past seizures were described by 35 respondents. Virtually every seizure type and every anticonvulsant was represented. There was no apparent connection between the occurrence or the nonoccurrence of seizures, or any aspect of anticonvulsant treatment, with behavior problems or with SIB.

Sleep

Sleep problems were very common: Although 38 respondents described no problem with sleeping, 23 said that the sleep pattern was variable, 19 said that the child was up frequently, 14 had difficulty in sleeping, had insomnia, or slept too little; 5 children were said to sleep too much, episodes of sleep apnea were reported for 4, and 18 more reported some variant or another of sleeping problem (83 yes; 38 no).

Eating

Appetite problems were also common, as one might expect in children with reflux and esophagitis, and other gastrointestinal conditions. The problems were variable appetite (24), diminished appetite or anorexia (18), excessive eating (5), and some other variant of positive (16) (63 positive respondents in all).

Personality

We inquired after personality traits, using the broadest strokes, and based on personal observations of CDLS children. Eighty-three of the children were described as "affectionate"; 57 were said to prefer sameness and routines, 51 were described as sensitive, 35 as easy to frighten, and 29 as easy to startle.

Behavior Problems

With respect to "behavior problems" in general, 64 were said to have had current or past difficulties compared to 14 who never had. Fifty-seven of the children had been aggressive at one time or another. Other problems described were hyperactivity (18), defiant, oppositional, and noncompliant (14), destructiveness (14), temper tantrums (13), anxious or easily upset (8), irritable or dysphoric (7), screaming (5) and withdrawal (4).

No fewer than 88 respondents had current problems with SIB; 10 more had past, possible, or rare SIB, and 33 were reported as having had none. SIB was reported to occur when angry (53), when frustrated (32), when sick (30), when unreasonable demands were made (22), for attention (18), or in response to pain (8). The pattern of SIB was occasional (28) or frequent (21) or rare (4), but rarely constant (3). It was explosive in 17, cyclic in 14, and unpredictable, without discernible pattern, in 19. Seventy-one of the respondents described their children as having a high threshold to pain, 17 a low pain threshold, and 29 a normal pain threshold.

The most common topography of SIB was self-biting (27), hitting or slapping (20), hair-pulling (15), head-banging (11), picking (10), scratching (5), and gouging (5). Virtually every other form of SIB was also represented in the list: eye-gouging, pulling at tissues, bruxism, rubbing, poking, cutting, and rectal digging. Restraints, which were usually personal or soft ties, had been used for 34 of the subjects.

In terms of physical injury as a result of SIB, there were no reports of self-mutilation to the degree one sees in connection with the Lesch-Nyhan syndrome, nor has the author ever seen such a case. Parents reported relatively mild injuries like scratches (10), scars (9), bruises (8), bites (8), cuts (7), sores (5), infections (5), hair pulled out (4), and two damaged tear ducts and one broken nose. Not a trivial list, by any means, but not in a league with Lesch–Nyhan.

The SIBQ is a 25-item questionnaire that is divided into four sections: 5 questions about SIB, 9 about other behavior problems, 4 about elements related to

TABLE 8.1. SIBQ[a] Scores for CDLS patients and a comparison group.

SIBQ SCORES	CDLS-1, current ($n = 122$)	CDLS-2, worst ($n = 121$)	Mentally retarded, current ($n = 520$)
SIB	3.6±4.6	6.7±6.9	0.8±2.4
Behav	8.0±6.9	12.4±9.5	3.0±5.0
Perf	5.9±4.3	7.3±4.8	3.1±3.4
Emot	5.9±6.1	10.8±9.5	3.0±4.9
Total	23.4	37.2	9.9

[a]The Self-Injurious Behavior Questionnaire (SIBQ) is divided into four subscales. The first (five items) is directly concerned with self-injurious behavior (SIB); the second (nine items) with behavior problems like aggression and hyperactivity that often occur in SIB patients; the third (four items) with elements of classroom or workshop performance like inattention and compliance; and the fourth (seven items) with affective symptoms like irritability and agitation.

Each item is rated on a 5-point scale, from 0 ("not a problem") to 4 ("severe problem"). There are 25 items in all, and the maximum score is 20 for SIB, 36 for behavior problems, 16 for performance problems, and 28 for emotional problems. (A copy of the SIBQ is appended at the end of this volume).

classroom or workshop performance, and 7 related to mood and affect. The subjects were rated at their worst, and as they had been over the previous week. The mean item scores for each of the SIBQ factors are given in Table 8.1.

For purposes of comparison, we have included "normative" data on the SIBQ in Table 8.1. These data are from a survey of 520 mentally retarded residents of the Orange Grove Center in Chattanooga, Tennessee, a community-based program. The SIBQs were rated by classroom teachers or by workshop supervisors on the basis of the client's behavior and performance over the preceding month. It is apparent from Table 8.1 that the CDLS cases had much higher scores than the community group (which included only 1 CDLS case and no Lesch–Neschan cases). Because the comparison group was not by any means a control group, however, a statistical comparison was not made of the data.

It is widely believed that difficult behaviors in CDL patients develop, or grow more severe, when the patients are adolescents. Parents were asked, therefore, when difficulties with SIB first developed and when the difficulties grew so severe that they sought professional consultation. The distribution of responses is given in Table 8.2. The largest group, 39 of 86 respondents, reported that SIB first began at ages 2, 3, or 4 years. The largest group, 17 of 49 respondents, reported that the problem of SIB became severe at ages 5 to 8.

The distribution of SIBQ scores by age, however, presents a slightly different picture (Table 8.3). When parents reported on the child's current status, problem scores for SIB, behavior, emotional dysregulation, and poor performance were

TABLE 8.2. Age of onset of SIB[a]

Age (years)	SIB began (n)	SIB a serious problem (n)
1	9	2
2	16	5
3–4	23	6
5–6	9	7
7–8	10	10
9–10	5	3
11–12	5	4
13–14	4	5
15–16	2	1
17–18	3	6
20+	0	0

[a]These data are based on information from 86 respondents who answered the question, "At what age did the problem (SIB) begin?" and on data from 49 respondents who answered the question, "At what age did SIB become a serious problem?" In response to the first question, 39 of 86 (45%) reported that the problem began at ages 2, 3, or 4; in response to the second question, 22 of 46 (49%) reported that SIB became a serious problem at ages 3 through 8.

TABLE 8.3. SIBQ scores at different ages

A. SIBQ scores based on current status.[a]						
n	Age	SIB	Behav	Perf	Emot	Total
30	0–5	2.8	6.5	3.0	5.3	17.7
33	6–10	2.9	9.2	6.2	5.6	23.9
28	11–15	3.8	7.7	6.1	6.6	24.1
16	16–20	**5.9**	7.7	7.6	**6.8**	27.9
6	21–25	2.3	**10.5**	10.8	4.2	27.8
7	26–30	4.0	8.4	8.1	6.7	27.3

B. SIBQ scores based on patient status, at his or her worst.[a]						
n	Age	SIB	Behav	Perf	Emot	Total
30	0–5	4.1	8.5	7.1	5.4	23.2
33	6–10	5.4	11.3	8.3	6.6	25.9
27	11–15	7.1	12.9	12.8	8.9	41.6
16	16–20	**11.5**	15.7	15.9	**9.3**	**52.4**
6	21–25	4.5	18.7	16.3	6.5	46.0
7	26–30	9.3	16.7	12.4	6.7	45.0

[a]In both A and B, it is seen that the highest scores are given to patients between the ages of 16 and 25.

highest in patients ages 15 to 30. The same was true for problem scores, based on how the patient was during his or her most difficult period.

Scores on the "current status" SIBQ were positively correlated with age for SIB ($r = .29, p = .002$), affect ($r = .25, p = .008$) and total score ($r = .25, p = .009$). Score on the "at his worst" SIBQ were positively correlated with age for SIB ($r = .30, p = .001$), behavior ($r = .22, p = .02$), affect ($r = .20, p = .03$), and total score ($r = 0.27, p = .005$). Although only a small amount of the variance in SIBQ scores therefore can be attributed to age alone, the common lore appears to be correct. Although SIB begins during the first decade of life, behavior problems increase as the children grow older, and they are at their worst during the second and third decades.

Medications

We asked if medications had ever been used for SIB or for other behavior problems. Eleven subjects had been on stimulants, methylphenidate, or dexedrine, but drug treatment improved hyperactivity in only 2 of the 11, and in the others it had either made the problem behaviors worse, or had caused anorexia, irritability, mood swings, or depression.

Sixteen had been treated with neuroleptics, but there were only three positive reactions, one only slight. In most of the cases, the behavior had grown much worse, or there were intolerable side effects like dystonia. Seven had been treated with antidepressants; 3 of 5 had done slightly better on imipramine; 1 subject had no effect on desipramine; and in 1, fluoxetine helped at first and then the effect disappeared.

In seven subjects, anticonvulsants had been prescribed for the behavior problems, independent of seizures. Carbamazepine and phenytoin had actually helped in three of these cases.

Thirteen were treated with tranquilizers or sedative-hypnotics. One of 4 responded to chloral hydrate. The antihistaminics helped in 2 cases; benzopdiazepines in 1 of 5; and buspirone in 1 of 2. Propanalol was tried twice, and did not work well in either case. L-tryptophan calmed one child and helped him to sleep better.

Contrasting Data

This is a survey of relatively young people who are living at home with their families. Does that introduce a degree of bias? Of course it does, but the appropriate question is whether the sample bias is such that it invalidates the results of the survey. To address this question, we should consider two groups: CDL people described in the literature, and older CDL people who are currently residing in residential institutions.

We examined our computerized tardive dyskinesia monitoring system (TMS) database (Gualtieri, in press) for cases of CDL at the mental retardation centers where we provide neuropsychiatric consultation on a regular basis. There were at the time of this survey six facilities with a total of 1440 mentally retarded clients; all were state-supported residential institutions. There were only 4 diagnosed CDL cases in the entire database, a number roughly equivalent to the number of Prader–Willi cases, but considerably fewer than the number of cases with tuberous sclerosis, phenylketonuria, Down's syndrome, or fragile X. (There were no Lesch–Nyhan cases in the database).

The four CDL cases were two males, aged 23 and 51, and two females aged 22 and 35. Their behavioral records were reviewed. Three of the four had previous difficulties with SIB, two of the four with intermittent agitation, and one with noncompliance and insomnia. Two had previously been treated with neuroleptic drugs. None of the four was currently on neuroleptics or any other psychotropic medication, and none of the four had current behavior problems sufficiently severe to warrant even a behavior program, let alone a psychoactive drug.

The author's personal experience with CDL, then, through the Foundation and in his consultation practice is considerably different from the experience that is cited in the medical literature. In 1971, for example, Shear et al. described two cases, one 5 and one 6 years old, who had severe self-mutilation; in one case, aversive behavioral treatment was necessary, and in the other, all the teeth were removed to prevent further self-mutilation. That same year, Bryson et al. (1971) reported four CDL cases at a state residential facility (ages 18, 15, 16, and 16) with long-term, persistent self-mutilation. They all had been treated, however, over the long term with neuroleptics, phenytoin, and barbiturate anticonvulsants. In 1973, Greenberg and Coleman described 11 CDL patients, aged 10 to 30 years, at state residential facilities. All had long-standing behavior problems, especially hyperactivity, destructiveness, aggression, and SIB. All had received long-term treatment with neuroleptics and/or anticonvulsants (considering the year, probably phenytoin and phenobarbital). In 1979, Andrasik et al. described a 22-year-old CDL man with chronic aggressive behavior who had multiple hospital admissions and long-term treatment with a variety of psychotropic drugs, especially neuroleptics.

How is one to reconcile the experience of this author with what these others have described? Selection, for one thing. What Shear, Bryson, Greenberg, and Andrasik were concerned with, and the points they were interested in emphasizing, were behavior problems, so naturally they wrote about CDL patients with behavior problems. We have no idea how many CDL patients they also saw who had no behavior problems at all, or had only mild, transient behavior problems.

On the other hand, all the patients they described who had long-standing, persistent behavior problems also had a long history of institutionalization and treatment with neuroleptics and/or sedative anticonvulsants. Is it possible that these elements—institutionalization, inappropriate medication—may have aggravated what was, to begin with, a relatively mild problem?

Behavior in the Cornelia de Lange Syndrome

CDLS is a syndrome with a behavioral stereotype, but SIB is not its most important element, nor is aggression, hyperactivity, or autism. CDL children are affectionate and sensitive, easy to frighten or to startle, and they prefer routines and predictability. They are temperamental, to say the least, and they are prone to SIB and other behavior problems when they are angry or frustrated or sick or in pain, or when demands are made on them, or when their routine is changed. Because they are temperamental, such occasions do not arise infrequently.

The behavior problems of CDLS children are SIB, aggression, destructiveness, and attention-seeking. Like their problems with appetite and sleeping, these behaviors are variable, not consistent. The children (and the adults, to a lesser degree) are given to good and bad times. They are not compulsively self-injurious, like Lesch–Nyhan patients, and very few of them have the scars and deformities of compulsive self-mutilation.

If one were required to select three words to describe the behavioral stereotype of CDLS, the author would choose immature, hypersensitive, and dysrhythmic. What are perceived as behavior problems, especially in the young CDLS patients, are the kinds of behaviors one associates with 2-year-olds. And if there is a trait that distinguishes CDLS children from normal 2-year-olds, it is that they are very temperamental. They are hypersensitive, given to strong reactions to ordinary stimuli and to prolonged reactions to stressors that are only transient. They are dysrhythmic, given to cycles of positive and negative affect, and given to irregularity in vegetative behaviors (eating and sleeping, for example) and in emotional response.

Immaturity

CDLS patients are small and immature, and many of the behavior problems that they do have, like hyperactivity, or "into everything," are explicable in terms of the exploratory behavior that one sees, for example, in normal children who are 2 or 3 years old. Even their problems with hyperactivity, aggression, tantrums, and sleep dysregulation are more similar to the problems of young children than they are to the problems of other neuropsychiatric patients.

Well, they may be immature, but is that any more than a truism? Is there something practical to be gleaned from that observation? In fact, it is a practical observation, with implications for pharmacotherapy, behavior management, and prognosis.

CDLS children seem to respond to psychoactive medications rather like very young children, with some occasional benefit from antihistaminic sedatives or methylphenidate, but with a variable response overall to medications, and a risk of side effects or of paradoxical response that is usually equal to the chance of benefit. One is familiar with the difficulties in treating preschool children with psychoactive drugs, as hyperactive children with stimulants, for example or autistic children with neuroleptics. The failure of consistent response is what characterizes those people, and the same problem seems to afflict CDLS children.

Self-injurious behavior is not unknown in normal infants, and head-banging, for example, may be a problem parents bring to the pediatrician. The appropriate management advice in such cases is to look for a medical condition that may be making the child uncomfortable, to find an alternative way to stimulate or to comfort the child, to limit the damage the infant is able to do to himself with padding or soft restraints, and to avoid hysterical overreaction. The risk of ignoring SIB in such infants is that physical damage may occur, or that the problem may turn from a transient event into a prolonged bad habit.

One should handle SIB in young CDLS patients in almost exactly the same way. Look for a medical cause, like otitis, esophagitis, UTI, or seizures. Find more appropriate ways to soothe or to stimulate the child. Rely on redirection and on soft restraint as primary methods of behavior management. Examine the environment of the child, to determine whether there are continuing stressors in his or her life that are provoking the self-injurious behavior. Stay away from psychoactive medications that are as likely to aggravate the problem as they are to improve it.

As a general rule, SIB in a CDLS child is, first, the expression of pain, discomfort, frustration, or dismay. It is therefore an attempt to communicate, or to resolve another problem. The appropriate treatment is exactly what the child would have you do, that is, to get rid of the primary problem.

Thus, the element of immaturity as a cause of SIB leads naturally to a series of commonsense approaches, and it is precisely these approaches that have been most successful, we have found, in our many conversations with parents of CDLS children.

The idea of immaturity conveys the notion of a prolonged physiological event. But we do not mean to suggest that the problem of SIB in the CDLS is entirely a "normal" or a physiological event. There are circumstances, after all, in which psychopathology can be expressed as an extreme variant of a normal process. There are also circumstances in which a normal variant may be transformed into a pathological event. An example of the first is childhood hyperactivity, or mild learning disabilities, where "pathology" is expressed in terms of a statistical deviation from normal. An example of the second is aggression, an extreme variant of normal assertive behavior that may become habitual; habitual aggression may, in turn, have secondary consequences. It is the secondary events—loss of social rewards, failure to develop appropriate skills, exposure to environments that are harsh and ungiving—that serve to reinforce the habit, to give it a new life of its own and yield a pathological outcome.

One may contend therefore that the behavior problems of CDLS children represent an extreme variant of immaturity, and a variant that may be reinforced unwittingly to the point that it becomes habitual and pathological.

"Temperamental"

The observation that CDL children are "temperamental," that is, hypersensitive and dysrhythmic, is also something that has practical implications.

The first implication is for prediction. It should be expected that the children will have behavior problems at one time or another, and one should be prepared to deal with those difficulties when they arise. Their management, unfortunately, is usually labor intensive, but that is how it is. There is no escaping it. When they are having a bad time, they require a lot of hands-on attention and management.

On the other hand, but by the same token, the untoward behaviors of CDLS children should be expected to resolve by themselves after a while. Bad times follow good times, but good times also follow bad times. That should lend some encouragement, at least, to parents and teachers who have to cope with the bad times. The arduous work of behavior management will be rewarded, one might expect, by a period of calm and compliance.

The second implication is for attribution. Although one must look for a physical or an environmental stressor when a child begins to have behavior problems, one must understand that there is not always a cause or a precipitant. People who are hypersensitive and dysrhythmic may experience periods when their threshold is so low that even the normal stimuli of day-to-day life are intolerable grievances. It is as if the kid wakes up with a hangover some mornings. The regular noises of the classroom may be jarring on such days; the failure of immediate gratification may be interpreted as a major frustration; a momentary lapse in normal interaction may be perceived as an intolerable slight. During such periods, it is futile to expect to find a clearly defined precipitant, or even a satisfying explanation for the misbehavior.

The third implication is for prognosis. The temperamental attributes of CDL children lead one to expect they may be vulnerable to pathological transformation if their difficulties are not handled, gently and appropriately, early on. They seem to be given to habits, forms of self-stimulation like rubbing or gentle tapping or picking; these same motor programs may be adapted to use in the service of controlling anxiety, frustration, and pain. Because they are dysrhythmic, there will be times when their threshold for frustration is low and even normal day-to-day events may evoke an extreme response.

If the SIB they have in such circumstances is handled harshly, with aversives, for example, or by ignoring the child's distress, or by administering a drug that may cause sedation, dysphoria, or akathisia, then there is the risk of turning a transient phenomenon into a persistent pattern of pathological behavior. The suggestion, then, is that SIB in CDLS represents a minor phenotype, or a proclivity, that may interact with circumstances in a particular way, and thus become a major difficulty.

Obviously, there is no experimental evidence to support this contention, and so the author has relied on observation, intuition, and evidence from other neuropathic conditions, as well as from the results of the CDLS questionnaire. In terms of evidence from other neuropsychiatric conditions, the two models that may be germane are from the study of recurrent affective disorder, in which it is believed that repeated episodes may, over time, grow more frequent and more severe (Post et al., 1982b); and from the study of epilepsy, in which it is known that a seizure focus may, over time, stimulate the formation of a mirror focus (Morrell, 1985). Both of these phenomena have been ascribed to a mysterious process known to neurophysiologists as "kindling," (Wada, 1977).

The idea, then, is that behavior problems in CDLS patients are likely to be recurrent and self-limiting, and that if they are treated gently, and without recourse to treatment measures that carry their own risk of damage, they can be controlled and they will not be permanently disabling. The idea may be wrong or it may be right, but is not a mischievous idea. It should encourage optimism and gentleness in the prescription of behavior treatments and pharmacotherapy, and that is never a bad way to begin.

Alternative Constructions

The alternative ideas about behavior problems in the CDLS are, in fact, less well supported by empirical data, and they may also be dangerous in their own way. For example, one alternative idea, and one that is widely believed, is that all CDLS people will have severe behavior problems, especially when they are adolescents and adults. This is a dangerous idea, because it is wrong—we have many CDLS patients who are adults, and who do not have behavior problems—and because it lends a degree of pessimism, a negative set of expectations, to parents and teachers who deserve to be guided by optimism and a positive outlook. It may even lead to the adoption of extreme treatment measures, like institutionalization or neuroleptic treatment.

The second alternative idea is that some CDLS patients will have severe behavior problems and a dire outcome; permanent institutionalization in behavior-disorder units, long-term drug therapy, persistent problems with agitation, aggression, and SIB. Of course, it is an idea that may well be correct, but it is impossible to disprove. And unless there is some way to predict exactly who these individuals will be, it is not a particularly useful idea.

Is it possible to know how many such incorrigible cases there are? How are they to be distinguished from CDLS patients whose difficulties are the consequence of tardive akathisia (Barnes and Braude, 1985) or chronic institutionalization? The author would feel more tolerant of this alternative idea if he had met one CDLS, anywhere, whose problems were in fact incorrigible and debilitating, or not possible to ascribe to an external influence.

The foundation of understanding the behavioral difficulties of CDLS children is not in terms of a neuropathic or a psychopathological model. It is much simpler than that.

The guiding principles for understanding and for managing the behavior problems of CDLS people are these: First, look for a medical cause; second, look for an environmental stressor; three, manage with gentle restraints and creative redirection; and four, understand that the onerous requirement of a labor-intensive behavioral approach will be rewarded by recovery, personal growth, and a diminished likelihood of future episodes.

Pharmacotherapy

It is appropriate to consider how this formulation speaks to the issue of pharmacotherapy, because so many CDLS patients are treated at one time or another with psychoactive drugs. It is also appropriate to consider whether the behavioral stereotype of CDLS may have a neurochemical basis. If there were a way to render these patients less sensitive and less temperamental, less dysrhythmic and more compliant, their management and their education should be that much improved.

If one were to rely on the survey data, one would conclude that no medication or class of medications has been predictably useful in alleviating SIB or other behavior problems in CDLS patients, and that this line of reasoning, therefore, is futile. Stimulants and neuroleptics have been used most frequently, with more cases, in each instance, of drug-related deterioration than of drug-related benefit. It appears that stimulants like methylphenidate may occasionally reduce hyperactivity, but sometimes it is at the price of mood swings, irritability, and increased SIB. The survey does not even contain a hint of what may be successful pharmacotherapy for SIB or for other behavior problems in CDLS.

Is it likely that some new medication may prove useful for CDLS? That is possible. There are many new pharmacological approaches to behavior disorders in the developmentally disabled, and most have never been tried in CDLS.

One would begin such an approach around an hypothesis, for example, that CDLS patients were affectively unstable, that their behavioral phenotype could be a partial variant of affective disorder. They might therefore respond to antidepressants or to lithium. A more concise hypothesis might focus on the occurrence of aggression and self-injury, perception of disordered threshold for the perception of pain, affective instability, and variability in appetitive function, especially sleeping and eating, and postulate a disorder of serotonergic regulation. Clearly, these are psychological functions one associates with serotonergic neurotransmission.

There is a case report of low levels of the serotonin metabolite 5-hydroxy indole-3-acetic acid (5-HIAA) in the amniotic fluid of one CDL case (Lacourt et al., 1977) and there is also a case report of successful serotonergic treatment for a self-injurious CDL child with low baseline whole-blood 5-hydroxy tryptophol (O'Neal et al., 1986).

What makes this proposal more interesting is the new availability of serotonergic drugs, like trazodone, fluoxetine, and clomipramine, and the new approach to cotreatment with more than one serotonergic drug [e.g., L-tryptophan, trazodone, lithium, the so-called serotonin cascade treatment (Hale et al., 1987)]. Buspirone is a novel and atypical anxiolytic that may be useful for some developmentally disabled patients, and it is, in contrast, a mixed serotonin agonist/antagonist (Ratey et al., 1989).

There are a spate of new psychoactive medications that may be useful for CDL, although their administration cannot be associated with any concise hypothesis, or even a vague one. Drugs like amantadine (Chandler and Gualtieri, in press 1990), the calcium channel blockers (Walsh et al., 1986), beta blockers (Ratey et al., 1986), and acetazolamide (Hiroshi et al., 1984) have been reported effective in isolated cases of SIB.

One is decidedly less sanguine about the continued use of present drugs, which have had their day and have not proven to be especially helpful. The stimulants, when they are used for hyperactive CDLS youngsters, should be monitored carefully, because they may increase irritability and SIB. When they are used, one may wish to consider cotreatment with L-tryptophan (Chandler et al., 1989) or using, instead, a postsynaptic dopaminergic drug like amantadine (Gualtieri et al., 1989).

It remains the author's opinion that neuroleptics are contraindicated for the treatment of CDLS patients. Their clear pattern of affective instability puts them at high risk for serious neuroleptic side effects like tardive dyskinesia (Gualtieri et al., 1986c) and tardive akathisia (Barnes and Braude, 1985). It is entirely possible that many of the severe cases of SIB in CDL patients reported in the literature are cases of tardive akathisia.

There is also the null hypothesis, that for CDLS patients there is no effective drug and no medical treatment anyway, now or in the future, that will correct their underlying intensity and sensitivity. That may well be the case, but it should be set aside for now as a null hypothesis. It should not prevent the occasional trial of a pharmacological probe in a CDLS patient who is going through a particularly bad time. There is nothing wrong with experimenting with some of the new alternatives. Something may be found to work. If we can find such an agent, the next step will be a controlled clinical trial.

Until there is a pharmacological alternative, assuming there will ever be one, one has, for treatment, gentle forms of behavior management, developmentally appropriate programming, structure, stability, and family support. Those are the keystones for now. They are labor intensive, and frustrating sometimes, but they seem to work, and they have no side effects. One has the intuition that if we emphasize these several keystones, and if we avoid drugs with behavioral toxicity, aversive behavioral measures, and institutionalization, that long-term misbehavior will not be a problem in CDLS.

CHAPTER 9

Autism

The word autism describes a constellation of behavioral attributes that are really quite diverse. In fact, the borders are so obscure that no one can be sure where the center is. Beyond the definitions that are given for the syndrome, there is little one can say for autism as an homogeneous or a biologically meaningful disorder. One can speak, and some people do, about the "medical treatment" of autistic people, but that has not been an intelligent approach to the problem.

The intelligent question is what one proposes to treat with a psychotropic drug; not "autism," certainly. That target is simply too broad. It is appropriate, rather, to speak in terms of the behavior problems that arise in people who are autistic, and then about the treatments that are likely to be effective.

Autistic people are a diverse, heterogeneous group, whatever dimension one may choose to study. Autistic individuals vary widely in clinical presentation, developmental level, etiology, associated disorders, and prognosis. Autism may be genetic, or congenital, or acquired. If acquired, the cause may be infectious, traumatic, metabolic, structural, autoimmune, or something else. Onset is usually in early life, but that could be infancy, or early childhood, or later on. The children may be intellectually retarded or brilliant, or somewhere in between. They may have seizures or not, they may have behavior problems or not, they may be verbal or not. . .

There is no element that is universal to the syndrome, no irreducible factor, no single point of departure. The deficit in *communication* is hopelessly broad, and overlaps with other developmental dysphasias. The deficit in *relatedness* is the one element that is likely to improve when the child grows up (Wing, 1969; Wing and Gould, 1979). To understand autism with the idea of rendering treatment, one must appreciate its diversity, and disenthrall oneself from the idea that it is a unitary biological entity. There is only the autistic individual, with unique, individual requirements.

Parts of this chapter appear in substantially modified form in C. Thomas Gualtieri. Neuropsychiatric Treatment of Autistic People. Forum Medicum, Inc., 1990. Lesson Number Eight.

What Is Autism?

What we have traditionally referred to as autism may be understood, not in terms of definitions, which are limiting, but in terms of models, which are not limiting but heuristic. There are in the author's opinion two models that can shed light on the medical treatment of autistic people: One is from developmental medicine, and one is from experimental neuropsychology. The first addresses the diversity of the syndrome; the second, its specific features.

To build a model of understanding around a syndrome like autism, it is necessary to consider its *structure*; that is, how autism resembles other conditions in psychiatry and neurology, and how it differs; especially in terms of etiology, pathology, course, and response to treatment. In terms of the model from developmental medicine, it is suggested that the structure of autism is parallel, not to the "functional" psychiatric disorders, but to the structure of mental retardation.

The cause of the disorder is not always known, but when the cause is known, it is a genetic, metabolic, toxic, hypoxic, infectious, or autoimmune insult to the brain. The same etiological factors that may cause autism *cum* mental retardation in one individual may cause mental retardation *sans* autism in another.

The onset of the disorder is, like mental retardation, in infancy. The course is static, that is, not given to dramatic deterioration or improvement. Although autistic children are known to be extremely variable in behavior and cognitive performance, the course of the disorder is not ordinarily given to relapses and remissions, with intervening periods of normal function, as are most of the psychiatric disorders.

Autistic people are almost always mentally retarded. The severity of their disorder parallels the severity of the mental handicap, and prognosis is determined by the degree to which they are retarded, not the degree to which they are autistic (Bartak and Rutter, 1976). The prevalence of the disorder is highest in the most severely retarded. Not all autistic people are retarded, of course, but not all Down's syndrome people are retarded either, nor is everyone with the Lesch–Nyhan, or fragile X, or Cornelia de Lange syndromes.

In terms of the developmental model, autism is a static encephalopathy. The spectrum of severity is relative to the extent of the causative encephalopathic event. While there *may* be some unique neuropathic substrate to the syndrome, as we explain further on, it is probable that the identification of neuropathic lesions will correlate better with the degree of mental handicap than with the degree of autism.

The psychopharmacology of autism also resembles the psychopharmacology of mental retardation. There is no drug treatment for mental retardation but there are drugs to treat the psychiatric syndromes and target behaviors that occur in retarded individuals. The same is true for autistic individuals, as we shall describe.

In terms of etiology, neuropathology, course, and outcome, it is clear that autism has the structure of mental retardation. It is, then, a mental retardation *variant*, and this model accounts for the diversity of the syndrome. The second model, from experimental neuropsychology, allows one to account for its *uniqueness*. Autism, after all, may be a concept that is derivative from mental retardation, but it is not identical to it. It is therefore necessary to consider the source of its distinction. Is there a biological definition that is distinct?

The first possibility is a genetic definition. A cogent argument may stem from the twin study published by Folstein and Rutter in 1977, which generated a "permissive" hypothesis of autism. Folstein and Rutter described a proclivity to dyslexia and developmental dysphasia in the families of autistic children upon which was superimposed, in the afflicted individual, a neuropathic insult. It was the latter that caused mental handicap, but the former that evoked the unique phenotype of autism (Folstein and Rutter, 1977). The model is important, insofar as it describes an interaction between genetic proclivity and acquired lesion. But it does not suggest that autism is a "genetic" disorder, in the sense that it has an established pattern of Mendelian inheritance, or that is associated with a specific chromosomal abnormality, or a specific gene.

The potential for a neurochemical definition is less attractive. It is hard to fit autism to a unitary neurochemical model, because no one neurotransmitter system can be bent to explain all its various elements. The neurochemical correlate that has been described most frequently, elevated peripheral levels of serotonin (Hanley et al., 1977), says nothing about central serotonin metabolism in autistic brains. Further, in light of our understanding of the role of central serotonin neurotransmission, it is hard to reconcile the known functions of that system to the symptoms of autism (Meltzer and Lowy, 1987).

It is more likely that the unique features of autism are neuropathic in origin, rather than neurochemical or genetic. Current research has been oriented toward the interesting discovery that some autistic individuals show neuroradiographic evidence of cerebellar hypoplasia, and this is consistent with a newly developing appreciation of the role of cerebellum in a variety of cognitive functions, such as language, learning and memory, emotional behavior, and complex motivated behaviors (Murakami et al., 1989). It is difficult at this time to really appraise the importance of the finding, because the comparisons have been made to normal control subjects rather than to people with equal degrees of mental handicap. Thus it is hard to know whether the neuropathic finding is, in fact, specific to autism; and, if it is, whether it is a primary event, or an event that is secondary to a primary lesion elsewhere in the central nervous system (CNS) a manifestation of diaschisis.

The most cogent neuropathic model is from experimental neuropsychology, the Kluver–Bucy syndrome (KBS) (Kluver and Bucy, 1939). The KBS is a monkey preparation with interesting behavioral concomitants related to surgical resection of the temporal lobes, including the uncus, the amygdala, and the rostral hippocampus. It is described, at greater length, later in this chapter.

Autistic people do not exhibit all the characteristics of KBS monkeys, of course, such as hyperphagia, hypersexuality, and emotional indifference; but neither are the neuropathic events that lead to autism so precise or anatomic. KBS monkeys are amnestic, and this feature does not necessarily characterize autistic people. On the other hand, humans with acquired partial KBS are known to have severe communication deficits, short attention span, distractibility, and echopraxia, and these are typical symptoms of autistic patients. The KBS model is supported by neuropathological studies of autistic people that have demonstrated deep temporal lobe abnormalities (Hauser et al., 1975).

The KBS model is not particularly helpful in directing pharmacological intervention, although it is useful for the design of behavioral programs, as we explain. In terms of psychopharmacology, the deep nuclei of the temporal lobe and rostral limbic lobe are so richly endowed with a host of neurotransmitter systems that it is not possible to base an argument for treatment on one particular neurotransmitter. What guides the psychopharmacology of autism is not a specific model like KBS, but a broad overarching model like mental retardation.

The Psychopharmacology of Autism

Neuroleptics

The idea once was that autism was infantile schizophrenia, and that therefore it was necessary to treat autistic children with antipsychotic or neuroleptic drugs. Low-potency neuroleptics like chlorpromazine were found to be too sedating, but clinical trials of high-potency neuroleptics like trifluoperazine, fluphenazine, and thiothixene seemed to be promising: "psychotic behavior" and hyperactivity were decreased, stereotypies were reduced, speech production improved, attention spans were longer, anergic children had more initiative, and withdrawn children were more related (Wolpert et al., 1968; Fish et al., 1969; Campbell et al., 1972; Engelhardt et al., 1973). This dramatic response to antipsychotic drugs, of course, affirmed the connection between autism and schizophrenia.

Then haloperidol took center stage; it is the most potent neuroleptic, a virtually pure D2-dopamine receptor antagonist. Haloperidol was not only effective in controlling negative behaviors, but it was also said to improve discrimination learning (Anderson et al., 1984) and the positive effects of behavior therapy (Campbell et al., 1978).

Then the issue of tardive dyskinesia (TD) was raised, and it was discovered that about 25% of autistic children treated with haloperidol developed early forms of TD after only about 2 years of treatment (Perry et al., 1985). And then came the neuroleptic malignant syndrome (Guze and Baxter, 1985) and tardive akathisia (Barnes and Braude, 1985). Within only a few short years, the salience of neuroleptic drugs to the treatment of autistic people was zero.

No one is proposing "antipsychotic" treatment for autistic people any more, and, in our view neuroleptic treatment is relatively contraindicated for developmentally handicapped patients in general. There may be times when a severely disorganized autistic person will require a neuroleptic, at least for a brief trial, but modern neuropsychiatrists usually try to avoid such measures (Gualtieri, 1988), and with a small degree of ingenuity one can usually arrive at a better solution.

There is no *rationale* for neuroleptic treatment in autism. Autism is not kin to schizophrenia. There is no evidence for dopaminergic hyperactivity in autism beyond the occurrence of stereotypies, which are by no means unique to autistic people. Neuroleptics never have induced more than short-term symptomatic improvement. In a mentally handicapped individual, or in an autistic patient, behavior deterioration when the neuroleptic dose is lowered might just as likely be a manifestation of tardive akathisia as the reemergence of a "psychotic process."

At this time, neuroleptics are relatively contraindicated for autistic people, and neuroleptic prescription should be reserved for very special circumstances, and then should be time limited.

Megavitamins

There was never much of a rationale for "megavitamin" therapy, either, but it seemed to work, at least for a while, and on the face of things it is safer than haloperidol. Or is it? High doses of pyridoxine, the "natural substance" that is the therapeutic core of megavitamin therapy, have been reported to cause peripheral neuropathy (Schaumberg et al., 1983; Dalton and Dalton, 1987). Water-soluble vitamins are supposed to "pass right through," but they are by no means free of toxic side effects (Alhadeff et al., 1984).

There have been a number of open as well as controlled studies to show that megavitamin regimes with pyridoxine can reduce problem behaviors and increase adaptive behaviors in autistic children, as we describe later. But one's interest in megavitamin therapy would be greater if the effect were stronger; if there were reason to believe that it corrected the cognitive delay that is the most handicapping element of the autistic syndrome; if it served to alleviate some of the severe behavior problems that occur in autistic people; and if one could be assured of its long-term safety. The author has not been entirely satisfied on any of these points.

Fenfluramine

Because high levels of the neurotransmitter serotonin were supposed to characterize at least some autistic people, it was natural to investigate the clinical efficacy of the serotonin antagonist fenfluramine, a diet pill and an atypical stimulant. In this vein, there had been unsuccessful trials of L-dopa (Campbell et al., 1976) and of lysergic acid diethylamide (LSD), of all things (Bender 1966). (But not of periactin, for some reason.) What was interesting about the fenfluramine idea was how quickly an uncontrolled clinical report grew to become a multicenter study. Critical judgment was suspended, it appeared, in the face of a "rational" treatment for autism. Fenfluramine was even said to "double the IQ score" of one autistic child (Geller et al., 1982). That alone should have raised some doubts.

As additional studies were reported, it became clear that fenfluramine is not very effective at all in the "treatment" of autism, although symptomatic improvement may be seen in occasional cases. Whatever benefit fenfluramine exerts is independent of baseline serotonin levels, so the idea of a "rational treatment" has fallen by the boards.

There is preclinical evidence to suggest that fenfluramine may be neurotoxic (Schuster et al., 1985). Until this last issue is resolved, it should not be prescribed, on a chronic basis, to anyone.

Naltrexone

The discovery of the opioid receptor in mammalian brain led to some wide-ranging speculations about what exactly the opiate receptor was for (Snyder, 1977). A series of very interesting experiments in rats led Panskepp (1979) to hypothesize that endogenous opiates mediated the social bond. Love and opium, according to Panskepp, are both potent rewards, and terribly addicting.

A cute idea if not compelling. There is room for doubt, however, about some of the inferential leaps that followed. Because autistic people have a profound deficit in social relating, scientists thought that they might have high levels of endogenous opiates (Panskepp, 1979). These persons could not respond to the rewarding climate of the social bond, because they produced all the endogenous rewards they needed on their own; or so went the argument. Not a very convincing one, in the author's view, but sufficient to advance treatment studies with opiate antagonists.

A similar rationale has been developed around the origins of self-injurious behavior (SIB), which is a common problem, as it happens, among autistic children. Unfortunately, the results of initial trials of naltrexone, for example, in autism (Campbell et al., 1988) and in SIB (Herman et al., 1987) have been equivocal. Whether that is because naltrexone does not block the appropriate opioid receptor, or because of some weakness in the theory, one cannot say.

In any event, if past experience with haloperidol, pyridoxine, and fenfluramine is any guide to what will happen with naltrexone, one can expect to read a spate of double-blind studies to prove that it works. Then the "treatment" will be abandoned altogether.

Psychopharmacology for Autistic People

Every once in a while a discovery in brain science captures the imagination. The left and right Brain is an example; there seems to be no end to speculating over the ramifications of *that* arrangement. Well, the endogenous opiate system is another. It has been called on to explain behavioral phenomena from jogging (Carr et al., 1981) to schizophrenia (Watson et al., 1978) to falling out of love (Panskepp, 1979). But we have no more idea why Providence put it there than we understand why He (She) gave us two hemispheres.

Neither do we understand autism—that is, so long as we try to formulate the disorder in unitary terms. When we ignore the facts of the matter, autism is a mystery, given to the wildest speculations. If on the other hand we accept the structure of the disorder as a variant of mental retardation, the mystery is more amenable to solution. Autism is an encephalopathy with various causes. The lesions are probably dispersed among the deep nuclei of the temporal lobe, especially the amygdala, the septum, and other limbic nuclei, and in the frontal lobes. In contrast to mental retardation, the encephalopathy of autism is more circumscribed; in addition to bradyphrenia, there is disconnection. The lesions are variable in extent, which explains the wide range of cognitive dysfunction, and variable in location, which accounts for the diversity of its behavioral attributes.

Autism may coexist with other neuropsychiatric syndromes, like epilepsy, Tourette's syndrome, intermittent explosive disorder, major affective disorder, and schizophrenia; that should not be surprising. All the neuropsychiatric disorders are known to overlap, in some individuals: Tourette's patients may be obsessional; epileptics may be explosive or psychotic; schizophrenics get depressed. The ideal of clearly defined neuropsychiatric entities is counterintuitive. It is antiphysiological. The brain is a conglomerate organ system, composed of many organs that live close together and that are poorly insulated one from the effects of one another. An hypoxic or a viral insult to one small nucleus is likely to effect others nearby directly, or indirectly, through mechanisms like kindling (Post et al., 1982b), diaschisis, or reciprocal inhibition or activation (Moscovitch, 1979). The behavioral deficits that arise from such an insult will necessarily vary from person to person, and from time to time, even within an individual's lifespan. Thus, an autistic child who is hyperactive and disorganized might develop a seizure disorder in adolescence, an explosive disorder in adult life, and then a case of early dementia.

That would be an extremely unfortunate autistic person, to be sure, but it is an illustrative case. Illustrative of how the practically minded neuropsychiatrist has to think; not in terms of autism, but in terms of behavioral or neuropsychiatric correlates of autism.

If we acknowledge that autism is a consequence of relatively circumscribed lesions in the deep frontal, temporal, and limbic lobes, then we must also acknowledge that these areas receive the projections of a host of different neurotransmitter systems. Therefore, it is unrealistic to speak in terms of a unitary chemical dimension to autism, or of a single chemical treatment for all or even most autistic people. It is necessary to define a specific behavioral element or a specific neuropsychiatric disorder that requires attention in an autistic individual, and then to direct treatment to that specific issue.

It has been our practice to treat behavioral syndromes occurring in autistic people largely as we would treat similar problems in mentally retarded people or in closed head injury patients. This is how it is done.

Epilepsy

Seizure disorders occur in a fourth or a third of all autistic people (Deykin and MacMahon, 1979; Olsson et al., 1988). Epilepsy may begin in infancy or during adolescence. The strong association between autism and epilepsy is one more piece of evidence in favor of a neuropathic basis of the syndrome in the temporal and frontal lobes, because these regions are much more likely to seize than the cerebellum, for example. The association should also raise one's suspicion, when dealing with an autistic person who has severe behavior problems, that a psychotropic anticonvulsant may be the appropriate treatment.

The notion of "subclinical epilepsy" is too obscure to discuss in this chapter, but it is increasingly apparent that some nonspecific behavior disorders have a paroxysmal structure that resembles epilepsy, and that they may respond very well to antiepileptic drugs (Monroe, 1982). Intermittent explosive disorder, with aggression or with SIB or both, may be a manifestation of "subclinical epilepsy"; that is an arguable point. The fact that such patients respond to carbamazepine or valproate is not (McElroy et al., 1987; Evans et al., 1987a). Other clues to behavior disorders that respond to the psychotropic anticonvulsants are disorders with wildly variable shifts in mood or behavior, "rapid cyclers," nocturnal episodes, or extremely stereotyped behaviors. One sometimes hears the term organic affective disorder used to describe such patients. Much as one abhors such labels, that is not a bad one, because it comes attached to some useful treatment ideas.

On the other hand, one sometimes sees autistic patients who had seizures early in life, but who have been seizure free for many years, and off drugs. Such patients might be referred with behavior problems—aggressive behavior, for example, or SIB, or wildly variable mood and behavioral states. In these cases, it is usually a good idea to begin treatment with carbamazepine or valproic acid. The idea is that the behavior difficulties may be related, in an obscure way, to the same focus that at one time led to overt seizures.

Self-Injurious Behavior

SIB may be more common among autistic people than among retarded people in general, perhaps because of the unique frustration a communications-handicapped person has in dealing with the world. But SIB is a nonspecific symptom that does not differ in its presentation among autistic people from other mentally handicapped people who are not autistic. It may be constant (compulsive SIB) or intermittent (paroxysmal SIB) or occasional (episodic SIB). Neither is the topography of SIB different in autistic people, nor the treatment. As a rule, the therapeutic approach is the same as described in Chapter 8.

Aggression

The aggression differential diagnosis of aggressive behavior in autistic patients is not different from SIB, and it is the same as in mentally retarded patients who are not autistic. In fact, many patients have aggression and SIB, and the treatments also overlap.

It should come as no surprise that neuroleptics are not very effective for the long-term control of severe aggressive behavior in any patient group, save schizophrenics. The effective treatments are the psychotropic anticonvulsants (carbamazepine, valproate, acetazolamide), the beta blockers, and serotoninergic drugs like lithium. If aggression (or SIB) occurs in the context of hyperactive-disorganized behavior, the treatment options should follow the recommendations given below.

Obsessive-Compulsive Behavior

Some autistic people are given to compulsive behaviors, rituals, and recurrent thoughts or ruminations. This may be especially true of high-level autistic people who are verbal, and whose speech may return ever and again to the same topics and phrases, often with a metallic, dysprosodic voice. "Preoccupation with sameness" is another autistic symptom that is sometimes interpreted as an obsession. The neuropsychiatric basis of these symptoms is discussed at greater length in Chapter 7 (this volume).

In spite of a superficial symptomatic similarity, there is no convincing evidence that these clinical features are an autistic manifestation of obsessive-compulsive disorder. If they were, one would expect them to respond to serotonergic antidepressants like clomipramine or fluoxetine, and they usually do not; they seem to respond to structure and to behavioral programming.

If, on the other hand, compulsive behavior is a means to stem the anxiety that comes from a bewildering environment, as panic may be the consequence of interrupting a ritual, then treatment with a beta blocker is indicated. (In high-level autistic people with panic attacks, a tricyclic or a benzodiazepine may be considered).

Tourette's Syndrome

Tourette's syndrome (TS) is a syndrome of chronic motor tics and coprolalia that occurs in people of normal intelligence, but which has also been observed in mentally handicapped individuals. It is a disorder that is sensitive to treatment with dopamine antagonists like haloperidol or verapamil; the latter is also a calcium channel blocker, and a drug that may have therapeutic effects in a number of unusual psychiatric syndromes (Gualtieri, 1988). It is a disorder that may be accompanied by obsessions and compulsions, or that may lead to severe depression.

The problem with TS is the quality of the treatment relative to the severity of the symptoms. Doses of haloperidol that are necessary to control the tics are often sedating, or produce untoward extrapyramidal side effects. Verapamil is a good substitute, except, in our experience, in severe cases (Walsh et al., 1986). TS does not seem to cooccur with autism with any special frequency.

Abulia

The word abulia means "lack of will," but it really refers to something else, as we have described in Chapter 1 (this volume). Some autistic people seem to lack initiative and drive. They are content just to sit, and they have little inclination to involve themselves in activities or pastimes. When they do, it is without energy and enthusiasm. Their only verbal production (if they can talk) is to complain, to whine, or to demur.

This is an interesting problem, one we occasionally encounter in head injury patients with lesions of the frontal convexity. It is also observed in head injury patients with striatal lesions, and the similarity to a cardinal feature of Parkinson's disease is probably not accidental. That is because treatment with direct (postsynaptic) dopamine agonists like amantadine or bromocriptine can be very helpful, at least in some cases.

Catatonia is sometimes observed in mentally retarded people, and some of the symptoms of catatonia, including posturing, immobility, and waxy flexibility, can overlap with abulia. In psychiatric patients, catatonia is more often a symptom of affective disorder than of schizophrenia (Taylor and Abrams, 1977). It is interesting, however, that treatment of catatonia often includes antiparkinsonian drugs like amantadine (Baldessarini, 1977).

Affective Disorders

Do autistic people ever get depressed? In the sense of a melancholia, not the demoralization that comes of a lifetime of being misunderstood, or worse? Well, if they do, people have been reluctant to write about it.

We have seen autistic people who are prone to episodes of withdrawal and diminished interest in things; we have seen autistic people who are prone to episodes of severe emotional instability, and we have seen autistic people who appear to be manic. We have seen autistic people who might have organic affective disorders, both slow cyclers and rapid cyclers, and they have responded very well to conventional treatment with antidepressants, valproic acid, carbamazepine, and lithium. We have never encountered an autistic patient, however, who was genuinely melancholic.

Because there is no literature on antidepressant treatment for autistic people, one must be guided by the principles of treatment for other handicapped people with affective disorders (see Chapter 7, this volume). There is reason to believe that antidepressant drugs, as well as lithium, carbamazepine, and valproate, will increase in importance for autistic people with symptoms of affective disorder.

Anxiety, Agitation, and Panic

Anxiety and agitation are not uncommon symptoms in autistic children and adults. Anxiety is not a single thing, however, and one must learn to distinguish among its major variants:

1. Minor worry and repetitive questioning (perseveration)
2. Anxious rumination (obsessions)
3. Performance anxiety
4. Panic attacks
5. Disorganizing agitation of psychotic dimensions.

The treatment is really quite different, pharmacologically. States 1, 2, and 3 may be treated behaviorally or programmatically; the fourth and fifth states just listed usually require pharmacological intervention from the beginning.

It is unfortunate that more has not been written about the differential diagnosis of anxiety in autistic people; they may not be very prone to depression, but they clearly show a wide range of anxiety-related symptoms. Anxiety symptoms in autistic people may be spontaneous or related to circumstance. They may come in response to an unexpected change or to a demand that is impossible to satisfy. They may simply be pervasive and "endogenous."

It is hard to establish whether such individuals actually have what psychiatrists call a "panic disorder." In the past, most autistic patients who were anxious were said to be "psychotic" and were treated with neuroleptic drugs. That clearly ignores the complexity of the anxiety disorders, and the fact that specific treatments, with antidepressants, beta blockers, or the new anxiolytic buspirone, can be more rational, more effective, and much safer.

The major new advance in pharmacological management of autistic people is probably the use of beta blockers for patients whose behavior problems can be attributed to panic or anxiety. Autistic patients who are aggressive or self-injurious, or who tantrum when their routines are interrupted, may well be showing a form of panic disorder.

The other strong development is the discovery that buspirone may be useful in low-to-moderate doses for retarded people who are autistic, anxious, aggressive, self-injurious, or disorganized. Buspirone is a serotonin antagonist, a mixed dopamine agonist-antagonist, and an adrenergic drug. It has a favorable toxicity profile, compared to benzodiazepines and neuroleptics; it is not addicting, disinhibiting, or usually sedating (Ratey et al., 1988, in manuscript). It probably deserves a closer look as a potential treatment for autistic people with symptoms of anxiety.

Psychosis and Schizophrenia

We hardly ever use the term "psychotic" to describe the usual autistic symptoms (e.g., stereotypy, echolalia, self-stimulation, or sameness) or even the extremely disorganized behavior that characterizes some autistic children (see following). But the word is appropriate to apply to adults, especially high-level autists, who sometimes present with a manic or a schizophreniform psychosis and who may require the usual pharmacological management. We consider this to be the simple coexistence of two neuropsychiatric conditions; there is no evidence that autistic people are any more prone to schizophrenia, for example, than any other group of developmentally impaired people. On the other hand, schizophrenia may be overdiagnosed in autistic people with an affective psychosis or a severe panic disorder, because their difficulties in communication and relating may resemble at least some of the symptoms of schizophrenia.

In the diagnosis of severe psychiatric symptoms in developmentally handicapped individuals, schizophrenia should be considered to be a "default" diagnosis. It is usually a hard diagnosis to make; it often stigmatizing, and it carries no specific therapeutic recommendations. Neuroleptics, for example, are extremely toxic, and they are much more helpful for the "positive" symptoms (hallucinations, delusions, paranoia, agitation) than for the "negative" or deficit symptoms (withdrawal, anergia, problems with relating or communicating). In spite of this, as soon as the diagnosis is conferred physicians behave as if lifelong neuroleptic treatment were mandated.

It is always better to consider the alternative diagnoses when dealing with an autistic person who is clearly psychotic: brief reactive psychosis, affective psychosis, drug-induced psychosis, the psychosis of temporal lobe epilepsy, and the psychosis of dementia. With these alternatives come a very different treatment profile, and one that is usually more sanguine than neuroleptics.

Hyperactive or Disorganized Behavior

This is saved for last, because it is the hardest problem to solve, pharmacologically: hyperactivity, "into everything," hypermetamorphosis, impulsive behavior, distractibility and short attention span, self-stimulation and stereotypy, emotional lability, insomnia. This behavior pattern is most frequent in retarded autistic children, and has been in the past the occasion for treatment with neuroleptic drugs. That is a poor thing to do, but the problem is, what are the alternatives?

The answer is that there are quite a few alternatives, but they do not always work. Whether this is from the nature of the behavior disorder, or the age of the patient, one cannot say, although it is the author's suspicion that the latter is very important. It is not uncommon for hyperactive, disorganized autistic children to improve substantially as they grow up. Alternatively, their behavior problems may become more differentiated and thus more amenable to specific diagnosis and treatment.

The first approach is differential diagnosis: one looks for some entrée to treatment, much as one does for SIB, by examining the diagnostic alternatives: the possibility of an occult seizure disorder, of a panic disorder, or of a drug-induced syndrome; or by examining the treatment alternatives, by focusing on explosive-aggressive or self-injurious behavior. Thus, we have treated autistic children who were hyperactive and disorganized with psychotropic anticonvulsants, beta blockers, serotonin agonists, antihistamines, calcium channel blockers, and lithium.

Stimulant drugs like methylphenidate or amphetamine have no place in the treatment of hyperactivity in severely handicapped children. They usually are not helpful, and they may have behavioral toxicity, like agitation or disorganization. They are indirect dopamine agonists, in that they require an intact subcortical neuron to express a therapeutic effect.

We have found that direct (postsynaptic) dopamine agonists like amantadine and bromocriptine are preferable to stimulants in head injury patients who are agitated and disorganized (Chandler et al., 1988), and we have also found that they work well in selected cases of hyperactive, disorganized autistic children (Chandler and Gualtieri, in press). This may speak to the relevance of a postsynaptic agonist for the treatment of people with subcortical lesions, while presynaptic or indirect agonists would be preferable for higher level patients whose lesions are not so extensive but are confined to cortical tissue.

Our therapeutic confidence is higher when we meet an autistic patient who is older, and who has a more circumscribed behavioral disorder, than when we meet a young autistic patient who is hyperactive and disorganized. That is the bad news for parents and teachers. The high rate of tardive dyskinesia that occurs with neuroleptic treatment for such behavior is bad news for what has been the treatment of choice in the past.

When a problem is refractory to pharmacological intervention, like hyperactive disorganized behavior in autistic children, one must examine the source of difficulty. The psychology of the KBS would suggest that extreme degrees of exploratory behavior (hypermetamorphosis) are entirely expectable, indeed physiological, in an organism with profound derangements of sensory integration or memory. Thus, exploratory behavior would represent nothing more than a physiological compensation for a structural deficit. Treatments aimed simply at the motor aspect of that compensation, like the neuroleptics, will exercise only a limited effect. The direct-acting dopamine agonists are probably more physiological, because they are supposed to enhance cortical regulation of sensory and motor processes.

The KBS animals were also disorganized and hyperactive; a similar picture is sometimes observed during coma recovery, when head injury patients may also show signs of the KBS. Direct-acting dopamine agonists are quite helpful in the latter group, but their usefulness in developmentally handicapped patients is still an open question, although our preliminary experience is gratifying (Chandler and Gualtieri, in press).

Drug treatment, then, for hyperactive, disorganized autistic children will remain empirical—trial and error—for a while at least. That is not a satisfying conclusion, but it is more honest than trying to pretend that drug treatment for the autistic child is simply a question of finding the "magic key."

The Kluver-Bucy Syndrome

The Kluver–Bucy Syndrome (KBS) was first observed by Brown and Schafer in 1888 in a rhesus monkey after the removal of both temporal lobes. The monkey had been fierce and aggressive, but after the operation he was placid and indifferent. There were some other, peculiar behaviors:

> He no longer seemed to understand the meaning of sounds, sights, and other impressions that reached him. Every object with which he came into contact, even those with which he was previously most familiar, appeared strange and were investigated with curiosity. Everything he endeavored to feel, taste, and smell and to carefully examine from every point of view. Food was devoured greedily, the head being dipped into the dish, instead of the food being conveyed to the mouth by the hands in the way usual with monkeys. Memory and intelligence seemed deficient
>
> —*Brown and Schafer, 1888.*

These were the important elements of a syndrome that Heinrich Kluver and Paul Bucy described in 1937: profound emotional changes in the direction of a placid temperament, "psychic blindness" (Seelenblindheit), hypermetamorphosis (exploratory behavior), and strong oral tendencies. They added hypersexuality as a feature of the syndrome but they did not emphasize the loss of memory, an important element when the KBS occurs in human beings (Kluver and Bucy 1937, 1938, 1939).

Much has been made of the question whether a "pure" KBS does in fact occur in humans, although that is probably an irrelevant issue, because the KBS is a surgical preparation in laboratory monkeys. No surgical procedure in man is likely to be so mutilatory, and no pathological event is likely to be so surgical, as to convey the full range of KBS. But when extensive bilateral temporal lobectomies used to be done in human patients, with removal of the medial surface to include the amygdala and anterior hippocampus, virtually all elements of the KBS were observed (Terzian and Ore, 1955).

The effects of viral infections of the CNS, like herpes simplex encephalitis, may be localized to structures of the limbic cortices, owing perhaps to the unique antigenic property of the cells in that region (Levitt, 1984). Herpes simplex encephalitis is sometimes associated with sequelae that resemble the KBS (Esiri, 1982; Damasio and Van Hoesen, 1985; Bakchine et al., 1986). Cases of KBS have also been observed to follow brain trauma (Gerstenbrand 1983; Lilly et al., 1983), or toxic exposure (Sandson et al., 1988), or dementia (Lilly et al., 1983; Cummings and Duchen, 1981). KBS symptoms may be a transient correlate of coma recovery following traumatic brain injury (Gerstenbrand et al., 1983).

The KBS has been proposed as a paradigm for the study of cognition. It has been observed, for example, that bilateral amygdalectomy impairs the capacity of the organism to establish sensory cross-modal associations. The psychic blindness and hypermetamorphosis that characterize KBS is really a failure of information received on one channel to register in a meaningful way on other sensory channels (Murray and Mishkin, 1985). A failure in the capacity to form cross-modal associations creates the necessity for constant sensory stimulation, especially by the near receptors (taste, touch, and smell). This represents an attempt to strengthen the engram that would normally be reinforced by parallel sensory systems. The cross-modal failure also weakens the capacity of the organism to grasp the wider meaning of events beyond their capacity to stimulate one sensory channel.

The memory impairment of KBS is the consequence of bilateral (not unilateral) temporal lobe ablation (Scoville and Milner, 1957. Conjoint amygdaloid-hippocampal lesions are essential, it appears, to the development of dense amnesia (Mishkin, 1978; Zola-Morgan et al., 1982). It is instructive to consider precisely what kind of memory is lost as a consequence of such lesions.

Lesions on the medial surface of the temporal lobes are associated with loss of "declarative knowledge" but not "procedural knowledge" (Zola-Morgan et al., 1982). Declarative knowledge is the acquisition of new facts: what the name of a thing is, where it is hidden, and procedural learning is the acquisition of new skills or procedures: how to do something. In the classic experiment, the dense amnestic cannot learn a simple word list, but he can acquire the skill for mirror-writing.

This understanding of the psychology of the KBS may be an effective guide to behavioral and ecological treatment, for autistic patients, for example, and for brain injury patients during the phase of coma recovery. The fact that declarative memory is impossible following bilateral injury to amygdala and hippocampus suggests that behavioral treatments based on operant principles would tend to be minimally useful, while treatments that are based on the principles of classical conditioning should be the best way to proceed. Operant conditioning, or learning from contingencies or consequences, is analogous to declarative memory, and is therefore less suitable for the amnestic. Classical conditioning is based on the creation of associations by simple repetition; it is analogous to procedural learning, and is thus more suitable for the KBS patient.

The treatment of KBS patients would require, therefore, structure and sameness, repetition and familiarity. The use of contingency systems to cope with undesirable target behaviors would be less effective than proactive efforts to guide behavior into enduring and familiar channels or habits. The essence of the education of KBS patients should be in the acquisition of skills through constant repetition—or repetition as many times as their stamina and attention span can abide. Efforts should be made to minimize the occurrence of novelty. Untoward behaviors in the face of novel circumstances should be understood to represent a physiological, not a pathological, response. The capacity to learn from novel events is not a characteristic of amnestics.

The treatment of patients with severe traumatic brain injuries or with severe developmental disabilities is based on learning, or relearning. Learning in turn may be incremental, that is, based on the introduction of new material, or repetitious, based on the invariance of the exercise. In fact, most learning involves both elements. But for the sake of the paradigm, one should assume that the capacity for incremental learning requires an intact system for cross-modal association, and the functional anatomy of this system is in the nuclei of the medial temporal lobe. When this area has been damaged, or ablated, one is left with the capacity only for learning by repetition, only with the ability to acquire procedures.

The therapeutic environment of such patients should be based on ecology, not contingencies. It should be constructed like a finger exercise, and a finger exercise requires a keyboard that never changes. The expectation of flexibility is counter-therapeutic.

Understanding the psychology of KBS permits us to understand the meaning of certain symptoms, like hyperactivity. In the context of such profound cognitive deficits, hyperactive disorganized behavior, in young autistic children, for example, must be considered physiological, not pathological. One should assume a failure to develop channels of understanding, by virtue of short-term memory loss or cross-modal failure or both. There is a basic need to construct channels to bind and direct sensory input that the child is unable to satisfy. This in turn impedes the child's ability to inhibit behavior or to direct it in meaningful, consistent ways. The result is constant exploratory behavior. It is two things: in motive, a need to fill sensory channels that melt away even as they are formed; in result, a failure of behavioral direction along the course of such channels.

The KBS has not been nearly so useful a paradigm for psychopharmacologists. It has been suggested, for example, that carbamazepine, a "temporal lobe drug," may be effective in controlling the agitation and assaultive behavior that often occur in humans with KBS (Evans et al., 1987a). (The fact that many postcoma patients and autistic patients with KBS symptoms are far from placid affirms the notion that "pure" KBS is a rarity in clinical circumstances, and that the events that lead to destruction of medial temporal lobe structures are probably destructive to tissue in the frontal lobes and septum as well.) The pharmacological management of KBS variants in patients may begin with carbamazepine, and then the calcium channel blockers, but the author will hold out no great hopes for success. The wide swath of injury to brain regions endowed with multiple neurotransmitters militates against successful treatment for all or even most cases with any single drug. This is probably why, for example, it has proven impossible to develop a unitary pharmacological treatment for autistic individuals.

The neurochemical composition of the limbic cortices is rich and diverse, so it should come as no surprise that the practice of pharmacology is by no means advanced by Kluver's preparation. He was interested, after all, in the functional contributions of the brain structures that he asked Paul Bucy to excise. He was operating under the assumption that the method of finding out what a part of the brain does is to remove it and to see what happens. That was a good method for psychologists, but it is not particularly useful for psychopharmacologists.

Megavitamins

There is hardly a branch of psychiatry or of psychology that has not been oversold as a cure-all, or alternatively dismissed as quackery. That is an essential paradox to afflict any branch of the physical sciences that is not quite physical.

Psychotherapy, for example, is dismissed out of hand by people who say that it is not effective. Behavior modification, on the other hand, is in danger of proscription precisely because it *is* effective. The efficacy of psychiatric drugs can hardly be gainsaid, but there are people who claim they are effective only because they cause irreparable brain damage (Breggin, 1983). The IQ test is said to be instrumental only in damaging the course of young lives.

Such opinions seem to be unavoidable, and the intrinsic worth of the endeavor at hand seems to be irrelevant. They are the inevitable reaction, one must suppose, to the avowals of revolutionary significance that usually greet small advances in our field.

Even the giants of our profession have said or done foolish things. Charcot gave demonstrations of the neurological examination of hysterical patients. Skinner raised his infant daughter in a box. Gall, who was the one who really began the science of neuranatomic investigation, lapsed into phrenology. Carl Jung was the Shirley MacLaine of his time, and perhaps a Nazi as well. Wilhelm Reich was put into prison on a mail-fraud charge. And as for Freud, our generation will probably never agree whether he should stand with Charcot, who made one or two dreadful mistakes, or with Franz-Joseph Gall, whose legitimate scientific pursuits ultimately degenerated to a cultish fantasy.

There are two reasons why ours is a profession where quacks and mountebanks thrive. One is a prosaic reason, and the other is cosmic, so to speak.

The prosaic reason is this. There are no quacks around the treatment of gonorrhoea. There are no elaborate theories on the subject, either. There is only penicillin, and that works well enough, and there is no room for quackery. But for schizophrenia, or autism, or learning disabilities, or AIDS—anything that we cannot treat very well at all—well, these are fertile grounds for quackery.

The cosmic reason is like the existence of life on planets in distant galaxies. Any astronomer who can turn a phrase and who cherishes fame can promote a theory about life on planets in distant galaxies. And he can say anything he likes, because nobody can ever prove that what he is saying is wrong. The same is true for some of our psychological theories, especially theories of "personality development" or the psychodynamic origins of psychiatric disease. Say what you like, especially to patients; spin a good yarn, nobody can ever prove that what you are saying is wrong.

If you want to be a successful quack, pick an disease that is incurable. Better yet, pick one that will get better by itself. Or better yet, a disease that does not really exist at all.

Thus, patients with severe psychiatric illness and their families often fall prey to charlatans, or shall we say in kindness, sincere charlatans. And patients with very minor psychiatric disorders, or no psychiatric disorder at all, are treated ardently in hospitals and in private offices, especially if they have insurance. The treatments, of course, are justified in terms of theories about human nature and the course of psychiatric disease that are prosaic or cosmic or both. And often as not, it is hard to decide if the theories are sound or trifling, and if the treatments are worthwhile or trivial.

It is the same for developmentally handicapped children and for people who have sustained brain injuries. There is Doman-Delacato, for example, "patterning" treatment. There are injections with extracts of animal embryos. There is sea-sickness treatment for dyslexics. There are: vestibular stimulation, coma stimulation, sensory integration, perceptual training, cognitive remediation, and cranial electrostimulation. There are bioecology, food allergy, elimination diets, the Fiengold diet, and megavitamins.

This is not to suggest that the list of remedies is no more than a rendition of the absurd, because it is very hard to know if any proposed treatment is completely outré. A few years ago, for example, physicians were roundly criticized for treating patients with injections of vitamin B_{12}. In fact, this relatively innocent measure has largely fallen from favor. In 1988, however, it was suggested that patients with a wide range of nonspecific "neuropsychiatric disorders," including paraesthesia, ataxia, memory loss, weakness, hallucinations, fatigue, mood, and personality changes, responded favorably to injections of cobalamin (Lindenbaum et al., 1988). The strength of the argument was bolstered by serum assays of methylmalonic acid and homocysteine, which may be elevated in patients with subtle forms of B_{12}

deficiency, even in the face of a normal hemogram and serum cobalamin in the normal range (Marcell et al., 1985; Stabler et al., 1987). The weakness of the strategy, on the other hand, is the enormous expense of the two assays, which are by no means routine and run to several hundred dollars apiece. The price of a course of B_{12} is substantially less.

If one were to believe Lindenbaum's results, we should return to the old practice with B_{12} injections at the GP's office. In fact, Newbold (1989) proposed that physicians "test for vitamin B_{12} dependency disorders by giving trial injections of hydroxocobalamin" for the treatment of "many types of illnesses."

It must be very hard to tell the treasure from the dross, because dubious practices are, to this day, promoted from the loftiest seats of intellectual achievement. Within the span of only the past few years, one medical journal, a paragon of lucidity and Bostonian propriety, proposed laugh therapy for collagen-vascular disease, diet pills that double the IQ of autistic children, and an erudite review of the so-called borderline personality. Students at major universities spend vast sums of money and years of their lives to acquire the skills of the "neurodevelopmental examination" or of "play therapy" or of administering a "neuropsychological battery." They spend the rest of their careers passing these expenses on to their patients. An affliction with evaluations is an iatrogenic disease of handicapped people and their families.

Autism is a disorder that seems to be peculiarly vulnerable to the opinions of quacks and mountebanks. It fits the model perfectly, of course. It is extremely hard to treat, and even Itard threw up his hands after working with the Wild Boy of Aveyron for a number of years. On the other hand, it is a disorder that is occasionally given to spontaneous remission, and that gives rise to anecdotal reports of cures by psychoanalysis, parental devotion, fenfluramine, and megavitamins.

Autism was born with a theory that is, in retrospect, palpably absurd, the old notion of "refrigerator mothers." The most recent exposition on the subject, a wildly successful Hollywood production, actually maintained that institutionalization was the only proper recourse for high-level autistic people. In between, there has been every kind of gimcrackery, therapeutic and theoretical.

It hardly matters that psychiatry and psychology are laden with intellectual trinkets. That is not a new opinion, and it hardly deserves reiteration. It is more interesting to reflect that the orthodoxies themselves may be found to be spurious, on occasion, and that novel ideas of worth and merit may arise in the most curious places. Reading psychiatry with a view to learning about the brain is like reading Jules Verne to learn about space travel or nuclear submarines. Reading about the brain to try to understand the vagaries of human behavior is like reading a telephone directory. The first is interesting, if dated and inaccurate. The second is accurate, but dry, and it never really achieves the appropriate perspective. So, one should never feel inhibited from devoting some interest, at least, to ideas that are beyond the pale—for example, megavitamins.

The issue of "megavitamin therapy" for autism was first advanced by Rimland, who was drawn to the idea on the basis of correspondence with parents of autistic children from around the world. Many of them had suggested a role for vitamin treatment, and Rimland subsequently developed a megavitamin regime that emphasized treatment with vitamin B$_6$, pyridoxine. There appeared to be a positive response to this regime from patients he treated, by mail, from his unique vantage point at the Institute for Child Behavior Research in San Diego. Then there were a series of controlled studies that appeared to support his contentions (Rimland et al., 1978; Martineau, et al., 1981). Autistic children who were treated with pyridoxine, a multivitamin mix, and supplemental magnesium and calcium were observed to improve in a number of dimensions: they became more alert, attentive, and communicative, they were less irritable, hyperactive, and emotionally labile, and there was less self-stimulation, stereotypy, and self-injurious behavior.

It has been easy to dismiss megavitamin therapy as ineffective and ill advised, even in the face of Rimland's research, especially since reports of peripheral neuropathy following high-dose pyridoxine appeared (Schaumburg et al., 1983). There had been earlier claims for megavitamin treatment of schizophrenia (e.g., Pauling, 1974), and a round controversy over that idea. A task force of the American Psychiatric Association concluded that vitamin treatment was not helpful (APA, 1973). There have also been claims that vitamins and dietary supplements prevent tardive dyskinesia in schizophrenic patients (Tkacz and Hawkins, 1981); that they improve symptoms of childhood hyperactivity (Coleman et al., 1979); that they improve intelligence, growth, and myopia in mentally retarded children (Harrell et al., 1981) and that they improve psychosis in children with the fragile X syndrome (Lejeune et al., 1981). None of these "findings" have stood up to replication; therefore the autism data should also be discounted.

We made one clinical trial of the megavitamin treatment for autistic children. The results were not impressive, but there were a few patients (6 of 15) who seemed to improve: less moody, less hyperactive, fewer tantrums, more attentive, more play, increased appetite, decreased self-stimulation, increased spontaneous speech, more cooperation, and improved general health (Gualtieri et al., 1981). Of course, any degree of improvement in patients at the Neuropsychiatry Clinic should be applauded. Our patients have always been a singularly truculent lot, refusing to respond to the treatments handed down by the luminaries, and probably out of spite. When we did a study of piracetam, the "no-otropic" drug for dyslexic children, ours was the only site, of five, where the placebo treatment actually worked better than piracetam (Evans 1986). Our attention deficit disorder (ADD) adults never responded to stimulants quite so dramatically as Paul Wender said that they did (Gualtieri et al., 1985), and we never found that methylphenidate blood levels corresponded to anything at all (Gualtieri et al., 1984). We seemed to have an "institute of negative results" for a while, a problem one may attribute, in retrospect, either to the singular clarity of our vision or alternatively to the mulish stubbornness of our patients.

So, the fact that some of the autistic children actually improved at least to a degree when they were treated with pyridoxine, and the fact that virtually every other study that has addressed the issue has had the same result, leads one to suspect that there may be gold, not dross, somewhere. Perhaps it would be worthwhile to pick it up and begin again.

It is not outlandish to propose that some aspect of vitamin therapy might be beneficial to developmentally handicapped people. There are other conditions, for example, that seem to respond favorably to pyridoxine. There are so many such conditions, in fact, that may respond favorably to vitamin B$_6$ that one smells a rat. But perhaps there is a common thread.

Pyridoxine dependency is a rare cause of infantile convulsions. Seizures respond well to pyridoxine administration and recur when supplementation is interrupted. The seizures probably result from depletion of the inhibitory neurotransmitter gamma-amino butyric acid (GABA), which is produced when the holoenzyme— glutamic acid decarboxylase (apoenzyme) plus pyridoxal phosphate (cofactor)— acts on glutamic acid (Rudman and Williams, 1983). Early treatment is necessary to prevent mental retardation, and B$_6$ supplementation must be continued indefinitely (Goutieres and Aicardi, 1985). Pyridoxine-dependent seizures are classified among the six pyridoxine-responsive genetic diseases (pyridoxine-responsive anemia, homocystinuria, cystathioninuria, hyperoxaluria, xanthurenicaciduria) (Mudd, 1971).

Isoniazid treatment is sometimes associated with niacin deficiency, or pellagra (Ishii and Nishihara, 1985). However, Brenner and Wapnir (1978) described a well-documented case of pyridoxine-dependent hyperactivity, irritability, and insomnia in a 3-year-old girl who had been treated with isoniazid. The child's blood level of pyridoxal phosphate was normal. However, the activity of enzymes along the kynurenine pathway appeared to be depressed, and tryptophan excretion following a tryptophan load decreased after treatment with pyridoxine. The metabolism of serotonin therefore seemed to be depressed, a consequence of drug-induced pyridoxine deficiency; presumably this was the neurochemical basis of her behavioral difficulties.

The serotonin hypothesis was supported by Coleman et al. (1979) who treated several hyperactive children with pyridoxine, and noted an improvement in behavior and an attendant increase in whole-blood serotonin levels. Pyridoxine is, after all, the cofactor for the l-aromatic amino acid decarboxylases that metabolize serotonin from tryptophan, and norepinephrine and dopamine from tyrosine and phenylalanine. A deficiency in B$_6$ will therefore impair the manufacture of monoamine neurotransmitters. Supplementation with B$_6$ could conceivably increase the functional availability of the monoamines.

A functional manifestation of the effects of pyridoxine on neurotransmitter metabolism is the effect on exercise-induced prolactin and growth hormone secretion. In normal volunteers, 600 mg of pyridoxine administered intravenously suppressed the rise in prolactin and enhanced exercise-induced growth hormone secretion, a dopaminergic effect (Moretti et al., 1982).

Estrogens and other steroid hormones compete with pyridoxal phosphate for binding sites and cause a redistribution of the cofactor among apoenzymes. By stimulating the activity of hepatic tryptophan oxygenase, high estrogen levels, for example in pregnancy or in women taking oral contraceptives, might increase the dietary requirement for vitamin B$_6$. Pyridoxine supplementation has been prescribed for symptoms of depression and irritability in women who are pregnant, or who take Oral Contraceptive Pills (OCP) (Brin, 1971; Leeton, 1974). Pyridoxine is also used to treat symptoms of the premenstrual syndrome (PMS) (Williams et al., 1985).

One may use the simple and sensitive measure of pyridoxine status, the assay of the vitamin-dependent red cell enzyme aspartate transaminase (or transketolase for thiamine or glutathione reductase for riboflavin), which are relatively stable and insensitive to the short-term effects of medication and diet (Carney et al., 1979). When such tests are administered to psychiatric patients, one may find evidence of impaired B6 metabolism, especially in postpartum depressives (Carney et al, 1979). [This observation, however, has not been affirmed by other researchers (Livingston et al., 1978).]

The neurological symptoms of pyridoxine deficiency include ataxia, irritability, depression, somnolence, diminished alertness, seizures, and abnormal head movements. Patients who are treated with pyridoxine may, paradoxically, *develop* symptoms of irritability or insomnia or aggressiveness (Gualtieri et al., 1981; Williams et al., 1985).

Patients treated with high doses of B6 may be prone to develop a peripheral neuropathy (Schaumburg et al., 1983). That has been attributed to the *neurotoxic* effects of pyridoxine, exercised selectively on the peripheral nervous system by virtue of limited passage across the blood–brain barrier; or the saturation of pyridoxal phosphate binding sites by biologically inactive pyridoxine; or some other element (Rudman and Williams, 1983). That, too, is at variance with reports of pyridoxine treatment for carpal tunnel syndrome and entrapment neuropathy (Ellis et al., 1976), a finding that has also been replicated, and that has also failed of replication (Scheyer and Haas, 1985).

Megavitaminists criticized the work of Schaumburg et al. (1983) on the basis of the extraordinary high doses of pyridoxine that were found to be associated with progressive sensory ataxia and profound distal limb impairment of position and vibration sense. The doses, they said, were far beyond the doses that they recommended (2–6 gm/day versus 250–750 mg/day). But there is also a report of neurotoxicity (paraesthesia, hyperaesthesia, bone pains, muscle weakness, numbness, and fasciculations) in women treated for premenstrual syndrome (PMS) with B6 in low doses (mean, 117 mg/day) for a prolonged period of time (2.9 years) (Dalton and Dalton, 1987). Pyridoxine-induced neuropathy, however, may be a function of secondary foliate deficiency (Wilcken and Turner, 1973), and the megavitamin people usually recommend supplemental B vitamins, foliate and magnesium, with the pyridoxine. Nevertheless, the risk of a low-dose pyridoxine neuropathy is disturbing. It suggests that no one should be treated with B6 without careful and enlightened medical follow-up.

It is ironic that the problem of toxicity should be the limiting factor in the development of a therapeutic use for one of the water-soluble vitamins, because they have always been advanced as "natural" treatments, free of side effects (Alhadeff et al., 1984). Nevertheless, there appears to be some clinical use for pharmacological doses of vitamin B6 with appropriate supplementation, at least for PMS and for mild depressions associated with pregnancy or oral contraceptive use.

The proper approach to vitamin therapy, from the point of view of medical orthodoxy, is the definition of specific pyridoxine-sensitive syndromes. It is clear that pyridoxine is not effective for epilepsy, but it is the treatment of choice for pyridoxine-dependent epilepsy. It is not an effective antidepressant, but it is the treatment of choice for mild depressions that stem from secondary pyridoxine deficiencies in patients who are pregnant or who take OCP. Pyridoxine is not a treatment for autism. Is it possible that there are pyridoxine-sensitive patients who are also autistic?

But it takes a long while before a pyridoxine-sensitive syndrome enters the literature, especially because most of the good neurochemists are into recombinant DNA these days. If we were to wait for the chemical definition of new syndromes to justify treatment interventions, we might all become therapeutic nihilists, and we might lose the opportunity to investigate promising treatments. The fact is that pyridoxine is, in theory at least, a monoaminergic drug. It is also GABAergic, and it regulates the metabolism of sphingosine, nicotinic acid, and the sulfur-containing amino acids.

One has the intuition that there are pyridoxine-sensitive mental patients; one only has to intuit who they are. They are probably people with problems with irritability, affective instability, depression, aggression, and self-mutilation. They may be overrepresented among the developmentally handicapped, because early, diffuse injury to developing brain structures might be expected to disrupt the development of neuromodulatory transmitter systems like GABA and the monoamines.

The argument against vitamin therapy is that dietary supplementation has no functional impact on metabolism of neurotransmitters because the availability of coenzymes is never the rate-limiting step, except in the face of a clear deficiency. So, the fact that pyridoxine is the agent of a particular neurochemical reaction does not mean that it will exercise a therapeutic effect at that locus. On the other hand, it might, and that is the rationale for megavitamin therapy.

It is not quackery. If it is, it is sincere quackery. It is something that deserves some scrutiny. Compounds that exercise potential effects on neurotransmitter metabolism always deserve a second look.

CHAPTER 10

Tardive Dyskinesia

The first report of tardive dyskinesia (TD) in mentally retarded people treated with long-term neuroleptics was published in 1975 (Paulson et al., 1975), and there were several subsequent reports over the next few years (Gualtieri and Hawk, 1980; Kalachnik et al., 1984). This was about 20 years after the disorder was first described by European psychiatrists (Schonecker, 1957; Uhrbrand and Faurbye, 1960), but it was contemporary with the development of serious concern about TD among American psychiatrists.

It was not until the publication of the American Psychiatric Association Task Force Report in 1979 that the weight of medical concern was directed to the problem of TD, even for the mentally ill. It was not until 5 years later that the problem gained widespread publicity, lawsuits began to multiply, and the second APA Task Force on Tardive Dyskinesia was assembled. Since then, the problem of TD has become a major issue for physicians who treat chronic patients, for administrators and makers of public policy, and for research scientists in psychiatry and neuropharmacology. The development of an antipsychotic drug that does not cause TD is a prime area of psychopharmacological research, an effort that has not met with notable success to date, clozapine notwithstanding.

It is possible that recognition of TD as a serious, potentially debilitating side effect of neuroleptic treatment has been responsible for the dramatic decrease in neuroleptic prescription in retarded people (Gualtieri and Barnhill, 1988), although other factors have probably played a more central role: the community movement, deemphasis of the medical model, renewed emphasis on behavioral and developmental programming, and new attention to alternative pharmacological treatments. Nevertheless, the problem of TD has been the red flag around which adherents have rallied to reduce the unnecessary prescription of neuroleptic drugs and to improve neuropsychiatric care for retarded people.

In 1968, the national rate of neuroleptic prescription to retarded people was about 50% (Lipmann 1970) and in 1978 (Sprague and Baxley, 1978). It fell to about 30% in 1985 (Hill et al., 1983), based on surveys of institutionalized people. However, TD remains a serious problem, because substantial numbers of retarded people continue to be treated with neuroleptics, and movement of retarded people from institutions into the community is often associated with an increase in neuroleptic prescription. TD is also a problem because the disorder itself is complex and confusing, and there is still a great deal to learn about it.

The enlightened view of TD in mental retardation is that it is a major hazard to the public health. It is widely believed that neuroleptic drugs are relatively contraindicated in retarded people, just as their long-term use is relatively contraindicated in children, brain injury patients, and the elderly. When neuroleptic prescription is considered, the treatment decision must be made with great care; formal TD monitoring systems are essential to quality care. Drug withdrawal trials or gradual dose reductions should be undertaken at appropriate intervals to test for occult or covert TD and to determine whether continued drug treatment is necessary. It is accepted opinion that any patient whose behavior problems are so severe as to warrant neuroleptic prescription should have a concomitant behavioral program with longitudinal behavior analysis.

The Prevalence of Serious Neuroleptic Side Effects

Tardive Dyskinesia

Estimates of TD prevalence published in the psychiatric literature have varied wildly in the past, largely as a consequence of idiosyncrasies in measurement and definition. The "average prevalence" of TD based on 33 studies reported from 1970 to 1979 was 24% (Kane and Smith, 1982). This is the figure psychiatrists seem to prefer, for example, when they are talking to medical students or to families. But the true rate varied, depending on the clinical population: from 12% among outpatients in a Veterans Administration clinic, to 13% in an acute psychiatric hospital, to 36% in a state hospital, to 67% among state hospital patients over 65 years old. The cumulative incidence of TD in psychiatric patients is said to be about 5% at 1 year, 10% at 2 years, 15% at 3 years, and 19% at 4 years (APA, 1991). There is said to be a 40% cumulative rate of TD in adult psychiatric patients after 8 years of exposure to neuroleptics (Saltz et al., 1989).

One important aspect of the TD problem, and one that is important to reiterate, is that maintenance neuroleptic treatment may mask the presence of the disorder. Therefore, any prevalence estimate will necessarily be influenced by the patient's medication status. A true prevalence rate can only be determined from the study of drug-free patients. In one survey of psychiatric patients on neuroleptics that were without signs of TD, new signs of TD emerged in no fewer than 34% when they were subsequently withdrawn from neuroleptics (APA, 1991).

There have been three survey reports of TD prevalence in mentally retarded populations, all conducted in residential facilities. In the study by Paulson et al. (1975), the prevalence was 20%. In the study by Gualtieri et al. (1986c), the prevalence of persistent TD was 34% and the prevalence of transient withdrawal dyskinesia was 29%. In the study by Kalachnik et al. (1984), the prevalence of TD was 45%. The latter two studies evaluated patients after neuroleptic withdrawal; in the first (Paulson et al., 1975), patients were examined who were currently on neuroleptic drugs, so the 20% figure is likely to be an underestimate. The TMS (computer monitoring system for TD, see below) data presented toward the end of this chapter agree with the 45% rate of Kalachnik et al. (1984).

One cannot argue that the estimate of TD occurrence in retarded people is inflated because they are given to a wide range of abnormal movements, even in the absence of neuroleptic treatment. The assessment of dyskinetic movements in severe to profoundly retarded people may be problematic, because the patients may not cooperate with the examination procedure. On the other hand, Gualtieri et al. (1986c) reported acceptable interrater reliability data using the AIMS exam in this population, and the study by Kalachnik et al. (1984) actually arrived at its prevalence rate by subtracting the basal rate of dyskinesia in drug-free controls.

In a unique prospective study of haloperidol treatment for autistic children, most of whom were mentally retarded, the incidence of TD after 6 to 30 months follow-up was 25% (Perry et al., 1985). The dyskinesias that arose were transient, however, as one might expect in young patients treated with low doses of neuroleptic for a relatively short period of time. On the other hand, the fact that an early form of TD arose in *one-fourth* of treated patients means, to the authors at least, that neuroleptics are relatively *contraindicated* in this group.

In the face of such extraordinary figures, one is compelled to warn patients on long-term neuroleptics that the development of TD is a likely event. On the other hand, it is also appropriate to assure patients that TD can be prevented by judicious use of neuroleptic drugs and by careful and knowledgeable medical supervision. After all, the highest rates of TD are found in public institutions for the mentally ill and the mentally handicapped, where drugs have been used in lieu of programming and where medical supervision is sometimes less than optimal. If neuropsychiatric care is available, neuroleptics can be used in low-to-moderate doses and for a sustained period of time, and the level of risk is probably acceptable—assuming, of course, that the drugs are only prescribed for the most severe and debilitating behavioral disorders.

The issue of TD prevalence rates obscures a more important issue, the requirement to distinguish between the prevalence of severe and debilitating cases of TD and the prevalence of relatively mild cases, between persistent cases and cases that will only last a few months or a year or two. Prevalence rates from 25% to 33% should ordinarily be cause for alarm. But if only a few of those cases are severe and persistent, and if most are mild or self-limiting, then the problem is manageable. If severe cases can be prevented by careful monitoring, then physicians will have the right to reassure patients and their families.

On the other hand, if severe and persistent cases comprise a significant fraction of the population of TD patients, then draconian measures will be required to reduce neuroleptic prescription. Most psychiatrists would say that severe cases are only a small minority of TD patients, and we have never argued with that contention. But when the issue is put to the test, severe TD variants have been observed in more than one-fifth of all diagnosed TD cases (Davis and Cummings, 1988)

Tardive Dyskinesia Variants

"Classic" TD refers to irregular choreoathetoid movements occurring predominantly in the buccal-lingual-masticatory (BLM) musculature and the distal extremities. It is the most common manifestation of the syndrome (93% of TD cases). Tardive dystonia is characterized by sustained contractions of skeletal musculature; it has been found to account for 26% of all TD cases referred to a movement disorder clinic. (Tardive dystonia is discussed further under the heading "Malignant Tardive Dyskinesia.") Tardive akathisia is also discussed later; it is estimated to comprise 18% of TD cases. Tardive Tourette's syndrome is characterized by motor and phonic tics (5% of cases) (Davis and Cummings, 1988).

Extrapyramidal Reactions

TD is a late extrapyramidal syndrome associated with neuroleptic treatment, as distinguished from the early extrapyramidal symptoms, or "EPS." These, of course, are pseudo-parkinsonism, acute dystonia, and akathisia. Acute EPS are sometimes quite severe, but they are time limited, and are easily treated by reducing the neuroleptic dose, by trying an alternative neuroleptic, or by prescribing an anticholinergic or amantadine (for pseudoparkinsonism), diphenhydramine (for dystonia), or propanalol (for akathisia). The EPS are common side effects, especially when high doses are prescribed.

Acute EPS can be a major problem if the treating physician is not alert to their sometimes subtle manifestations. This is frequently the case with neuroleptic-induced akathisia. The symptoms of akathisia can be subtle, and may be easily confused with some of the target behaviors for which the neuroleptic drugs are prescribed to begin with: restlessness, irritability, fidgeting movements, pacing, dysphoria, and an inability to sit still. The prevalence of akathisia is usually set at about 20% of neuroleptic-treated patients, although more recent studies have indicated much higher prevalence rates (Barnes and Braude, 1985).

Even the structure of neuroleptic-induced akathisia is different from other acute EPS. It does not respond well to anticholinergic treatment, it is likely to appear late in the course of treatment, and it may be a prodrome or an early manifestation of TD (Barnes and Braude, 1985). In fact, tardive akathisia, which can persist after neuroleptic withdrawal, is a particularly troublesome variant of the TD syndrome (Munetz and Cornes, 1983; Stahl, 1985).

Other little-known EPS include akinesia (Rifkin et al., 1975) and aphonia (Behrman, 1972). Neuroleptic-induced EPS are at least as common in mentally retarded people as in other patient groups (Carter, 1983).

Neuroleptic Malignant Syndrome

Neuroleptic malignant syndrome (NMS) is a devastating, sometimes fatal neuroleptic side effect arising early in treatment, especially with high-potency drugs. The symptoms are muscular ("lead-pipe") rigidity, mental state changes (e.g., delirium), and autonomic changes (hyperthermia, hypertension, tachycardia), accompanied by elevation of the whole blood cell count (WBCC) and the serum creatine phosphokinase (CPK). If the disorder is not recognized promptly, and if proper treatment measures are not instituted immediately, the patient may die of renal failure. Treatment is neuroleptic withdrawal, fluid replacement, and dantrolene or dopamine agonists (e.g., bromocriptine). It is said that NMS occurs in 1% to 2% of neuroleptic-treated patients and that 10% to 20% of cases are fatal (Keck et al., 1987). That estimate is probably too high to be true, but there is no denying that increased familiarity with this extraordinary syndrome leads to increased recognition.

Although NMS is most likely to occur early in treatment, it may arise at any point, even when the patient is on a stable maintenance dose (Guze and Baxter, 1985). Risk factors include a state of psychomotor agitation before neuroleptic treatment, high doses of neuroleptics that are increased rapidly, and intramuscular administration (Keck et al., 1989). Other risk factors are the use of high-potency neuroleptics, and patient-related variables, such as a dehydrated or physically exhausted state or a previous history of neuroleptic toxicity. It is incredible that a side effect so severe, and presumably so common, went unrecognized for so many years (Levenson, 1985).

NMS is a major problem for nursing personnel, because the key to successful treatment is early recognition and a high index of suspicion. Any neuroleptic-treated patient with rigidity and mental state changes should be reported to the attending physician immediately as a medical emergency, and neuroleptics should be withheld until an examination can be done and the appropriate laboratory tests can be drawn. The fact of NMS requires special training for nurses who tend to neuroleptic-treated patients, and, naturally, careful monitoring by physicians who are familiar with the syndrome. NMS, more than any movement disorder, has spelled the future of neuroleptic treatment; neuroleptics are not routine treatments to be administered by primary care physicians with no special training in psychopharmacology.

Tardive Akathisia

Akathisia is taken from the Greek word that means "not to sit still." I don't know why the Greeks happen to have a word that means "not to sit still."

Akathisia is a syndrome of intense restlessness and dysphoria that is encountered in Parkinson's disease, or following traumatic brain injury (TBI), or as a consequence of drug treatment. Acute akathisia is a side effect of neuroleptic treatment, but it may also occur with antidepressants.

Tardive akathisia (TDAK) refers to a variant of TD that is entirely behavioral, characterized by extreme motor restlessness and dysphoria. It is a "tardive" side effect because it comes on late in the course of treatment, as does TD. The symptoms may arise on maintenance doses, or when the dose is lowered, or after neuroleptics are discontinued. They usually persist for a long time after neuroleptics are withdrawn.

People with akathisia are miserable. They feel as if they were crawling out of their skin, and they have to pace constantly just to win a small degree of relief. They are irritable, unhappy, and emotionally unstable. They are so unhappy, and they find it so hard to understand what is happening to them, that they may erupt in explosions of aggressive, destructive, or self-injurious behavior. They may be described as hyperactive, disorganized, or psychotic. In other words, they may develop, as a consequence of long-term neuroleptic treatment, irreversible symptoms that are identical to the problem behaviors for which neuroleptics were originally prescribed.

The term *akathisia* was coined by Haskovec in 1902 (Haskovec, 1902, 1903; Barnes and Braude, 1985). Bing adopted the term during the 1920s to refer to the "muscular impatience" that was associated with Parkinson's disease and other disorders of the basal ganglia (Bing, 1939; Stahl, 1985). Ekbom described restless movements of the legs that might arise spontaneously in some people [Ekbom's or "restless legs syndrome" (RLS)] (Ekbom, 1944); RLS may also be an akathisia variant.

In 1954, the term was applied to symptoms of motor restlessness resulting from treatment with neuroleptic drugs (Steck, 1954). The prevalence of neuroleptic-induced akathisia has been estimated at about 20%, although the figure may range as high as 45% (Barnes and Braude, 1985). Akathisia may arise early in the course of neuroleptic treatment, when it is considered to be one of the acute extrapyramidal syndromes (EPS); or it may arise late in the course of treatment, when it may coexist with tardive dyskinesia. Simpson (1977) described late-onset akathisia, frequently associated with tardive dyskinesia, as "virtually untreatable."

The connection between akathisia and tardive dyskinesia is not entirely clear. It is thought that early akathisia may predispose to TD, or that akathisia may evolve into TD, or that "tardive akathisia" may be a variant of the TD syndrome, just as tardive dystonia is a TD variant (Munetz and Cornes, 1983). More recent publications seem to accept the idea of tardive akathisia (Barnes and Braude 1985; Stahl, 1985) as a TD variant, as a purely behavioral manifestation of neuroleptic toxicity.

Akathisia, then, refers to an early side effect of neuroleptic treatment, and its structure is that of the other acute extrapyramidal side effects, pseudo-parkinsonism and dystonia. It remits when the neuroleptic dose is lowered or when neuroleptics are discontinued, and it may be treated successfully with beta blockers or with other drugs (but usually not anticholinergics). Tardive akathisia is a late-onset manifestation of neuroleptic toxicity, and it has the structure of TD: It gets worse when the dose is lowered, it may persist after the drugs are withdrawn entirely, and it is not very responsive to drug treatment.

The treatment of akathisia, acute or tardive, is with beta blockers (Yassa et al., 1988a; Ratey et al., 1985; Lipinski et al., 1984) or with clonidine (Adler et al., 1987b; Zubenko et al., 1984a). The frequent success of such drugs in the treatment of akathisia suggests an effect of chronic neuroleptic blockade on noradrenergic neurotransmission. Neuroleptics are known to increase cerebrospinal fluid (CSF) and brain levels of norepinephrine; the mechanism may be presynaptic dopamine blockade, a neuroleptic effect that has been determined to increase norepinephrine release, at least in laboratory animals (De Keyser et al., 1987).

Lorazepam or clonazepam may also be used, with only occasional success; benzodiazepines may even be used in conjunction with beta blockers. There have been reports of successful treatment with codeine and propoxyphene (Walters et al., 1986), that we have been unable to confirm, and with buspirone (D'Mello et al., 1989), which we have. Another possible treatment is amantadine (Borison and Diamond, 1984).

As in severe cases of TD, the only effective treatment may well be reinstitution of neuroleptics, especially atypical neuroleptics like molindone, thioridazine, or clozapine, and then a very gradual withdrawal over time. Such a withdrawal may be "covered" with simultaneous treatment with beta blockers or clonazepam.

For a long time, we had been concerned with the possibility of a behavioral analogue of TD (Gualtieri and Guimond, 1981). It was reasonable to believe that a syndrome of abnormal involuntary movements that arose from irreversible damage to neurons in the corpus striatum would also have behavioral and neuropsychological concomitants. After all, other diseases of the striatum, like Parkinson's and Huntington's, are accompanied by severe psychological symptoms; and virtually every study that has addressed the issue has discovered neuropsychological impairments in patients with tardive dyskinesia (Gualtieri and Barnhill, 1988). The problem was in proving the point. When one was looking at a population of patients with severe cognitive and behavioral impairments to begin with, how could one possibly demonstrate that neuroleptics, over the long term, made things worse?

The issue is by no means settled, but a consensus is growing around the idea of tardive akathisia that never really developed around the ideas of "supersensitivity psychosis" or "tardive dysmentia." But that is all we have: clinical consensus, not unequivocal proof that there is such a thing as tardive akathisia.

Nevertheless, when we became familiar with the idea, we grew convinced of its validity, and we found that it could explain many difficult clinical situations encountered in our practice with mentally retarded people. Patients, for example, who really never responded very well to neuroleptics to begin with, but who grew much worse after they were withdrawn. Patients whose behavior deteriorated sharply after their neuroleptic dose was lowered beyond a certain point, but who remained difficult and uncontrollable even after the dose was returned to what had earlier been a therapeutic level. Patients whose symptoms of TD were accompanied by high levels of hyperactivity and restlessness, who were extremely dysphoric when neuroleptics were withdrawn, and who never could be treated effectively with any pharmacological agent.

Our conviction that tardive akathisia was a real issue has been supported by clinical observations in our neuropsychiatry practice in North Carolina, and by consultations at residential facilities in Tennessee, Louisiana, Colorado, California, and Idaho. It seemed that the association of motor restlessness (independent of dyskinesia) and dysphoria was very common in retarded patients after long-term neuroleptic treatment. Most of the time, these symptoms were accompanied by dyskinetic movements characteristic of TD, but in some cases they arose in the absence of dyskinesia. In our surveys, the prevalence of tardive akathisia was no less than 14% of all retarded patients treated with longterm neuroleptics (Gualtieri, 1990). These numbers compare to the prevalence figures cited above, and to the 18% figure in psychiatric patients cited by Davis and Cummings (1988) and to the prevalence rate of 7% in mentally handicapped people generated by Ganesh et al., (1989).

The only akathisia rating system that existed when we began our investigations had been developed by Barnes and Braude (1985) and included these elements:

Subjective Complaints

Lower limb paraesthesia
"Inner restlessness"
Inability to remain still
Inability to keep legs still
Associated distress
Examination: Sitting

Fidgety arms/hands
Fidgety legs/feet
Shifting position
Inability to remain seated

Examination: Standing

Rocking from foot to foot
Walking on the spot
Other purposeless movements
Inability to stand still (walking or pacing)

Examination: Lying

Fidgety feet/legs
Truncal movements
Inability to remain lying

The problem with using this system for evaluating retarded patients should be clear, because an essential element of diagnosis had to do with the patient's verbal communication of an internal feeling state. It was also clear that the distinction between restlessness, fidgeting movements, hyperactivity, stereotypy, and chorea must be extremely difficult to make with any degree of confidence. We developed an alternative system, (the TDAK, see Appendix), and which lists all the symptoms that arise in retarded people that may be confused with akathisia. The TDAK Rating Scale incorporates the AIMS exam, and so is useful for monitoring for TD as well as TDAK, and we routinely use it now in place of the AIMS.

We also have a companion scale, the MABS (Movement and Behavior Scale), which is directed to behaviors that may be associated with TDAK, such as insomnia, that are apparent to direct care staff but which may not be apparent during a physical examination (see Appendices).

Risk Factors for Tardive Dyskinesia

Patient-Related Risk Factors

Three patient-related risk factors are clearly associated with increased risk for TD: age, sex, and affective disorder. A fourth, preexisting "brain damage," may be associated, although the data are by no means certain. As a general rule, a risk factor that is linked to a higher likelihood of developing TD will also be linked to severity and to persistence.

The risk factor most consistently identified with the development of TD and with severe persistent TD is age. Elderly patients are more prone to the disorder, an effect that is probably independent of cumulative neuroleptic dose or the duration of neuroleptic exposure (Smith and Baldessarini, 1980; APA, in press). It is possible that this association is related to the age-related decline in dopamine neurons in the striatum, an idea that is strengthened by the spontaneous occurrence of buccal-lingual dyskinesias in elderly patients who have never received neuroleptic drugs (Waddington and Youssef, 1985).

Some neuropathic syndromes are given to premature aging and dementia. In cases of Down's syndrome, for example, or in postencephalitics, or post head injury patients, this risk factor may be operative while the patient is still comparatively young.

It appears that females are at greater risk than males to develop TD, and that severe forms of the disorder are likelier to occur in females (Kane and Smith, 1982). This may speak to estrogen-related dopamine sensitivity (Hruska and Silbergeld, 1980). Nicotine can also sensitize the dopamine receptor, so tobacco addiction must also be counted among the risk factors for TD (Yassa et al., 1987). Clinical lore holds to the ironic contention that TD is more likely to occur in patients who do not respond particularly well to neuroleptic treatment, but whether this is related to high dose treatment, to frequent dose changes, to conjunctive treatment, or to some other factor is not known.

More recently, it has been discovered that patients with affective disorders are peculiarly vulnerable to "malignant TD" (Gardos and Casey, 1984). This is very important for treatment of retarded people, among whom affective disorders tend to be underdiagnosed. If it is true that mania and depression present in this population as behavior problems, and are treated with neuroleptics instead of more appropriate drugs, then the risk of severe TD is going to be higher than it ought to be.

Whether preexisting "brain damage" may actually predispose to TD, or to severe and persistent TD, is not known, although it is an important question for practitioners who deal with mentally retarded patients, demented patients, or patients with neurobehavioral sequelae of traumatic brain injury (Gualtieri, 1988). Prescription of neuroleptics has always been high in these groups (Gualtieri and Barnhill, 1988).

Risk Factors Related to Treatment

Several factors related to treatment with neuroleptic drugs have been associated with increased risk of TD, but only one, early development of extrapyramidal symptoms (EPS), has won wide acceptance on the basis of controlled experiments.

Results from the New York Longitudinal Study suggest that patients who develop TD are more likely to have EPS early in their treatment (Kane et al., 1984). The association does not appear to be related to treatment with selected neuroleptics with a low proclivity for EPS, but rather that patients who are prone to early extrapyramidal reactions are at greater risk for TD by virtue of some unique pharmacodynamic tendency (Jeste et al., 1984).

If concomitant anticholinergic treatment is associated with TD at all, the effect is probably mediated by the occurrence of early EPS. That is, patients who develop early EPS are more likely to receive anticholinergics; the former confers risk, not the latter.

One would think that neuroleptic dose has something to do with the development of TD, but the clinical literature is equivocal. Cumulative neuroleptic dose was found to be associated with severe TD in one study of retarded patients (Gualtieri et al., 1986c), but not in studies of schizophrenics and other psychiatric patients. It is likely that there is no linear association between cumulative dose and TD, but that a minimum cumulative dose is necessary to evoke the phenotype in patients who are vulnerable to TD, by virtue of other risk factors. The importance of idiosyncrasy cannot be minimized, because some patients have been known to develop TD after short-term treatment with very low neuroleptic doses, while others seem to be free of the disorder even after years of high-dose treatment.

There does not seem to be a particular neuroleptic that is less likely to cause TD, or conversely one that is more likely. There has been some recent commentary on the new atypical antipsychotic drug clozapine, which has a very low incidence of acute EPS. It has been said that long-term treatment with clozapine does not cause TD. Of course, when haloperidol was first introduced, it was said that it did not cause TD, either. The data for clozapine are better than the data for haloperidol, but not by much. One should reserve judgment.

An appreciation of TD risk factors is essential to clinical treatment, because it allows the physician to recognize cases that require very careful monitoring, more frequent neuroleptic withdrawals or at least dose reductions, and a more aggressive approach to identifying pharmacological alternatives. The informed consent process should address the patient's individual vulnerability to TD. To reiterate, then: established risk factors for neuroleptic-induced TD are advanced age, female sex, smoking, affective disorder, early EPS, and possibly "brain damage" and cumulative neuroleptic dose.

Biological Mechanisms

The prevailing view of the pathophysiology of TD is that chronic blockade of striatal D2-dopamine receptors leads to a state of denervation supersensitivity, and that the abnormal movements are a manifestation of dopamine hypersensitivity (Ananth, 1982). Support for this idea is from animal studies (rats, cats, primates) in which chronic neuroleptic administration is known to increase the number and density of striatal dopamine binding sites (e.g., Creese et al., 1977), to elicit behaviors like gnawing or rotation that are mediated by dopamine (Fjalland and Nielsen, 1974), and to cause choreoathetoid movements that are typical of TD (Weiss and Santelli, 1978). The abnormal movements of TD are topographically identical to dyskinesias that characterize other hyperdopaminergic states: Huntington's disease, Tourette's syndrome, and L-dopa-induced dyskinesias (Stahl et al., 1982).

The dopamine supersensitivity hypothesis is not sufficient to explain the phenomenon, however. For example, the dyskinesias that arise in animal models of TD are early onset and readily reversible. With prolonged neuroleptic administration, the dopamine receptor hypersensitivity actually disappears (Casey and Gerlach, 1986). In human postmortem studies, TD patients are not found to have D1 or D2 hypersensitivity (Waddington, 1984), nor do they show CSF or neuroendocrine indices of dopamine sensitivity (Casey and Gerlach, 1986). The supersensitivity hypothesis may underlie the occurrence of transient or "withdrawal" dyskinesias, but the pathophysiology of persistent unremitting TD is unknown (Tarsy and Baldessarini, 1977).

If receptor supersensitivity cannot be held to account for cases of severe and persistent TD, then it is necessary to consider alternative hypotheses. The fact that the disorder can be irreversible, refractory to treatment, and occasionally associated with continued deterioration even after drug withdrawal (Fahn, 1985) leads inevitably to the idea that neuroleptics may exercise, in some patients at least, a cytotoxic effect. Although there is no direct evidence to support this idea, it is known that neuroleptics may be cytotoxic to hematopoietic and to hepatic cells (Munyon et al., 1987). Occasional reports of postmortem findings in TD patients have demonstrated neuronal degeneration in the substantia nigra (Christensen et al., 1970) and caudate nucleus atrophy (Hunter et al., 1968; Pandurangi et al., 1980). Nielson and Lyon (1978) observed cell death in the corpus striatum of rats given long-term treatment with neuroleptics. Neuroleptic treatment has been found to retard recovery from brain injury in rats (Feeny et al., 1982).

The relative cytotoxicity of eight neuroleptics on five different test systems was measured by Munyon et al. (1987). Thioridazine, chlorpromazine, trifluoperazine, fluphenazine, and thiothixene were found to be the most cytotoxic; haloperidol and loxapine less so, and molindone the least. (Molidone and loxapine have not been described in connection with many severe cases of TD at all, although that may be a function of their recent introduction and limited range of prescription.) Because neuroleptics are metabolized into many active compounds, it is conceivable that some individuals are prone to relatively higher levels of a unique neurotoxic metabolite, or that in some individuals such a metabolite is likelier to cross the blood-brain barrier. These would be the people who go on to develop severe and unremitting TD, even after only a few months of treatment. If this idea is speculative, it is not trivial, because the discovery of such a process would lend a rationale to preventive monitoring and a clue to pathogenesis.

Diagnosis

The diagnosis of TD requires more than the simple administration of a rating scale like the AIMS or the DISCUS. Those are only screening instruments, useful because they can be reliably administered by a nonphysician and because they raise the level of staff consciousness concerning TD. But they are complements to the neurological examination and the process of differential diagnosis, not a substitute for it.

The first step in diagnosis requires a thorough description of the patient's abnormal movements, including a topographic analysis of the distribution of dyskinesia and an accurate description of its nature. The topographic categories are orofacial, buccal-lingual-masticatory (BLM), truncal (or axial), centrifugal (i.e., involving the extremities), and holokinetic (i.e., all over). The different types of dyskinesia are choreoathetoid, dystonic, myoclonic, ballistic, and tic-like movements (so-called "Tardive Tourette's syndrome").

Topography and dyskinesia interact in relatively predictable patterns. Choreiform movements are often centrifugal, while dystonic movements are more commonly axial in distribution. The area of distribution is significant, because severe TD may sometimes have a total body distribution and thus render the patient incapacitated by virtue of holokinetic movements. Movements that are circumscribed in area are not so likely to be incapacitating, unless they are dystonic, or unless they involve the oropharyngeal or respiratory musculature. These elements are essential for determining the severity of TD and may also aid in the prediction of outcome. Severe and persistent TD is most often associated with mixed types of movements with a generalized distribution, or with dystonic movements with a more local distribution.

The next step involves the process of differential diagnosis. The topography and classification of dyskinesia do not establish diagnosis. Indeed, many other movement disorders may resemble TD. Stereotypies and manneristic behaviors are common in severely retarded and autistic patients. These movements may be suppressed by neuroleptics and reemerge when the drug is reduced in dose or discontinued entirely. Such movements are usually more complex than those seen in TD, and are usually stereotyped in quality. Nevertheless, TD coinciding with stereotypies may pose a diagnostic problem.

The differential diagnosis of TD includes Tourette's syndrome, choreoathetosis attendant on cerebral palsy, Huntington's disease, Wilson's disease, and other disorders of the basal ganglia; Hallovoerden–Spatz disease (dystonia); familial dystonia and chorea; ballistic movements related to vascular disease; and other drug-induced dyskinesias, for example, those related to phenytoin (Chadwick et al., 1976), carbamazepine (Jacome, 1979), valproate, tricyclic antidepressants, or stimulants. Dyskinesias may arise spontaneously in elderly or in demented patients. Idiopathic calcification of the basal ganglia is associated with dyskinesia and other neuropsychiatric symptoms (Muenter and Whisnant, 1968; Cummings et al., 1983).

Other causes of movement disorder include Sydenham's chorea, systemic lupus erythematosis, and some encephalitides. Disturbance in thyroid and parathyroid function may be associated with dyskinesia (Jeste et al., 1984). The differential diagnosis of dystonia has been addressed most recently by Marsden (1988).

The evaluation of a patient with possible TD involves a series of steps to exclude alternative causes of dyskinesia, especially treatable conditions like Wilson's disease. A family history is very important. Laboratory diagnosis may rule out infectious, endocrine, metabolic, and degenerative disorders. Appropriate studies include a toxic drug screen, serum electrolytes, sedimentation level, ASO titers, thyroid and parathyroid studies, serum ceruloplasmin, LE prep, and antinuclear antibodies. Appropriate neurodiagnostic studies include computed tomography (CT) or magnetic resonance imaging (MRI), at least in selected cases. Calcification of the basal ganglia, iron deposition in the globus pallidus, or degeneration of the caudate and other subcortical structures may provide etiopathogenic evidence that can influence clinical decisions.

A thorough differential diagnosis is important, but the most important diagnostic element is, of course, a history of toxic exposure (to neuroleptics, or to other dopamine blockers like metaclopramide) and a high index of suspicion on the part of the treating physician. A patient with dyskinesia and a history of neuroleptic exposure has TD until proven otherwise.

Treatment

It is not easy to talk about the treatment of TD, because there really is no treatment that is reliably effective. The basic treatment is to withdraw neuroleptics, keep the patient drug free, and wait for the disorder to remit.

Patients with choreiform TD may respond to drugs that influence gamma-aminobutyric acid (GABA) neurotransmission like clonazepam, baclofen, or valproic acid (Fahn, 1987). The timing of treatment may be important, because some TD patients progress to a severe dystonic form of the disorder that is usually resistent to pharmacologic treatment (Gardos and Cole, 1987). Drugs that deplete presynaptic dopamine like reserpine or tetrabenzamine may be helpful, but they can exacerbate affective illness in vulnerable patients (Fahn, 1983; Asher and Aminoff, 1981). Patient response to acetylcholine agonists is variable. Physostigmine provocation has been advocated as a screening procedure to identify patients who will respond to cholinergic precursors (Casey and Denney, 1977; Moore and Bowers, 1980). Clinically, acetylcholine agonist treatment approaches have been disappointing, and side effects have limited their utility (Gelenberg, 1979).

Tardive dystonia differs clinically from idiopathic forms of dystonia, yet it may respond to similar treatments. In dystonia, physostigmine tends to increase the severity of abnormal movements. Anticholinergic drugs have been helpful, but their clinical utility is limited by the occurrence of memory impairment, agitation, and delirium (Lang, 1986). Dopamine-depleting drugs may be helpful in 10% to 12% of patients with dystonia (Kang et al., 1986). Dopamine agonists like L-dopa and amantadine may be effective in a similar percentage of dystonic patients (Stahl and Burges, 1982). The use of GABAergic drugs has been of limited benefit. As a treatment of last resort, a combination of atypical neuroleptics, dopamine agonists, and anticholinergic drugs may be required.

The Course of the Disorder

It is a mistake to classify TD as "irreversible," because long-standing TD patients may experience remission even after several years. It is better to classify TD as "transient" or as "persistent" and to specify precisely how long the movement disorder has in fact persisted.

What proportion of patients has TD that remits after only a few weeks or a few months, and what proportion persists for years? Although that is an important question, it cannot be answered on the basis of direct research. The persistence of TD may be masked by continued neuroleptic treatment, and most TD studies in psychiatric populations have been done in schizophrenic patients who are treated with neuroleptics even after TD is diagnosed.

In elderly patients, TD is usually a persistent disorder, while in studies of children treated with neuroleptics the remission rate is very high (Gualtieri et al., 1984b; Perry et al., 1985). Although persistent cases are not unknown, they are rare (Gualtieri et al., 1980a). There is an age-dependent decrease in dopamine neurotransmission that may interact with neuroleptic neurotoxicity to cause severe and persistent forms of TD in elderly patients, and this same element could conceivably confer a measure of protection to young people (Waddington and Youssef, 1985). Of course, children also tend to be treated with low doses of neuroleptics for shorter periods of time, and they metabolize drugs more efficiently. The relative persistence rates for TD in young and old patients may be a pharmacodynamic phenomenon, or it may simply be related to prescription habits.

It is possible that even transient TD in early life may set the stage for neurodegenerative changes in later years; admittedly a speculation, but one that is based on some established models of the evolution of neuropsychiatric disorders— postencephalitic parkinsonism, the late neuropathic sequelae of poliomyelitis, late-onset psychosis following traumatic brain injury, and the putative kindling psychosis of temporal lobe epilepsy (Gualtieri and Barnhill, 1988). There are all models of early CNS insult followed by late deterioration in function. It is possible that some patients who have had transient TD in early life will develop encephalopathic changes when they are old. The question is, will we ever know?

In retarded people, one study reported TD in 25 of 38 individuals who were withdrawn from neuroleptic treatment, but 13 of 25 had transient TD that remitted within only a few weeks (Gualtieri et al., 1986c). A subsequent study of a subgroup of that original sample who returned to neuroleptic treatment, and who were withdrawn from neuroleptics a second time 3 years later, demonstrated progressive TD in 5 patients and TD that had actually decreased in severity in 4 patients; the former had been treated with high doses of neuroleptics, the latter group with low doses (Gualtieri and Barnhill, 1988). Although this was only a small study, it suggests that patients with TD may continue on neuroleptics, if they absolutely have to, so long as the dosages are kept low.

Paulson et al. (1975) reexamined a group of retarded people 4 years after a neuroleptic withdrawal trial and found that 6 (of 15) had persistent TD with no change in severity, 5 were more severe, and 4 had actually improved.

If one can make any surmise from these small studies, it is that TD is persistent in some substantial fraction (one-third or two-thirds) of retarded patients who have the disorder, that persistence is to be measured in years, but that remission may occur with time and judicious management. How does this surmise square with the results of TD research in other patient groups?

The research data from studies of schizophrenic adults are contradictory and hard to interpret. In one study of TD patients maintained off neuroleptics, no appreciable symptom reduction was noted after 12 months (Glazor et al., 1984). In another, Yassa et al., (1984) reported a 2-year follow-up: 66% of the TD patients showed no change, 18% improved, and 16% grew worse over time. In a 5-year follow-up study by Chouinard et al., (1986), the annual, remission rate in TD patients was 5.5%; this was outweighed by an incidence rate for new cases of 8.4%. In contrast, there have been several reports to suggest that TD remits far more often than it persists (Casey, 1985; Yagi and Itoh, 1987; Quitkin et al., 1977; Casey et al., 1986; Wegner and Kane, 1982), even if neuroleptic treatment is continued. Exactly how substantial the "substantial fraction" is, then, of those who have persistent TD, remains an area of surmise.

Well-controlled epidemiologic studies of the course of TD are extremely hard to do, because the recruitment of a large number of subjects will necessarily include patients on neuroactive drugs that may influence the course of the disorder, patients who will drop out for one reason or another, and patients with degenerative CNS disorders. As a consequence, research attention is turning in the direction of case-control strategies. It is assumed that at least some patients will have long-term persistent TD, and that others will remit. The relative proportions are irrelevant; the key to the strategy is accurate assignment to one group or the other. The next step is to identify clinical elements that are associated with persistence, and to replicate the finding. This is the hard part. First, clinical elements from the medical history will be hard to discover, especially in chronic patients who are institutionalized. Second, subject variance will conspire against a successful replication. But the strategy is important; if reliable information is attainable, it can be used to guide programs for TD prevention.

A first attempt at this strategy was published by Gardos et al. (1987). They found that generalized dystonic and athetoid movements characterized a more malignant and persistent form of TD. They also reported that severe and persistent TD patients displayed a variety of axial and centrifugal movements, with BLM choreoathetosis early in the clinical course and a gradual evolution to dystonia as the disorder progressed. Males were more commonly affected with severe and persistent TD, and the duration of treatment was relatively short (less than 1 year). Gardos et al. concluded that patients who develop severe and persistent TD have a unique vulnerability to neuroleptic-induced movement disorders, and that this could be defined in terms of the TD risk factors discussed earlier, especially age, early EPS, and affective disorder.

Malignant TD

The severity of TD is defined in terms of persistence, the nature of the dyskinesia, and the degree to which it afflicts the patient's behavior and compromises the activities of his daily life. The disagreement over relative rates of persistence is mirrored in controversies about relative severity, or whether patients with TD are even much bothered by their disorder. There is little to be gained from a reiteration of these arguments.

The consensus developing among psychopharmacologists is that TD may sometimes be a malignant disorder, rapid in onset and extreme in its consequences. It seems that some patients are uniquely vulnerable to severe and persistent TD; that they can develop the disorder after only a brief course of low-dose neuroleptic treatment; that their TD is extraordinarily debilitating; and that dystonia and akathisia are its likeliest manifestations. Patients with so-called malignant TD (MTD) tend to have affective disorders to begin with (Gardos and Casey, 1984). They are often young, and their disorder is persistent and refractory to treatment. They are rarely if ever anosognosic for the disorder. This is a very serious problem (Burke et al., 1982).

There are only estimates of the relative prevalence of severe forms of TD. The most recent survey, based on 100 TD cases seen at a movement disorder clinic that were probably a seriously afflicted group to begin with, reported 23 severe manifestations of the disorder: persistent bruxism (1 case), masseter or lingual hypertrophy (3), sustained involuntary tongue protrusion (6), incomprehensible speech arising from dysarthria (2), spasmodic dysphonia (2), anterior cervical spondylolisthesis (1), palatal dyskinesia with secondary sinus pain (1), respiratory stridor with laryngospasm (2), and disabling dystonic posturing (5) (Davis and Cummings, 1988).

MTD is the reason neuroleptic-treated patients should be examined regularly, at least every 3 months. Nurses also, or parents or house parents, should be trained in the early recognition of TD. Patients with affective disorders, with affective symptoms, or with family histories of affective disorder should not be treated with neuroleptics except in extraordinary circumstances.

The authors have had occasion to attend many mentally retarded patients with MTD. The frequency of this extreme drug effect, and its prevention, are central to current TD research.

Behavioral and Cognitive Manifestations of Tardive Dyskinesia

Are the manifestations of neuroleptic toxicity limited to dyskinesia, or can neuroleptics exercise a toxic effect on other brain systems? In 1979, Davis and

Rosenberg raised the question of a "limbic equivalent of TD," that is, behavioral toxicity as a consequence of neuroleptic-induced changes in mesolimbic dopamine receptors. In the same year, Famuyiwa et al. reported more intellectual deterioration in neuroleptic-treated patients with TD than in non-TD controls (Famuyiwa et al., 1979). Two questions then were posed: whether neuroleptic treatment could lead to behavior deterioration, and whether neuroleptics could cause dementia. In other words, whether "higher cortical functions" might be damaged, much in the same way that motor control systems were damaged. One may imagine the excitement and dismay this question has raised—in fact, much heat and little light; it is a difficult point to prove, one way or the other.

Cases of "supersensitivity psychosis" have been described by Chouinard and Jones (1980) (who coined the term), by Sale and Kristall (1978), and by Caine et al. (1978). These were neuroleptic-treated patients who developed a dramatic, rapid-onset psychosis as soon as neuroleptics were withdrawn; the psychosis was held to be a consequence of neuroleptic treatment, not simply the reemergence of a preexisting disorder. The psychiatric community has not found this contention particularly believable (APA, 1991), although it would be imprudent to dismiss it out of hand.

There is near unanimity, however, on the issue of dementia, because virtually every study that has researched the issue has found an association between TD and signs of dementia or so-called negative symptoms of schizophrenia. When TD patients are compared to similar patients who do not have TD, clear evidence of cognitive dysfunction is almost invariably demonstrated in the TD group (Edwards, 1970; Wilson, I.C. et al., 1983; Struve and Wilner, 1983; Wolf et al., 1983; Collerton et al., 1985; Waddington et al., 1985; Wegner et al., 1985; Goldberg, 1985; Thomas and McGuire, 1986; Gilleard and Vaddad, 1986). What is at issue is how to account for the finding. The usual explanation is that patients with preexisting neuropsychological deficits are more vulnerable to the neurotoxic effects of neuroleptic drugs. The alternative is, of course, that neuroleptics cause cognitive decline in some patients; that neuroleptic treatment may cause subcortical dementia (Gillead and Vaddad, 1986) or frontal lobe syndrome (Wilson, I.C. et al., 1983). This idea is supported by a recent PET study that demonstrated long-term neuroleptic effects on brain glucose metabolism in schizophrenic patients, in the direction of decreased metabolism in the frontal lobes ("hypofrontality") and enhanced metabolism in the corpus striatum (Szechtman et al., 1988).

Neither alternative is savory to physicians who treat retarded patients, elderly patients who are demented, or head injury patients. Either preexisting encephalopathy is a risk factor for the development of TD, or it is a risk inherent to long-term neuroleptic treatment. It might seem like an academic exercise, therefore, to try to resolve the issue; in either event, neuroleptics should be administered by experienced psychopharmacologists, and only in grave clinical circumstances when alternative treatments have been tried and have failed.

It is possible, however, to shed at least some light on the question. A cogent argument on behalf of neuroleptic-induced dementia may be made on the following basis.

The argument for a behavioral or a cognitive analog of TD is usually predicated on the assumption of neuroleptic toxicity to limbic or to cortical dopamine projections. The weakness of the argument is that such damage has never been demonstrated to occur. It is known, however, that neuroleptics can cause irreversible changes in striatal dopamine systems. Yet one does not require an extrastriatal locus for neuroleptic toxicity to support the occurrence of behavioral or cognitive changes. The corpus striatum is responsible for much more than motor control; it is a complex organ that mediates a wide range of complex human behaviors (Divac, 1963; Buchwald et al., 1975). No disease that afflicts the striatum is known to have only motor symptoms; Parkinson's disease and Huntington's disease are two examples of striatal pathology with far-ranging psychological consequences. A neurotoxin, therefore, that impairs striatal function should be expected to have behavioral and cognitive effects. The burden of proof should reside with those who maintain that long-term neuroleptic damage is absolutely confined to the domain of motor control.

That is just an argument, and it is not necessary to guide one's actions with respect to neuroleptic treatment. The occasional occurrence of neuroleptic side effects like akathisia, NMS, and TD is sufficient to invite the most extreme caution in the prescription of these drugs to human beings, and to limit their use only to the most severely afflicted patients. On the other hand, the growing acceptance of the idea of tardive akathisia, characterized not by dyskinesia but by dysphoria and motor restlessness, indicates that psychiatrists are finally coming to accept the idea of a behavioral equivalent of TD.

Neuroleptic Nonresponders

Neuroleptics have a high rate of success as "major tranquilizers" for the acutely disturbed patients. This rapid effect in patients who are acutely agitated, psychotic, or assaultive is one of the greatest contributions of modern pharmacology. There is no substitute for chlorpromazine or haloperidol, in the emergency room, for the psychotic patient; for the hospitalized demented patient who is pulling out IV lines or screaming all night; for a violent patient who is dangerous and uncontrollable. Unfortunately, this rapid effect in the acute clinical circumstance is sometimes translated into a long-term treatment program that may not be necessary or that may be counterproductive. Worse, the reliability of this "tranquilizing" effect may be mistaken for universality. In such circumstances, neuroleptics are reliably effective, but they are not *always* effective. There are such persons as neuroleptic nonresponders. In fact, there are patients with severe behavior problems whose clinical condition may be *aggravated* by neuroleptic treatment.

It is important to remember that there are even some schizophrenic patients whose disorder grows worse with neuroleptic treatment. In rare cases, psychosis may even occur as an *effect* of neuroleptic treatment (Chaffin, 1964). Neuroleptics can cause dysphoria (Singh and Kay, 1979), panic (Bachmann and Modestin, 1987), phobia (Mikkelson et al., 1981), and depression (Moller and von Zerssen,

1982). Although acute behavioral toxicity to neuroleptic treatment may not be common, it is by no means uncommon. Not only may some patients fail to respond to neuroleptic treatment, but some patients, even diagnosed schizophrenics, may actually grow worse with the drugs.

Virtually every physician who has treated mentally handicapped patients has noted cases in which neuroleptic treatment exercises no benefit, but the drugs cannot be withdrawn because behavior deteriorates when they are. This is a peculiar variant of neuroleptic toxicity that has not appeared in the literature. The authors are at a loss to explain the phenomenon, although they are beginning to suspect that at least some of these patients have tardive akathisia.

Alternatives to Neuroleptic Treatment

Years ago, it was reported that most retarded patients who were withdrawn from neuroleptics could be managed drug free, or on nonneuroleptic psychotropics (reviewed in Gualtieri et al., 1986b). The situation may now be somewhat different, because many mental retardation programs have instituted periodic trial withdrawals for neuroleptic patients, and those who continue to be treated with neuroleptics often have severe behavioral problems or diagnosable psychiatric conditions. There does seem to be an irreducible minimum number of retarded people for whom some form of psychotropic drug treatment is necessary.

The problem case is not a well-established neuroleptic responder whose target behaviors are in complete remission, who can be maintained on low doses, who is carefully monitored, and who has not developed any neuroleptic side effects. The problem cases are people with TD, or people who require very high neuroleptic doses, or who are only partial responders to drug treatment. If such patients cannot be properly managed in the drug-free state, what are the alternatives?

Clearly, the answer to such a question depends on the nature of the patient's condition, and it is not appropriate to enumerate the long list of neuropsychiatric disorders and behavioral aberrations that can afflict mentally retarded people, along with the various treatments that are indicated. On the other hand, it is appropriate to at least allude to the various approaches that are currently under investigation; the interested reader must be advised to pursue the matter not only in the mental retardation literature, but in medical journals that are devoted to neuropsychiatric studies of other patient populations: certainly, the "orthodox" psychopharmacology journals, but also the literature that is developing around treatment for behavior disorders in the demented elderly, victims of traumatic brain injury, epileptics, and children. Psychopharmacology for retarded people is best appreciated as part of the wider field of psychopharmacology for special populations. In this field, research attention is increasingly turned towards the therapeutic potential of the psychotropic anticonvulsants, beta blockers, lithium, new antidepressants, opiate antagonists, calcium channel blockers, cholinergics, angiotensin-converting enzyme inhibitors, and dopamine agonists (Gualtieri, 1988).

When patients are unable to tolerate neuroleptic discontinuation, the clinician should attempt to find alternative treatments. Patients with epilepsy might do well when withdrawn from behaviorally toxic anticonvulsants like phenytoin or phenobarbital and with substitution of psychoactive anticonvulsants like car-bamezepine or valproic acid (Evans and Gualtieri, 1985; Gualtieri, 1988). Both drugs are perfectly good anticonvulsants, and they are known to have positive effects in patients with mood disorders, episodic aggression, and other behavior disorders related to mental retardation or to neurological disease. Even patients without epilepsy can profit from these drugs, and they are sometimes helpful in the management of selected patients with explosive self-injurious behavior (SIB) or aggression (Gualtieri 1989). Lithium may also be a viable alternative to neurolep-tics, for example in aggressive patients with emotional lability (Chandler et al., 1988). Patients with cyclic or episodic behavioral disturbance may also respond to lithium. Antidepressants may be helpful for patients with mood disorders, and the rapid development of new antidepressants with novel neurochemical mechanisms of action holds certain promise; antidepressants that influence serotonergic neurotransmission may aid in the management of hyperactivity, emotional lability, or SIB. Beta blockers like propranolol have proven beneficial for patients with hyperactivity, explosive-aggressive behavior, social phobias, or intense reactions to environmental change. There is evidence that beta blockers may be helpful for some cases of SIB (Ratey et al., 1986). Amantadine, a dopamine agonist with antiparkinsonian effects (and also an antiviral agent), has been helpful in the management of emotionally labile and hyperactive-disorganized patients (Chandler et al., in press). Calcium channel blockers like verapamil and nifedipine are reported to be effective in the treatment of affective disorders, psychosis, and Tourette's syndrome (Dubovsky, 1986; Walsh, 1986). Angiotensin-converting enzyme inhibitors like captopril, developed originally as antihypertensives, may have positive mood effects in depression, and may also prove helpful in the management of pathological water intoxication, of all things (Deiken, 1986). Opiate antagonists like naltrexone may eventually prove helpful in the management of some patients with SIB, hyperphagia, or polydispsia (Kathol et al., 1986; Sandman et al., 1983).

The point is that neuropsychopharmacology is a field that is developing extreme-ly fast, and many of the new agents hold promise for patients with severe behavior disorders attendant on static or even progressive encephalopathy. There are, right now, a host of useful alternatives to neuroleptic treatment; in years to come, there will be many more. The challenge is to develop systems for new drug evaluation in special populations such as retarded people. It is not wise to estimate new drug utility and safety entirely on the basis of clinical research that is done in other patient groups. We have been down that road once before, and the consequences were tragic.

Tardive Dyskinesia Policy and Recommendations

For the first 25 years of the psychopharmacology era, neuroleptics were virtually the only psychoactive compounds prescribed to mentally retarded people. It is natural, therefore, in light of our dreadful experience, that current policy towards psychopharmacology in mentally retarded people should be characterized by extreme caution, skepticism about the potential benefits of drug treatment in general, safeguards against drug overuse, and agency-wide drug monitoring programs. These safeguards, coupled with the current emphasis on behavioral and developmental programming in community-based facilities, are all to the good. They guarantee that pharmacological interventions can be made not simply to mute the individual's legitimate behavioral and emotional responses to neglect and humiliation, but rather to treat specific neuropsychiatric disorders. Insofar as we have been able to meet the ideals of our movement, we are thus empowered to take advantage of this fabulous new technology. To the degree that we fall short, to that degree is medical practice diminished in its scope and power.

The untoward experience of years of neuroleptic overuse is drawing to a close as a new era of intelligent and sensitive neuropsychiatry comes upon us. Yet the consequences of the neuroleptic experience will be with us for a long time to come. It will still be necessary to keep the issue of TD alive, to monitor patients carefully, and to take careful stock of the scars that will persist. It is good that TD monitoring systems are de rigueur, and that nurses and physicians are trained to detect abnormal movements, and to take at least some steps in coping with them. But it will be necessary to establish a new level of TD detection, one that incorporates the new concern over severe neuroleptic syndromes like MTD, tardive dystonia, tardive akathisia, and the neuroleptic malignant syndrome. It is also necessary to develop methods that will prevent these catastrophic events, or that at least will mitigate their consequences.

TMS: A System for Prevention and Control

It is not outlandish to think of drugs as if they were microbes that can sweep through populations like an epidemic. The drug is a microbe, and the unwitting physician is the vector. There is a wave of treatment, and then a wave of morbidity attendant on the treatment. The wave passes, and some broken lives are left in its wake. The neuroleptic era was such an epidemic.

Like microbes during a plague, treatment epidemics do the most damage to vulnerable populations. In the 1950s and 1960s when the neuroleptic era began, mentally retarded people were the most vulnerable population. They were treated like animals. They were oppressed and mistreated in so many dimensions, they were systematically dehumanized, and they were uniquely vulnerable to the most mean-spirited ideas. The ideals of normalization, of community living, and of a respectable, gainful life were remote, and they would have seemed unrealistic to most professional people. If they were difficult to manage, well, they needed a tranquilizer, and the more sedating it was the better. No one would have supposed that most of their management problems were owing to the circumstances of their lives.

It is the very definition of a plague: neuroleptic drugs, the agent; physicians, the vector; ignorance, inhumane environments, and an attitude of pervasive nihilism, the setting events.

It is important to reflect on the role of the medical community in permitting this epidemic to occur. It is a bitter shadow of the immortal Semmelweiss, who also noted the responsibility of physicians for spreading an epidemic of puerperal sepsis. The birth of psychopharmacology was by no means free of stain, and the present epidemic of tardive dyskinesia and of tardive akathisia, especially in mentally handicapped people, is one of those stains.

Today we know that a new technology cannot be engrafted on a professional community that is unprepared for its consequences. When neuroleptics were first introduced, psychiatry was a field devoted to interpersonal psychotherapy, and the idea of medical psychiatry was remote. On the other side, neurology was dominated by a spirit of therapeutic nihilism. When the first psychotropic drugs were introduced, psychiatrists and neurologists were in no position to understand their proper administration, or to offer guidance to general physicians in the proper use of complicated compounds like the neuroleptic drugs. The prevailing standards of care were as unequal to the challenge of psychopharmacology as they had been to the challenge of psychosurgery 20 years earlier (Valenstein, 1986).

The appropriate measure to take in the face of a technology that has been out of control is to develop a technology to contain it. But that requires more than just research and training. It also requires a degree of social organization. To control an epidemic, one needs more than a vaccine against the agent and trained physicians to treat the victims; one also has to deal with predisposing events that render a population vulnerable.

So, to correct the problem of psychotropic drug misuse among mentally handicapped individuals, we shall need more than new research and new physicians. One needs new technology to ensure the quality of psychopharmacological practice. The TMS (Tardive Dyskinesia Monitoring System) was developed as a technology to organize and control the use of psychopharmaceuticals, a way to ensure quality of care for large numbers of people in a most efficient and cost-effective manner.

The Development of TMS

We developed the TMS originally as part of a research program that was investigating the prevalence and course of severe TD in retarded people. Its origins were in monitoring patients who were ultimately intended to enter research protocols. But the system had to be designed to monitor the quality of neuropsychiatric care as well. It was a self-serving decision with an air of mutuality; there was really no way to do honest research in a facility until the basic neuropsychiatric requirements of patients and professional colleagues were first addressed.

But then the development of microcomputer technology for psychopharmacology monitoring and quality control became an end in itself. It was no longer just a way to advance the goals of a research project. What began as a research tool, to advance small, specific questions, grew into a method with much broader application. Our computer monitoring system for tardive dyskinesia research (TMS) began as a quick fix to facilities that might one day participate in research protocols, and as such it was a partial success. But as a method for addressing a much more entrenched problem, as a way to guide good neuropsychiatric practice, it has had greater success.

The TMS is a fully portable personal computer- (PC-) based quality control system that can identify problem areas in psychopharmacology and develop strategies for their solution. It is capable of monitoring the success of a consultation arrangement, making consultants accountable for the outcome of their work. It is particularly good for developing skills in psychopharmacology in primary care physicians, who are after all the ones who usually prescribe psychotropics and anticonvulsants in mental retardation programs. The TMS was first used in a small, university-based neuropsychiatry clinic that specialized in the care of patients with developmental disabilities and traumatic brain injuries. It has since been applied in nine regional residential centers in seven states, and in one community-based program in an eighth state.

The TMS begins with a neuropharmacology database, a spreadsheet that incorporates demographic and clinical data and all the pertinent information about psychotropics, target behaviors, psychiatric diagnoses, side-effects monitoring, seizures, anticonvulsants, and blood levels. On the basis of a baseline review of current practice at a facility, one may appraise the quality of care and areas that require further attention.

The TMS generates summary statistics known as control codes. Control codes are numbers, or indices, that quantify the quality of neuropharmacological practice. Because the same control codes are developed at many different facilities, the TMS has the capacity to define practice norms, comparative data from one facility to another.

One simple control code is the CONRATE, or percentage of residents currently on neuroleptics:

CENTER :	FV	WR	OG	FS	PR	LL	NI	KN	MD
CONRATE:	29	22	07	19	60	22	23	18	28

Because the national rate for neuroleptic administration in retarded people is about 25% (Hill et al., 1983), it appears that most of these programs are in good shape, except for PR, which has an extraordinarily high rate of neuroleptic use. Neuroleptic reduction at that facility has therefore become a major priority.

A simple code like the CONRATE does not tell the whole story, however. One should evaluate the nature of the clients who are referred into the center from the surrounding community. In three of the centers, we did a TMS review for new admissions over the previous 2 years.

CENTER:	FS	LL	MD
CONRATE:	19	22	28
CONRATE, new admissions:	56	26	77

New admissions to the Centers were likelier to be on neuroleptics than people who had been resident there. Thus, the facilities had to contend with an influx of patients on neuroleptic drugs, and this is something that would tend to keep its CONRATE high.

One may use control codes to evaluate neuroleptic treatment in terms of daily dose, defined as chlorpromazine equivalents (CPZEQ) in milligrams per day, by the method of Davis (1976).

CENTER:	FV	WR	OG	FS	PR	LL	NI	KN	MD
CPZEQ:	417	487	247	277	758	514	369	347	369

Another way to do the same thing is by using the Neuroleptic Dose Index (NDI), the number of residents on high (600 mg/day) or ultrahigh (1000 mg/day) neuroleptics, divided by the total number currently on neuroleptics. Lower numbers are better:

CENTER:	FV	WR	OG	FS	PR	LL	NI	KN	MD
NDI:		.24	.10	.29	.50	.25	.27	.16	.26

The NDI is more like a median statistic, and CPZEQ is a mean. Together, they give a good appraisal of the quality of neuroleptic dosing at a given facility.

The Withdrawal Index (Windex) is a measure of efforts at the facility to reduce unnecessary neuroleptic treatment. It is the number of residents currently on neuroleptics divided by the number of residents who have been successfully withdrawn from neuroleptics at the Center:

CENTER:	FV	WR	OG	FS	PR	LL	NI	KN	MD
WINDEX:	—	—	4.1	1.04	—	4.8	—	23	1.48

At KN, only a very few residents have been successfully withdrawn. At FS, they have been able to withdraw almost as many residents as they have continued on neuroleptics.

The TDRATE and the AK(athisia)RATE vary wildly from one place to another, by virtue of different patterns of neuroleptic treatment and the intensity with which the existence of TD and TDAK is investigated:

CENTER:	FV	WR	OG	FS	PR	LL	NI	KN	MD
TDRATE:		.37	.36	.53	.00	.14	—		.46
AKRATE:		.08	—	.14	.00	.02	.00		.15

Places with very low rates simply have not been monitoring properly. The rates from OG, PR, and MD have been checked and double-checked, and they alone are valid representations of the frequency of TD and TDAK.

There is also a PSYRATE, the percentage of clients on all psychotropic medications, and PSY/NL, the percentage of clients on psychotropics who are on neuroleptics. The latter code describes the degree of reliance on neuroleptics:

CENTER:	FV	WR	OG	FS	PR	LL	NI	KN	MD
PSYRATE:	.33	.26	.09	.34	.65	.27	.31	.24	.40
PSY/NL:	.87	.86	.77	.56	.93	.82	.75	.76	.70

The heaviest reliance on neuroleptics was at PR. The most energetic effort to discover pharmacological alternatives to neuroleptics was at MD.

The Polypharmacy Index is the number of residents on more than one psychotropic divided by the number of residents on only one:

CENTER:	FV	WR	OG	FS	PR	LL	NI	KN	MD
PPI:	.61	.33	.29	.16	2.93	.31	.54	.32	.90

A lower number is better, although the statistic may be elevated, as at MD, by virtue of activity toward reducing neuroleptics and finding pharmacological alternatives.

REVA/C stands for review Anticonvulsant therapy. The REVA/C rate is the percentage of people on anticonvulsants who require special review, by virtue of anticonvulsant polypharmacy or continued reliance on archaic anticonvulsants (phenobarbital, mysoline, phenytoin, mebaral, ethosuccimide, bromides).

CENTER:	FV	WR	OG	FS	PR	LL	NI	KN	MD
REVA/C:		.49	.79	.65	.97	.90	.68	.86	.53
A/Ci:		1.07	2.5	2.19	3.6	2.35	2.59	2.32	1.88

The A/Ci, or Anticonvulsant Index, is a number composed of the sum of points for anticonvulsant polypharmacy added to points for archaic anticonvulsants. A lower number is better. It is not likely that anyone will ever achieve a better A/Ci than WR, where the consultant neurologist pursues monotherapy with a zeal that borders on fanaticism. Poor old PR has as much difficulty with anticonvulsants as it does with neuroleptics.

The original TMS created a view of neuropharmacology practice at a center at a point in time. It was good for identifying areas that required special attention, and for comparing one facility to another, with respect to control codes. But it was not good for serial evaluations, because it was only a spreadsheet, not a serial record.

Son of TMS

The second generation of the TMS, which was introduced in 1990, moved from the confines of spreadsheet monitoring to the wider domain of the computerized medical record. It has 15 screens instead of only 1, and it includes all the essential information for medical and psychological management of chronic patients in residential facilities, or, more important, in community-based programs. Rather than an appraisal at one point in time, it contains data from serial records over the years. It is an entirely self-contained system that is based in the pharmacy and networked to the medical clinics and the administrative offices. Patient data can be printed out as individual records, for medical review, or as summary reports for groups of patients for quality assurance monitoring. The system can be run by anyone who has a small degree of computer literacy; it does not require a special consultant.

The development of a self-contained system that can be used to monitor psychiatric care in community-based programs is increasingly important. As the deinstitutionalization movement gains strength, there has been, in some communities, an increase in the use of psychotropic drugs, especially neuroleptics. Patients are being looked after by community physicians, and they are usually general practitioners who do not have the requisite skills for handling complicated neurobehavioral problems. There seems to be less tolerance of deviant behavior in some community-based programs. And it is much harder to monitor the quality of psychopharmacological services in small, widely dispersed populations with local physicians who have only a small amount of time to devote to Medicare patients.

The second TMS was designed to monitor, to record essential medical and behavioral information and seizure data, and also to provide on-line information about psychotropic drugs and their proper use. It has a built-in intelligence, which is updated quarterly. So, you enter data on the record, and the record talks back to you.

It uses conventional software (DB4) that can be reprogrammed by anyone who cares to learn the system. Programmers can expand the screens to include additional data, and they can write new report formats.

It is PC based, so there is no major investment in a micro- or a mini- that will be obsolete before it is up and running. If you buy a modem, you can use the PC you have at home to access the system. And because there is no big investment required in software development, either, and because the system can be integrated with other systems, it can be built up incrementally, and networked as far as one chooses. And it takes advantage of off-the-shelf software and hardware from prominent manufacturers (e.g., IBM™), who are not likely to fold anytime soon; spare parts should not be a problem.

CHAPTER 11

Three Neuropsychiatric Conditions of Childhood

The constraints of composing a book like this pose an inevitable dilemma toward the end; one has to stop somewhere. At some point, it is necessary to encompass a subject with only a few strokes of a narrow pen. So must it be for the neuropsychiatric disorders of childhood—sufficient to discuss only a few topics that express some interesting principle, and leave to others the unenviable task of being encyclopedic.

That is a shame, because there is much to say about the neuropsychiatry of childhood. Much that has been said, about the learning disabilities for example, and "childhood depression," and most recently about obsessive-compulsive disorder, may be misleading or erroneous. As a rule, the expression of psychiatric conditions in prepubertal children is partial and imperfect, and the diagnostic process is at best an approximation. As a consequence, the pertinent literature likewise may be found to be partial and imperfect, and only an approximation of the truth.

As a rule, the response of children to psychopharmaceuticals is different from that of adults; in general, it appears to resemble the response of brain-injured patients and of developmentally handicapped patients. This, however, is an imperfect rule, and thus only partially true.

One would prefer to devote more attention to the rules that govern pediatric psychopathology and pediatric psychopharmacology, but one is mercifully restrained by the realities of space, time, and exhaustion with the task at hand.

The three conditions I have had the opportunity to consider are childhood hyperactivity, which is highly prevalent and a model in many ways for understanding of psychopathology in general; the Kleine–Levin syndrome, which is extremely rare but an interesting model for the atypical manifestation of affective disorders during adolescence; and rheumatic psychosis, which is neither common nor rare, but is if anything a hypothetical issue. It may be important, or it may be "blue sky."

Childhood Hyperactivity

The meaning of shapes that are not clearly identifiable is as important as the meaning of shapes whose outlines are clear.

—*Magritte.*

Childhood hyperactivity, or "attention deficit/hyperactivity disorder," is notable on several counts. It has had more name changes than Stalingrad. It is one of those medical conditions, like malaria and the gout, for which the appropriate treatment was established long before physicians had an idea what it was they were treating. Intense research interest in the disorder during the 1970s was predicated on a fallacy, the "paradoxical response" of hyperactive children (HAC) to stimulants. As soon as that myth was exposed, a whole community of neuroscientists who had been cultivating hyperactive rats and calming them down with amphetamine seemed to lose interest in the subject. The disorder fell from favor, at least among researchers. All that has happened recently is a couple more name changes.

Hyperactivity is more than an historical curiosity. It is a paradigm for a class of neuropsychiatric disorders that afflict large numbers of people to a mild degree and small numbers of people to a severe degree. It is a model for the spectrum of liability model that is drawn from behavioral genetics. It is a model "dysmaturation" syndrome, and a model for a class of frontal lobe pathology. It is a lesson in psychostimulant pharmacology, and an example of how not to explore the neurochemical basis of behavior. It is not really a psychiatric disorder at all, but a prototype for the mild developmental disabilities: how they may be misconstrued as psychiatric conditions. It is also a model of how misconstruction can impede the science of treatment.

The structure of childhood hyperactivity is well defined, but it is also quite variable. It is defined in terms of a few cardinal symptoms: locomotor hyperactivity, impulsive behavior, excitability and emotional immaturity, short attention span and distractibility, inefficiency in work performance. Problem behaviors are first noted in infancy, although they may not be remarked as such, and they continue through childhood with the possibility of abatement at any time.

There also appears to be a small group of HAC who have "pervasive" symptoms; they tend to have other developmental or neurological problems as well, their symptoms are less amenable to drug treatment or to behavioral programming, and the outcome is a life of relative handicap (Menkes et al., 1967). In such cases, one is often able to identify a neuropathic cause, or at least a concomitant.

The much larger group of HAC are normal kids with a relatively benign disorder and with problems that wax and wane with the vagaries of development, but with a good response to treatment and a long-term prognosis that is really quite favorable (Weiss and Hechtman, 1986). For most cases, no etiology or associated neuropathic feature is ever identified, but there is often a family history of similar problems.

The stimulant response in HAC remains one of the most gratifying experiences in psychopharmacology. It is a function of presynaptic dopamine agonist action on regulatory frontal lobe structures. But the pattern of drug response has a peculiar economy: the most to those who need it least. Patients who respond best to stimulants are those who have relatively mild conditions, and severe cases, especially retarded HAC and other neuropathic cases, respond poorly. The degree to which an individual deviates from the stereotype of a high-IQ, middle-class kid who comes from a stable home and has no concomitant pathology, to that degree will the stimulant response diminish.

The model that is proposed here for childhood hyperactivity is, in fact, a conjunction of models. The principle is one of multiple perspectives. It derives from the belief that no one system or point of view can be brought to bear on or to account for all the dimensions of the problem. It is idle to posit a unitary explanation, such as "arousal" or "attention" or "frontal lobe dysregulation," for a disorder of brain and behavior. There must be a conjunction of views: genetic, pathological, ecological, neurochemical, and neuroanatomic. If the model is valid, one should expect that the correct view from one perspective will lead, naturally and smoothly, to the next perspective, and that all the points of view will be not only consistent but also interrelated and mutually supportive. The model should address all the important elements of the problem: etiology, neuropathology, neuropharmacology, psychology, and treatment.

It is the completeness of our understanding of childhood hyperactivity that accounts for its current importance. As a clinical problem, it probably does not require much more in the way of research attention. As a paradigm for understanding certain other neuropsychiatric disorders, however, it deserves a great deal of attention.

The Genetic Model

Childhood hyperactivity is conceptualized as a constellation of personality traits. The phenotype is broad and widely distributed in the population; the prevalence may be as high as 5% of the school-age population. Problems like hyperactivity and attention deficit are so prevalent, and manifest such extreme diversity, that they can only be conceptualized as variants of the human character. Hyperactivity and attention deficit are human traits that are themselves composed of traits, like impulsiveness and excitability, locomotor hyperactivity, sustained and selective attention deficits, and so on.

Hyperactivity tends to run in families, but the pattern of inheritance has never suggested a Mendelian model. The default opinion, and probably a correct one, is that the disorder is "polygenic." That means that there are multiple sites in the genome that contribute to the phenotype, and that the phenotype is expressed only when a certain quantity of such genes are present and operative in concert. It is assumed that these "polygenes" are normally distributed in the population (Carter, 1965; Gualtieri and Hicks, 1985a). Polygenetic inheritance is a pattern that characterizes the inheritance of other human traits, such as IQ or height.

When one considers that the distribution of genes for Hyperactivity and related deficits is probably normal, then there must necessarily be a group of people who have a substantial genetic load, and they are the people who are going to express

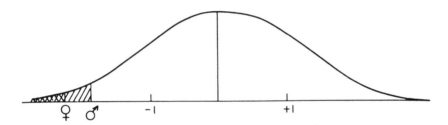

FIGURE 11.1. Normal distribution of polygenes for attention deficit/hyperactive disorder (AD/HD): variable threshold of expression by sex.

the phenotype. The threshold for expression may vary, however, with the circumstances; the threshold for detection may also vary, depending on diagnostic fads and custom.

For example, if hyperactivity is at all similar to other neurodevelopmental disorders, it is likely that the threshold for expression is lower for boys than for girls; that boys require fewer "hyperactivity genes" than girls to express the disorder. If the polygenetic model is correct, with a variable threshold for expression by sex, then one may make certain predictions about hyperactivity:

1. More boys will be afflicted than girls.
2. When girls are afflicted, they will be more severely so.
3. Girls will have more afflicted family members than boys.
4. Hyperactive fathers will have hyperactive sons; hyperactive mothers will have hyperactive sons and daughters.

The threshold of expression by sex is confounded, however, by the phenomenon of selective identification by sex. (Boys are more likely to be referred to professionals for evaluation and treatment of deviant behavior. There is also, then, a threshold of detection difference.) The model is presented in Figure 11.1. It is a presumptive model, and there are only a few studies to support it, but it gives rise to testable hypotheses. It is largely supported by extrapolation from studies of other neurodevelopmental disorders. A polygenetic model with variable threshold of expression by sex has been proposed to account for sex differences in the occurrence of certain congenital malformations (Carter, 1965), dyslexia (Lewitter et al., 1980), conduct disorder and sociopathy (Cloninger et al., 1978), stuttering (Garside and Kay, 1964), autism (Tsai and Beisler, 1983), pyloric stenosis (Carter, 1965), and cleft lip and palate (Woolf, 1971).

The polygenetic model is useful, however, as more than a genetic hypothesis. It may be expanded to include other factors that can play a role in the genesis of the syndrome. Other elements, nongenetic elements, may be included on the normal curve, which would read on the abscissa: genes and environmental factors that contribute to the phenotype. And the threshold for expression need not be determined by sex alone. Other elements may contribute to where that threshold lies;

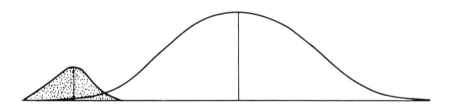

FIGURE 11.2. "Two-stage" model for "attention deficit/hyperactive disorder" (AD/HD) temperamental and pathological variants.

especially environmental factors like social perceptions, classroom expectations, racial prejudice, or other issues that we discuss further on.

The fundamental belief that underlies this model is that the clinical "symptoms" of hyperactivity are in fact elements of human personality. There is a genetically permissible range of expression for the various traits that comprise human personality, and for any given trait, there will be a certain proportion of the population that will express a certain amount of deviance. That deviance may be defined in terms of pathology, and it is not surprising that physicians prefer to define human variability in such terms. After all, that is their currency. Shoe salesmen define deviance in terms of feet that are too big or too small to fit the available selection of shoes. They are neither right nor wrong in so doing; they are simply behaving like shoe salesmen.

The Two-Stage Model

The occurrence of symptoms of hyperactivity in patients with other neuropathic problems, such as mental retardation or epilepsy, and the severity of their symptoms suggest that the "normal distribution" model is not sufficient to capture the entirety of the clinical syndrome. This leads to a second model, derived from the study of intelligence and mental retardation.

Intelligence is also a human trait that is normally distributed, and it seems to be determined, at least in part, by polygenes. For the sake of argument, let us assume that there is a genetically permissible range of intelligence, in terms of IQ, from 40 to 160. But that normal distribution does not account for a "pathological bump," an excess of cases with severe and profound deficits in intelligence (i.e., IQ below 40). Their handicap may be genetically impermissible, but it happens anyway. It occurs as the consequence not of a genetically permissible range of human variability but of some severe neuropathic event, like encephalitis or anoxia, or some severe derangement of the genome. The model is well known in the study of mental retardation, where it is possible to distinguish between "inherited" and "pathological" conditions; it is presented in Figure 11.2.

The relationship between "temperamental" and "pathological" hyperactivity probably follows this two-stage model. On the left tail of the normal curve is the large group of HAC with a benign disorder and no associated neuropathy. To the left of the tail, and overlapping it to a degree, is a small group of HAC who have significant neurological, developmental, or psychiatric pathology. The problems they exhibit are attributable only in part (if at all) to polygenes that code for hyperactivity traits. They are attributable to an underlying neuropathic disorder.

Now, this is a conceptual model that speaks to the two sides of hyperactivity: the high-prevalence, mild disorder with a generally good prognosis, and the low-prevalence, severe disorder with a prognosis that is determined not by the behavioral symptomatology but rather by the nature of the underlying neuropathic event.

The two-stage model suffers from the weakness of dichotomy; the idea that clear and unequivocal divisions can be drawn on the basis of constructs like "pervasive" versus "situational" hyperactivity, or "temperamental" versus "neuropathic." It is not to pretend, for example, that one form of the disorder is brain based and physiological while another form is personality based and therefore nonphysiological. The two-stage model is an addendum to the genetic model. Both models speak to the origins of hyperactivity. The genetic model represents that this disorder lies at the far edge of a continuum of permissible temperaments; the two-stage model represents that for certain cases the origin of the disorder is discontinuous, or neuropathic. For the first, pathology is defined in dimensional or quantitative terms; for the second, it is stated in categorical or qualitative terms.

The Frontal Lobe Hypothesis

The etiology of the disorder, therefore, is polygenetic, or it is neuropathic. The second issue, then, is the pathologic anatomy of the disorder. What is the functional neuroanatomy of hyperactivity? We have proposed that it is localized to the orbitofrontal cortex, the rostral pole of a diffuse axial brain system that mediates cortical arousal and regulation.

The frontal lobe hypothesis is not necessarily a neuropathic model. The basis of the hypothesis is the contention that regulation of attention, locomotor activity, impulse control, and emotional response is a frontal lobe function, and that deficits in frontal lobe function may be manifest as symptoms of hyperactivity. Deficits in frontal lobe function may be pathological, the consequence of a lesion, for example; or they may be developmental, the consequence of a dysmaturation in frontal regulatory systems. The development of the frontal lobes is a long and arduous process; the myelination of frontal neurons, for example, is not completed in humans until the fifth decade of life. It is an amusing irony to reflect that frontal lobe maturation is not complete until core rot has set in the rest of your brain.

Providence has not had a great deal of experience wiring structures as complex as the frontal cortex, so we ought to forgive the mistakes He (or She) has made along the way. It is natural to expect a great deal of interindividual variability, in the rate of frontal lobe development, simply by virtue of its complexity and its evolutionary novelty. When we speak of dysmaturation of frontal lobe development, we are alluding to nothing more than extreme variability in the rate of development.

The frontal lobe hypothesis of childhood hyperactivity is based first on the clinical similarity between hyperactive children and patients with certain frontal lobe syndromes: similar problems with excessive variability and dysregulation (heterostasis), distractibility and short attention span, locomotor hyperactivity, excitability and lack of impulse control. In both patient groups, the apparent paradox of concurrent symptoms of perseveration and distractibility is explicable in terms of a diminished capacity for self-regulation; they persist in inappropriate behaviors that feedback indicates is inappropriate (and which they can describe as such).

Both groups are also liable to various minor motor abnormalities in addition to excess motor activity such as clumsiness, problems with motor coordination and motor imitation, and associated or synkinetic movements. Both demonstrate striking deficiencies in various dimensions of impulse control, including low tolerance for frustration, low ability to delay gratification, antisocial behavior, delinquency, and impaired sphincter control. Defective impulse control may also be partially responsible for the notorious lack of planning and poor planning attributed to each group. Antisocial, or at least socially disapproved behavior characterizes both classes of patients: impulsiveness, undependability, destructiveness, and aggression. Both exhibit deficits in social interactions, in part a consequence of these impulsive behavior patterns. Interpersonal relating is probably influenced as well by another shared characteristic, disordered emotionality. The apparent lack of modulation of emotional response of both hyperactive children and patients with frontal lobe problems is indicated by their mercurial lability, varying in extremes from anhedonic depression to uncontrolled excitement (Gualtieri and Hicks, 1985b).

Additional evidence for the frontal lobe hypothesis is adduced from animal models of hyperactivity from frontal and striatal lesions and neurochemical lesions to the dopaminergic projections to striatal, limbic, and frontal cortex. The stimulant drugs are known to enhance dopaminergic neurotransmission, and the hypothesis can be called upon to explain the therapeutic benefit of stimulants in terms of an effect on rostral dopaminergic projections. Stimulants like methylphenidate and amphetamine are also known to improve behavioral and cognitive deficits in closed head injury patients with frontal lobe lesions (see Chapter 3, this volume). Thus, the frontal lobe hypothesis may provide a basis for understanding the neurochemical basis for stimulant response.

The hypothesis is that childhood hyperactivity is a dysregulatory or a heterostatic disorder. The excessive intrasubject variability of hyperactive children in autonomic, electrocortical, and behavioral response is also found in frontal lobe patients. It is appropriate to propose that structures on the orbital surface of the frontal lobes are essential for the coordination of various somatomotor and visceromotor activities. This area is unique in that inputs from virtually all bilateral sensory systems converge; it constitutes the major neocortical representation of limbic output; and it constitutes the rostral end of a powerful descending, inhibitory, and synchronizing system. Afferent information from all parts of the body and "affective marking" would be a prerequisite for the coordinating role of a cortical center that regulates many levels of the neuraxis (Gualtieri and Hicks, 1985b).

Direct support for the frontal lobe hypothesis is obtained from regional cerebral blood flow studies by Lou and colleagues (Lou et al., 1984) and, more recently, from positron emission tomography (PET) scan studies by Zemetkin at the National Institute of Mental Health (NIMH).

The frontal lobe hypothesis is consistent with the polygenetic model of hyperactivity, because it may be held that maturation of such a complicated system is necessarily prone to substantial interindividual variation, and that the individual rate of maturation of frontal lobe regulatory systems is under polygenetic influence. It is also consistent with the two-stage model, which suggests that some cases of hyperactivity are a consequence of a neuropathic process involving the orbital surface of the frontal lobes.

The frontal lobe, or heterostatic, hypothesis is also consistent with the next model of childhood hyperactivity, the ecological model, and it speaks to the basis for behavioral management of hyperactive patients. If the disorder is indeed a function of dysregulation of behavioral response, then its manifestation will inexorably be decided by the degree to which the environment confers stability and structure on the one hand, or instability and disruption on the other. Patients with frontal lobe lesions are notoriously vulnerable to sudden unpredictable changes in set, to which they respond in extreme fashion. When their world is well ordered and predictable, they are stable, and their deficits may not be apparent at all.

The Neuropharmacological Model

This model, of course, is in the currency of modern psychiatry; defining disorders in terms of specific and unitary neurotransmitter abnormalities. In childhood hyperactivity, there is an extensive literature on this topic. Hypotheses concerning the neurochemical basis of the disorder are derived from three sources: (1) the known neurochemical effects of drugs that are effective in treating the disorder; (2) neurochemical lesions in laboratory animals whose behaviors mimic the symptoms of the disorder; and (3) measures of neurotransmitter metabolites in the urine, blood, and cerebrospinal fluid (CSF) of patients with the disorder. Research in the latter two areas have led to hypotheses of childhood hyperactivity as a disorder of serotonin, norepinephrine, or of dopamine metabolism, and in each instance the abnormality has been held to be a functional deficit or, alternatively, an overproduction state.

The neuropharmacology of childhood hyperactivity has been well covered in the literature, so there is no need to dwell on the subject here. There has been no definitive finding from all the research that has been done, so one's judgment must be guided by two elements: the neuropharmacology of the anatomic substrate, and the neuropharmacology of the drugs that work well for the symptoms of the disorder. There is concurrence from both sides. Midbrain projections to the orbitofrontal cortex are monoaminergic, especially dopaminergic; and drugs for hyperactivity are monoaminergic, especially dopaminergic. Dopamine agonists work because they enhance tonic control of frontal lobe regulatory systems.

The therapeutics of hyperactivity may be influenced by the locus of the anatomic deficit. Presynaptic or indirect agonists, like the stimulants, are most useful for "high-level" HAC and for head injury patients with minor lesions of the frontal lobes, the "postconcussion" syndrome. In contrast, patients with extensive subcortical damage, for example, severe head injury patients or hyperactive children who are mentally retarded, do poorly on stimulants, but they do well with postsynaptic or direct dopamine agonists like amantadine or bromocriptine.

The Ecological Model

This paradigm is also a necessary derivative of the polygenetic model, with a variable threshold of expression of the phenotype. We have suggested that sex may be one element that determines placement of the threshold. The explanation for differential expression by sex is an issue we have addressed on earlier occasions (Gualtieri and Hicks, 1985a). Sex, however, is not the only feature external to the disorder that may influence occurrence. The very definition of the disorder in terms of normative expectations of standards of behavior and classroom performance for children suggests that norms and expectations will necessarily influence syndrome recognition. The notion of "situational" hyperactivity suggests that certain situations may evoke the phenotype, while other situations may serve to mask it.

The threshold of expression, therefore, is also a threshold of perception and of attribution. It is a threshold past which a given environment will evoke the symptoms. In practical terms, it appears that an unstructured classroom setting, with only a minimum of individual attention and a heavy load of individual responsibility, will move the threshold of expression to the right, that is, in the direction of identifying more cases as pathological. Life circumstances that are full of instability and lacking in external supports, and academic requirements that are intellectual rather than practical, will also shift the threshold to the right.

An educational system that emphasizes normative achievement and a high degree of conformity to standards of behavior will likely discover greater numbers of children with a "psychiatric disorder" which is defined in terms of nonnormative behavior and achievement. That does not mean that the disorder is contrived or imaginary, only that the terminology is wrong. The appropriate terminology is in terms of deviation from developmental norms, not psychiatric disorder.

If what we call the disorder of childhood hyperactivity or attention deficit is conceptualized as, in most cases, a normally occurring constellation of human traits, then we might do well to consider the traits that a culture values, contrasted to the traits it devalues. Sustained attention to dull repetitive tasks that are heavily laden with verbal information is valued by our culture, and scanning attention to a broad array of stimuli is devalued. The capacity to react to circumstances only after reflection and due consideration of social expectations is valued more keenly than the capacity to react quickly and decisively, with consideration only to exigencies of the moment. The capacity to subdue one's emotional response is valued more than the capacity to express it. The ability to mature at a rapid, normative rate, at least with respect to skills that are valued in the marketplace, is valued more than the proclivity to develop at a slow, idiosyncratic rate. When one defines as a disorder something that is usually nothing more than a developmental variant, one has to look very carefully at the cultural, political, and economic values of society as a whole. Such values define where we will place our thresholds of expression and detection; they define, in fact, that which we will detect.

The signal contribution of the developmental movement is to accept the normative definition of a disorder, but not to feel any compulsion to construct a pseudopathological framework around it. Rather, the thrust is to address the norms that render the disability handicapping. The thrust, therefore, is in the direction of treatment, and treatment is to conform the patient's environment to his or her native capacities.

In childhood hyperactivity, the first approach to treatment is to change the ecology of the hyperactive child. And here, the changes are very similar to what we also suggest for patients with frontal lobe lesions: a high degree of structure, feedback that is frequent and directive, removal from circumstances that are unstable or excessively stimulating, avoidance of rapid or frequent changes in set, and tolerance for a considerable amount of idiosyncratic behavior. In heterostatic disorders, like childhood hyperactivity and like the frontal lobe syndrome, the goal of treatment is to reduce the untoward consequences of dysregulation by giving the patient less that he has to regulate around.

Ecological treatment, then, is rational, insofar as it eliminates the firing points that evoke a pathological response. Stimulant treatment is also rational, in the sense that it addresses the problem of heterostasis, the problem that renders toxic circumstances that are really quite normal.

The ecological model may be recognized in terms of analogy, like the parable of the shoe salesman, or it may be defined in conceptual terms. The latter introduces the concept of a threshold. The shoe salesman will be more tolerant of deviance in foot size if he (or she) has an extensive inventory of shoes. A teacher will be more tolerant of deviant behavior in the class if he (or she) has more resources to bring to bear to cope with an unexpected or a difficult situation. The teacher's threshold may be exceeded early or late, depending on the reserve he holds. It is well known, for example, that the threshold for deviant behavior is much higher for little girls than for boys. The latter are referred sooner to a psychologist because teachers and parents are more apt to view their behavior as deviant. That is nothing more than a social norm, but it is translated, every day, into an operation that has medical consequences. The misbehavior of white children is more likely to be perceived as a clinical problem, the misbehavior of black children as a social or a criminal problem. The misbehavior of middle-class children is more likely to be perceived as a medical or a developmental issue, but the misbehavior of poor children is something for the probation officer.

A society that views education as a normative process will consider individual variation to be deviant; a society that considers education as a deeply individual process will view individual variation as something to be cherished and rewarded.

The Cumulative Model

The frontal lobe hypothesis of hyperactivity suggests that factors intrinsic to brain development will determine the expression of the behavioral syndromes. The pathological event that is intrinsic to childhood hyperactivity may be a structural lesion (rarely), or more commonly it may be dysmaturation, a failure of frontal lobe regulatory structures to mature at the same rate as that of most other kids.

There are a host of examples of dysmaturational events that can be interpreted as pathological, if one's view of human development is so inclined: head-banging in 1-year-olds; tantrums in 2-year-olds; stuttering in 4-year-olds; tics in 9-year-olds; hypersomnia or negativism or rebelliousness or risk-taking in adolescents. Hyperactivity and distractibility may simply be, in some cases, a normal developmental variant. It would be a dysmaturation that will clear as factors intrinsic to frontal lobe development take hold.

The ecological model describes how extrinsic elements determine the "course" of a "disorder." Poor schooling, lack of training, or a failure of support or of opportunity may all contrive to maintain or even to aggravate a developmental weakness. A child who might be perceived only as high spirited or impetuous in a classroom that is structured, orderly, and individual oriented might be perceived as hyperactive and impulsive in a large, noisy class where the major goal of instruction is to make it through the day. A child whose attention span is quite sufficient to tasks that engage his particular interests may be perceived as inattentive to work that is perceived as dry and meaningless. A dysmaturation that could remit if left to its own dynamic, with only a degree of support and guidance, can be misdirected and fixed in a pathological channel if it is the occasion of destructive influence.

In our studies of adults with residual symptoms of childhood hyperactivity, we discovered that the severity of the childhood disorder had little bearing on the outcome of the patient, but that other features, such as IQ and social class, had greater weight (Gualtieri et al., 1985). IQ, to some degree, can be considered an intrinsic feature, and social class can be considered an extrinsic feature. In other studies, researchers have established, for example, that hyperactive children with aggressive symptoms fare less well than hyperactive children who have no behavior problems at all (Loney et al., 1981). The problem with childhood hyperactivity as a "psychiatric condition" is that it carries no particular course or outcome; it does not have a life of its own.

The medical or psychiatric model of a disorder like hyperactivity would impute some intrinsic direction to the course of the disorder, a linear trend that is maintained by the pathological energy of the syndrome itself. If such an energy is to be had, it is proposed to be the dysmaturation of frontal lobe regulatory structures. But that is only the setting event; it does not capture the totality of an individual's clinical picture. The reality of the clinical picture, its complexity, the determinant of outcome, and the guide to treatment are not entirely the dysregulatory foundation of hyperactivity, but rather circumstances that lie beyond the boundaries of the syndrome. These are ecological, as we have described; personal issues, like family support, physical attributes, or an engaging personality; other clinical factors, like specific learning disabilities, aggression, low IQ; and social factors, like SES and race, the influence of friends and neighbors, the values and resources of the school.

It is nothing to paint a multifaceted image of the elements that contribute to the outcome of a human life. It is something your grandmother could tell you. The important feature, however, to this construction rests not simply with the accumulation of untoward elements, but rather with a proposal concerning their lawful array. It is suggested that a pathological outcome to childhood hyperactivity is a function of the accumulation of associated risk factors, and that the impact of their accumulation is exponential. That is, the consequences of two additional risk factors would impede the success of a hyperactive child by a factor of four; three factors, by nine, and so on. This is the model Rutter developed in the Isle of Wight study, where the likelihood of developing a psychiatric disorder was, in fact, exponentially related to the occurrence of external risk factors (Rutter et al., 1970).

The evolution of a disorder from childhood to adult life can hardly be understood in terms of fixed elements that capture all the variance. It is much more likely that outcome is determined by a combination of intrinsic and extrinsic factors that operate in additive fashion at low levels and exponentially at high levels of occurrence.

This is not simply a theoretical exercise, because it captures a fundamental principle of therapeutics. What is necessary is not a specific treatment for a disorder like hyperactivity, but a series of corrective measures directed against elements that may aggravate the symptoms, or turn awry the course of development. Successful treatment accepts the intrinsic limitations of the individual, and aims to correct these limitations pharmacologically. It also requires a diminution of extrinsic factors that will combine to impede the normal, intrinsic tendency of brain to self-correct.

The Algorithmic Model

The algorithmic model is the operative model. It is the question parents ask and it is what guides practitioners. It is the definitive response to the question, "Is this child hyperactive?"

This model considers childhood hyperactivity as an idea that is only a stage for specific action. The "diagnosis" speaks to a recommended course of remedy: parent education, school intervention, structured programming, and stimulant medication; all, if necessary, or only some. The rationale for all these steps is derived from the various models presented here: to remake the environment of the child, that is the ecological model; to structure his environment, that is the frontal lobe model; and to remedy associated deficits, that is the cumulative model. Stimulant treatment is rational because we believe that dopaminergic projections to frontostriatal systems are central to the pathophysiology of the disorder.

But the essence of the algorithmic model is that treatment is central. The diagnosis of childhood hyperactivity is nothing more than a suggestion that certain treatment steps will be successful while others will be inappropriate. And whether the treatments are "rational" or not, by the standards of the various models proposed, is beside the point. What counts about the treatment is whether it works. The algorithmic model is an empirical model.

The proliferation of models is satisfying to a practitioner, who must grow accustomed to individual variation and who indeed thrives on it in the art of practice. It is less satisfying to the scientist, who requires discrete hypotheses that can be disproved or supported. Considering a problem like hyperactivity from a single perspective has the advantage of generating experiments. Considering hyperactivity from a number of perspectives has the advantage of capturing the clinical reality of the situation. But the danger of proliferation is that it may simply capture idiosyncrasy and lead to obscurity.

It is easy to lapse into personal idiosyncrasy when one is considering the ecology of children, because we all have our painful memories of childhood, and most of us have occasion to visit the same miseries, or variants thereof, upon on our own offspring. We do this because we love them.

It is harder to express the concept of ecology in terms that are universally acceptable. One view of the ecology of American classrooms is that they are normative to a fault, that they exact conformity from creatures who are free by nature, that conformist expectations are too easily medicalized, and that strong-willed children are drugged into submission as a matter of course. The alternative view is that schools have grown so sensitive to children's individual needs, in the face of a demanding society, that they routinely screen students for even minor health problems, that even minor learning and attention deficits merit their special concern, and that they take pains to guarantee that appropriate treatment is conferred. The point is not to decide between these extreme points of view. The issue is to accept them as poles on a continuum; the truth is closer to one pole or another, depending on the school, depending on the child, and depending on the family.

The purpose of this exercise, which is to propose a conjunction of models for childhood hyperactivity, is not to erect a theoretical structure that will generate testable hypotheses but rather, to synthesize a theory from the large body of research already done in this area. The theory is designed to capture the essential elements of the syndrome, not in a reductionist way, but a way that captures the complexity and diversity of the clinical population.

Psychiatrists, quite naturally, have focused on behavioral symptoms ("diagnostic criteria"), and their success with drug treatment has impelled a concentration on the biochemical basis of the disorder. This has not been a necessary step in the evolution of understanding, it has been a sidetrack. It has turned our attention away from the need to formulate a different way of thinking about neurobehavioral disorders in terms of conjunctive systems. The idea that one can reconstruct a pathophysiological system from the study of symptoms and drug response is nothing more than a conceit. It is linear thinking, and it is just a loan from the organ pathologists of the nineteenth century: etiology $\rightarrow$ organ pathology $\rightarrow$ clinical presentation $\rightarrow$ outcome.

The foundation of neurobehavioral pathophysiology is not linear, it is multidimensional. The brain is not an organ, it is an organ system, and the interactions and interrelations among the organs of the brain are complex and ever changing. They are poorly insulated one from another, and they influence one another in ways that we understand only dimly. When we do learn something about the communication of organ systems in brain, we discover physiological processes like kindling and reciprocal activation and inhibition that are unlike those of any other organ system in the body. There is no limit to the difficulties that accrue to a simple organ-based view of the central nervous system: the redundant assignment of functions, left-to-right, up-and-down; assignment of function based on age and stage of development, or influenced by fatigue or stress; transfer of function from one area to another, in response to lesions or other factors; the fact that lesions can be passive—a functional area is simply subtracted from the array—or they can be active, poisoning the activity of other areas in a nonspecific and unpredictable way.

It is natural that scientists have tried to explain phenomena like hyperactivity in terms of old concepts and presumptions, just as generals always make plans to fight a war that is just like the last one. It is interesting, however, that a simple clinical problem like hyperactivity can be given to a degree of reinterpretation that is salient to a host of other neuropsychiatric disorders.

A society that views development as a process of moral imbuement will consider deviance as a sin. If development is a normative psychological unfolding, deviance is the occasion for reeducation. If development is a biological phenomenon, then deviance is the occasion for diagnosis and treatment. If development is simply an expression of the exuberant diversity of the human spirit, then deviance is nothing but occasion for admiration. The fact is that development is all of these things.

The Kleine–Levin Syndrome

The Kleine–Levin Syndrome (KLS) is a peculiar disorder that primarily affects adolescent males. First described by Kleine (1925), the syndrome is characterized by alternating episodes of hypersomnia and hyperphagia. Critchley (1962) included disturbance of mood and other appetitive functions as symptoms of KLS; the symptom list seems always to have grown with succeeding descriptions. The incidence of KLS is unknown, and fewer than 50 cases have been reported in the literature.

KLS patients present with acute onset of stupor, relative ease of arousal, irritability on awakening, and hyperphagia. Hypersexuality has been described in several patients, and seems to be associated with a generalized increase in other appetitive behaviors. Subsequent descriptions by Lewis (1926), Levin (1936), and Daniels (1934) corroborated a clinical picture of recurring hypersomnia (16 to 20 hours per day), awakening only for urination and defecation; excessive food intake; and mild confusion and mood disturbances ranging from euphoria to extreme irritability. These symptoms were in marked contrast to the patient's premorbid state of health. Powers and Gunderman (1978) added fire-setting as an associated symptom in a single case study. Orlosky (1982) added confusion, amnesia for the episode, (unspecified) movement disorder, delusional thinking, and auditory and visual hallucinations to the list of KLS symptoms.

In spite of the dramatic presentation, few positive findings have been reported on neurological examination. On the other hand, symptoms associated with KLS are commonly seen in other neurological diseases. Hypersomnia has been reported in connection with medial mesencephalic lesions (Culebras and Magnana, 1987), medial thalamic lesions (Jurko et al., 1971), posterior hypothalamic lesions (Ranson, 1939), and lesions that affect elements of the reticular activating system. Hyperphagia and mood instability have been reported in lesions of the hypothalamus (Reeves and Blum, 1969), orbitofrontal cortex (Cummings, 1986), and periventricular areas (Krahn and Mitchell, 1984).

In KLS, positive neurological findings are infrequent and are often confined to atypical cases. Popoviciu and Corforice (1972) reported a single case with modest enlargement of the third ventricle on pneumoencephalogram. In contrast, Furgeson (1986), Goldberg (1983), Thompson et al., (1985), Merriman (1986), and Orlosky (1982) reported no significant changes in the CT scan. To our knowledge, MRI, PET scanning, and quantified EEG analysis have not been applied to KLS. Kleine (1925) and Daniels (1934) reported that some KLS patients had an influenza-like illness before onset of the syndrome. Headache and fever were recorded, but there were no definitive signs of encephalitis. Critchley (1962), Takrani and Cronin (1976), Carpenter et al. (1982), and Merriman (1986) reported cases of KLS after viral encephalitis. Critchley (1962) described two cases with upper respiratory illness and headache preceding the onset of KLS.

Takrani and Cronin (1976) reported neuropathic findings that included neuronal loss, glial proliferation, and perivascular changes in the hypothalamus, amygdala, and anteromedial temporal cortex. Carpenter et al. (1982) described similar necropsy findings along with calcification of the thalamus in a single case. Merriman (1986), in a single case report of KLS in a 25-year-old man, noted CFS findings consistent with encephalitis.

The results of neurophysiological studies have been ambiguous. Merriman (1986) described nonspecific slow wave activity in a single patient with documented encephalitis. Critchley (1962) and Orlosky (1982) reported acute phase changes that included bursts of bilaterally synchronous 2- to 4-cycle/sec activity, consistent with sleep. There was no reported epileptiform activity.

Green (1970), Garland et al. (1965), Lavie et al. (1979), Elian and Bornstein (1969), and Thacore et al. (1969) reported a different set of EEG irregularities. Lavie et al. (1979) reported a male KLS patient whose EEG was characterized by "instability" in the sleep architecture. His second case was a female patient with sleep-onset REM activity reminiscent of narcolepsy. Kupfer et al. (1972) described a similar pattern of sleep-onset REM sleep during multistep sleep provocation. Elian and Bornstein (1969) reported paroxysmal episodes of high-voltage, 2.5- to 3.0-Hz activity during sleep episodes. The degree of EEG abnormality seems to be related to the duration of symptoms. Thacore et al. (1969) reported similar bursts of delta activity, but also noted bursts of 8- to 12-Hz activity alternating with slow-wave activity, activation of slow-wave activity with eye-opening, and a reduction in sleep spindles. The latter finding has also been described in patients with thalamic lesions (Culebras and Magnana, 1987).

On the other hand, Orlosky (1982) noted that polysomnographic studies of 30 KLS patients were consistently negative. In spite of this negative result, he recommended sleep polysomnography for KLS patients. Kupfer et al. (1972) and Lavie et al. (1979) supported this recommendation, especially in atypical cases, to rule out narcolepsy or sleep apnea. Sleep-onset REM activity is pathognomonic for narcolepsy but uncommon in typical cases of KLS. Sleep apneas might be confused with KLS on the basis of hypersomnia, but polysomnography should reveal episodes of apnea not present in KLS (Cuetter, 1985).

The results of neuroendocrine tests of hypothalamic function have been disappointing. Kleine (1925) initially described abnormalities in thyroid function in some patients. Later, Gilbert (1964) reported an atypical case of KLS in a female who had episodically taken thyroid extract for unclear reasons. Thyroid function in this case, however, was reported to be normal. This same patient displayed an increase in 24-hour urinary cortisol excretion that persisted after recovery. Thompson et al. (1985) measured cortisols, melatonin, and prolactin in a 17-year-old male with classical KLS symptoms. Serum levels of these hormones were obtained hourly during episodes of hypersomnia and after recovery. They reported that prolactin and melatonin were essentially unaffected by episodes of hypersomnia. Serial cortisols revealed a persistent disruption of diurnal secretion that persisted after recovery. Thompson concluded that this reversal of diurnal secretion represented a disruption in circadian rhythm, possibly involving the suprachiasmic area of the hypothalamus.

The existence of the syndrome is hardly in doubt, although few physicians have ever had the opportunity to attend a case. The association appears to be some nonspecific neuropathic event, but the nature of the event, or its localization, has never been clearly defined. In fact, there has never been a coherent theory of the disorder. If one were writing a textbook, one could not be sure exactly where it belonged. It is the author's opinion that it belongs in the family of affective disorders.

In 1988, a colleague and I described a typical case of KLS in a 14-year-old white male who presented with abrupt onset of hypersomnia (18 h/day), irritability upon awakening, and a ravenous appetite when he was not asleep. These episodes had followed several evenings of relative sleep deprivation. The patient was an average student with no specific learning deficits. The past medical history and the family history were unremarkable.

An EEG obtained during the active phase of his disorder showed no epileptiform activity. A cranial CT scan was within normal limits. A follow-up EEG during remission was normal. As the patient grew increasingly hypersomniac and disorganized, he was hospitalized, and it was necessary to initiate a short course of neuroleptics. To this, he developed severe extrapyramidal symptoms. A more detailed history of prodromal behaviors then indicated sudden onset of hyperactivity, euphoric mood, reduced need for sleep, hypersexual behavior, and a significant loss of previously adequate social judgment, before the onset of KLS symptoms. Lithium treatment was initiated and the response was dramatic. Over the ensuing week waking time increased and he was more alert and cooperative. He continued a steady improvement, maintaining stable lithium levels in the 1.0-1.2 mq/liter range.

The patient was followed for 2 years. He had two recurrences of hypersomnia and hyperphagia; both occurred in the early fall and followed a night of sleep deprivation. On both occasions, the patient had stopped his lithium to "see how I would do"; he relapsed within 2 to 3 weeks of drug discontinuation. Because the medication was restarted almost immediately, he never experienced a full-blown syndrome.

A short time later, we saw another case, a 14-year-old white boy who presented with a history of hypersomnia, hyperphagia, and irritability at age 13. The patient experienced episodes of hypersomnia (up to 15 hours/day), hyperphagia in which he ate continuously while awake, irritability, and aggression. He had a previous history of a mild closed head injury and of a sexual assault by an older male. The family history was positive for lithium-responsive bipolar illness. Before the onset of KLS, the patient had only a history of attention deficit/hyperactivity.

Diagnostic evaluations included two CT scans, an MRI, and repeated EEG studies. The EEG tracing revealed a preponderance of stage II sleep activity during an active stage of his illness. The MRI scan revealed a suspected lipoma in the quadrigeminal area, but follow-up studies did not suggest expansion. The patient displayed consistently normal neurological and physical findings. Neuroendocrine studies revealed a strongly positive DST with a 24-hour post-dexamethasone serum cortisol of 14.4 mcg/dl. The patient's initial response to dextroamphetamine was positive, with improvement in KLS target symptoms. After several days, however, he became increasingly irritable, aggressive, and hyperactive. Insomnia without fatigue was described in the hospital notes. These symptoms were short lived, and the patient was discharged for follow-up.

He continued to experience symptom breakthrough in spite of amphetamine treatment and subsequent hospitalizations for hypersomnia, hyperphagia, and intermittent aggressivity. Relapses occurred every 3 or 4 months. In response to the positive family history, the cyclical nature of his symptoms, and the limited response to dextro amphetamine, a trial of lithium was initiated. He showed an initial positive response to this approach, and there has been no recurrence of symptoms during a subsequent 1-year follow-up on lithium.

Thus, we had the unique experience of two young adolescent boys, both with the typical clinical presentation of KLS: one preceded by a brief period of hyperactivity, insomnia, and euphoric mood, and one by a mild head injury and a severe psychological stressor. Both patients were responsive to lithium treatment over follow-up for 1 to 2 years. The first patient had some initial symptoms suggestive of hypomania, but no family history of major affective disorder; the second patient had a strong family history of bipolar disorder, responsive to lithium, in two first-degree relations, and he had a DST that was strongly positive during an acute episode.

It is not unreasonable to suggest that KLS may be a peculiar variant of adolescent major affective disorder (MAD). Hypersomnia is known to be associated with the depressive phase of bipolar disorder (Hawkins et al., 1985) and episodic hyperphagia has also been described in MAD (Carlson and Strober, 1978). Other symptoms associated with the KLS that are known to occur in bipolar patients are hypersexuality, irritability, withdrawal, and intermittent aggression (Carlson and Strober, 1978; Bowden and Sarabia, 1980; Ballenger and Post, 1980; Ballenger et al., 1982; Manfredi et al., 1987).

Psychostimulants are the conventional treatments for KLS (Orlovsky, 1982); the rationale is that KLS is a disorder of "arousal" (Manfredi et al., 1987). Stimulant treatment, however, may not prevent recurrences of KLS (Jeffries and LeFebvre, 1973; Abe, 1977; Ogura et al., 1976), and they did not do so in our second case. On the other hand, successful treatments with lithium in KLS has already been described by Ogura et al. (1976) and by Abe (1977). It is our opinion that lithium should be considered the treatment of choice for recurrent KLS. In KLS patients who do not respond to lithium or who cannot tolerate the drug, treatment with the usual alternative drugs for bipolar disorder should be considered: carbamazepine, valproic acid, or clonazepam (Roy-Byrne et al., 1984; Chouinard, 1985; Schou, 1979; Lena, 1979). There are, however, to our knowledge, no reports of treatment trials with these drugs in KLS.

Of course, lithium response does nothing to finalize the diagnosis of MAD. Lithium has been helpful in the management of self-injurious behavior (Schou, 1979; Lena, 1979), violent and aggressive behavior (Schou, 1979), and other nonspecific behavior difficulties associated with brain injury or brain disease (Krauthammer and Klerman, 1978). By the same token, it is virtually impossible to establish a connection between two syndromes whose manifestations are entirely behavioral and whose underlying pathophysiology is unknown. The putative association between bipolar affective disorder and KLS is important only insofar as it may guide treatment for patients who would respond poorly to the usual treatments.

That, of course, is the necessary intellectual caveat one is compelled to dispense. In fact, it is important to have a theory for a disease; it must go somewhere in the table of contents. The KLS probably belongs among the major affective disorders, an atypical variant that arises in adolescence; adolescence is the time for atypical affective disorders.

Rheumatic Psychosis

The behavioral concomitants of Sydenham's chorea are usually mild: hyperactivity, mischievous behavior, emotional lability, impulsiveness, and emotional lability (Herskowitz and Rosman, 1982). Severe psychiatric symptoms are not very common, although affective and schizophreniform symptoms have been described, at least in the past, when rheumatic fever was more common than it is now. A generation of physicians, however, have been trained during an era when rheumatic fever and its complications have been a comparative rarity. Now, even as the disease seems to be making a return, it is easy to forget that the sudden onset of severe psychiatric symptoms may be no more than a complication of rheumatic fever.

We have had occasion to attend to children with recurrent episodes of "encephalitis," characterized by chorea, weakness, psychosis, and catatonia. The patients were referred as "functional" psychoses, but they probably had Sydenham's chorea and rheumatic psychosis. The diagnosis was supported by the clinical history and physical findings: choreiform movements arising soon after the occurrence of a febrile illness, with behavioral symptoms developing soon thereafter, characterized by catatonia, disorganization, and hallucinations. The ASLO titers were elevated. There was no other cause to be found for the dyskinesias and psychiatric symptoms. The premorbid history was clear, and the episode remitted sans sequelae. In one case, there was a previous episode identical in presentation and outcome.

In such cases, there may be no evidence of carditis. The clinical picture in our cases was consistent with the diagnosis of Sydenham's chorea, and no alternative diagnosis, either in psychiatry or in neurology, seemed as compelling. On the other hand, because the choreiform movements represented only a minor, transient part of the clinical picture, and because the mental state changes were really the most important aspect of the clinical problem, the diagnosis of "rheumatic psychosis" is probably more accurate.

It is known that rheumatic fever can present with psychiatric symptoms, absent carditis, and absent dyskinesia (Leys, 1946). But that fact is not common knowledge. In 1946, Duncan Leys wrote:

> Rheumatic psychosis of various types have been described by neurologists or psychiatrists in studies of psychosis of encephalitis, but does not seem to have been remarked by pediatricians (Leys, 1946, p. 448).

In Leys' article titled "Rheumatic Encephalopathy," three cases were described, "diagnosed...without hesitation as schizophrenic," all of whom were children who developed chorea following a febrile illness, with mental state changes similar to those observed in our cases. Leys also reviewed similar cases reported by Neal (1942), Wilson (1940), Winkelman and Eckel (1932), and Coombs (1912).

It is also pertinent to note that an early history of rheumatic fever has been reported with increased frequency in psychotic patients, and especially in catatonic patients, by Bruetsch (1944), Wertheimer (1957), and Wilcox (1986); the association is not specific, because similar findings have also been reported in patients with obsessive-compulsive disorder (Swedo et al., 1989). The existence of autoantibodies to subthalamic and caudate tissue in acute rheumatic fever was described by Husby et al. in 1976. This may represent the connection between the acute infectious reaction and the subsequent development of chorea and psychiatric symptoms.

In an individual case, one can only surmise that a patient's psychosis is rheumatic in origin; an elevated ASLO titre, for example, does not establish the diagnosis, it only affirms an exposure to the streptococcus. The diagnosis is only suggested by the overall clinical picture.

On the other hand, rheumatic psychosis is a real thing, it seems, although its existence has not been widely appreciated, even in the days when rheumatic fever was a common pediatric problem. If rheumatic fever is in fact growing in frequency (Bisno et al., 1988; Hosler et al., 1987), one may expect to see more of this clinical phenomenon. The occurrence of acute psychosis in a child or adolescent should be the occasion for a careful examination for other signs of rheumatic fever, and appropriate laboratory investigations should be undertaken. It is important to know whether the disease will resolve on its own, without recourse to psychiatric medications, and whether it is a psychotic disorder that can be prevented from recurring with prophylactic antibiotics.

CHAPTER 12

Behavioral Psychopharmacology

Psychopharmacology is an empirical thing, but that does not mean it has no principles. It is trial and error, and sometimes there are as many errors as trials. However, that does not diminish the *lawfulness* of the exercise. Therapeutic vision may be limited, but it is not blind.

Conventional psychopharmacology has been limited by two constraints: a theoretical base in Kraepelinian, nosological psychiatry, and the failure to develop a meaningful brain map. The first restraint has obscured the true, empirical base of psychopharmacology. The second has blinded practitioners and clinical scientists to its lawfulness.

Conventional psychopharmacology has pretended to follow existing "functional" psychiatric diagnoses. Drugs are defined in terms of the conditions they are prescribed to treat: antipsychotics, antidepressants, anxiolytics, thymoleptics. The premise is that diagnoses based solely on behavior are meaningful; the corollary is that drug actions are sufficiently understood in terms of the established psychiatric nosology.

To the neuropsychiatrist who practices behavioral psychopharmacology, it is clear that this approach is limited, if not fallacious. The established categories are occasionally useful, but only occasionally. The established treatments are sometimes effective, but not often enough. The diagnostic categories are sometimes useful, but sometimes not. The premise is weak, and the theory is limited.

The principles of behavioral psychopharmacology are, in contrast, deduced from observed phenomena; they are not induced from a theory of the organization of psychopathology. The principles of behavioral psychopharmacology are deduced from observations of events related to drug action, both in laboratory preparations and in clinical circumstances. No overarching theory guides the elucidation of these phenomena, nor has any general theory arisen from them. But the assembling of observed facts in behavioral psychopharmacology is sufficiently well advanced that one can draw laws and principles simply from the results of practice—principles and guidelines that in turn are capable of clearing the limited vision.

The first weakness of traditional psychopharmacology, then, is its enduring attachment to a Kraepelinian nosological system. The second weakness of the traditional approach is the absence of a meaningful brain map. There is, in clinical psychopharmacology, nothing of etiology, nothing of pathological anatomy, and very little of pathophysiology. The diagnoses are based on external behavior, and that is a notoriously unreliable guide to events in the brain. Behavior by itself is not an appropriate basis for medical diagnosis. Behavior is a measurable thing, that is all; it is not the high road to any place.

In behavioral psychopharmacology, the brain map has primacy, whether it is a map derived from established lesions, inferred lesions, animal models, or hypothesized dysfunctions on a neurochemical basis. One assumes that a specific behavior or a pattern of behavior, such as aggression or psychosis, may originate at any of several different sites, and may be fed by any of several different neurochemical processes. What is important is not the behavior, but the site of origin and the nature of the pathological process. To the degree this is understood, then diagnosis is a sound process and therapeutics may be rational. To the degree it is vague or ambiguous, then diagnosis and treatment are no more than hypothetical exercises. This view of behavioral psychopharmacology is inevitable in anyone who spends his or her career working with "special populations," like the people we have been talking about in the last 11 chapters. It is a view less clear to psychiatrists who work among traditional patient groups, in acute-care hospitals, for example, where the old categories still have some cogency. But it is a view, in the opinion of the author and many of his colleagues, that will achieve primacy even in traditional psychopharmacology before too long.

The study of "special populations" has always been a remote outpost in the history of psychiatry and psychopharmacology. The most interesting things have always seemed to happen in the center of the empire. But sometimes the news from a remote frontier is compelling, and sometimes it may announce changes that will shake the empire to its foundations.

Well, some day there may be interesting news from this remote outpost, but there is nothing world-shaking yet. The first 11 chapters may have contained some quaint provincial wisdom, but that, in the author's opinion, is all. What follows, by way of wrapping it up, is a series of pithy homilies about the craft of behavioral psychopharmacology. Not a "Hints from Heloise" for psychopharmacologists, because that formula has been preempted by Shader and Greenblatt. Not a "Whole Earth Catalog" either, because the "Neuropsychopharmacologists" do that every few years. More like "An Intelligent Woman's Guide to Socialism and Behavioral Pharmacology," with apologies to G.B. Shaw.

Therapeutic Trials Are Hypothesis Testing

The diagnostic process in neuropsychiatry, with its inherent limitations, does no more than set the stage for testing hypotheses. The clinical presentation raises a series of hypotheses about what might be amiss; the hypotheses are rank-ordered in terms of likelihood, and drug trials are oriented towards testing the validity of the hypotheses, in succession.

The key to this process is how the question is framed.

The question, "Is this child hyperactive?" is not a valid question. The appropriate question is whether the child's problems with hyperactivity, inattention, and disinhibition are sufficiently severe to warrant a drug trial; and, if so, will moderate doses of a stimulant drug lead to substantial improvement. If the "diagnosis" of hyperactivity is at issue, the hypothesis cannot be properly tested. That is because there is no definitive physiological test of "hyperactivity" as a medical condition. But if the "diagnosis" is simply an algorithm that suggests specific therapeutic steps, then it is a solid beginning point. The "diagnosis" becomes an hypothesis: Will stimulants work? And the hypothesis is testable.

The question about diagnosis is not a valid scientific question, because it cannot be validated except in terms of some dubious authority like a diagnostic manual or a rating scale. Questions about severity are answerable, because the answers may be based on observed phenomena. Questions concerning the success of a drug trial are answerable, because they are measurable.

Every clinical presentation leads to a series of hypotheses about what might be wrong with the patient and what might be done to alleviate the problem. The hypotheses may be rank-ordered in terms of likelihood or credibility. This is a form of differential diagnosis or, to be precise, differential therapeutics—drug trials, not as a means to affirm a diagnosis but rather as a way to affirm or to disprove an hypothesis.

A patient with explosive aggressive outbursts may be suffering the toxic effects of a drug, like phenobarbital for example, or a stimulant or a neuroleptic (akathisia). If that is so, then removing the drug should alleviate the problem. Or he may have an epileptiform disorder, even if neurodiagnostics are clear. In such cases, carbamazepine or valproate may be successful. Or he may have an affective disorder and respond to lithium. Or he may have a disinhibition syndrome, resulting perhaps from an old injury to the orbitomedial surface of the frontal lobes; here again the results of imaging procedures may be equivocal. In such cases, dopamine agonist treatment will usually be successful. And so on; the possibilities are ranked in order, and drug trials follow systematically.

It is not merely a semantic difference: to say, on the one hand, that a certain drug is indicated in light of the patient's diagnosis, or on the other hand that a certain drug might be successful, if we hypothesize that the patient's problems are a consequence of a particular process. It is not a semantic difference. It is the difference between posturing and honesty, between faith and science.

Theoretical Models Run in Parallel

The concept of parallel models is a point of view we first developed around the problem of childhood hyperactivity (Chapter 11), but it is equally useful in considering the wider issue of pharmacological treatment.

Hypotheses in support of a clinical drug trial are created from an idea that a "particular process" is operative and that the drug will affect that process in a particular way. The key, though, is to understand that the processes in question may themselves be understood in terms of a number of sources. It is possible to develop the idea that a conventional psychiatric process is operative: a major affective episode, a schizophreniform disorder, or a panic disorder. Alternatively, it is possible to base one's hypothesis on the presumption of a conventional neurological diagnosis; an autistic person who is abulic, bradykinetic, and lacks initiative and spontaneous expression may be regarded as parkinsonian and treated accordingly. A patient with explosive nocturnal episodes may be considered as if he were an epileptic, and treated accordingly.

Alternatively, hypotheses may be generated in terms of the supposed neuroanatomy of the problem; an explosive patient who is disinhibited may have an orbitofrontal lesion and may respond to dopamine agonists, while an explosive patient who is intensely emotional, afflicted with memories, and prone to peculiar sensations may have a temporal lobe lesion and respond to carbamazepine.

Hypotheses may be generated in neurochemical terms. A postconcussion syndrome may be conceptualized as a generalized monoamine deficiency; monoamine agonists are therefore likely treatments, and monoamine antagonists would be regarded less favorably. A compulsive self-injurer may be hypothesized as serotonin deficient and treated with serotonin agonists.

Neurochemical and neuroanatomic hypotheses may be joined, for example, when we speak of treating a mild head injury victim with an indirect dopamine agonist, while a severe head injury with extensive subcortical damage would require an indirect agonist (Gualtieri, Chanler Cooks & Brown 1989)

Hypotheses may be generated in terms of presumed pathophysiological processes, like the development of psychosis after a temporal lobe injury, which can kindle a schizophreniform disorder. The choice of a drug, then, might be made on its effects on the kindling process.

Hypotheses are sometimes generated in terms of a dichotomy between environmental and physiological "etiologies" to a problem. It is more appropriate to develop the idea in terms of a *threshold* of response to an environmental toxin (as it were) or in terms of the *amplitude* of the response to an environmental stressor, or in terms of the *duration* of the response. Drug treatment might be oriented, then, to raising the response threshold or alternatively to lowering the amplitude of the behavioral response or its duration. On the other hand, the stressors may be so toxic and the behavior response so inevitable that no medication short of anaesthesia would be appropriate.

No one body of information and no one theoretical base is sufficient to embrace the wide range of utility of the psychoactive compounds. The physician as hypothesis-generator requires a range of theoretical outlooks. The rank order of possible explanations usually includes elements from different points of view.

Behavior Is a Measurable Thing

The orientation of treatment is around specific behaviors, sometimes called "target behaviors," a convenient expression if somewhat dry and mechanical. The orientation is not to "treat" an "illness," because that would be presumptuous, presuming a degree of understanding that we rarely have. The idea is that treatment should be aimed directly at changing some unwanted behavior patterns. Indirectly, it is a test of the hypothesis concerning the origin of the behavior pattern. But the key is behavior change, and documenting that the change occurs.

The use of behavior rating scales and direct behavior observations is an essential part of this process. So is the use of a structured examination that repeatedly gauges the presence or absence of particular clinical elements. The behavioral psychopharmacologist has the equivalent of a graphic chart at the patient's bedside. It does not track the course of an illness; instead, it tracks the particular target behaviors that are of most concern.

In the treatment of self-injurious patients, one measures the course of treatment by tracking the occurrence of target behaviors, like the number of self-injurious outbursts within a period of time or the amount of time the patient can tolerate being out of restraints. The long list of pathological behaviors that cooccur with self-injury (self-injurious behavior, SIB) have been assembled in a rating scale, the Self-Injurious Behavior Questionnaire. Selecting between a rating scale, a direct observation system, or some other measure like a periodic examination or a structured interview depends on the nature of the clinical situation and its economy. SIB that occurs infrequently may be counted directly; SIB that occurs with great frequency requires an interval count, or a measure of time in and out of restraints; and SIB that cooccurs with many other symptoms is best handled using a rating scale.

Because psychopharmaceuticals are known to influence cognitive variables like memory and motor coordination, it has been proposed that serial neuropsychological testing be a component of all drug follow-up. This idea will win wider approval when there is a valid, reliable, and economical way to do serial neuropsychological testing.

There Is a Personal Economy to Consider

Practical therapeutics requires at least some understanding of the wealth of the system, its dynamics, and its resources. There is a personal economy to consider—the resources a patient brings to bear—and a wider economy,—the resources and limitations of the patient's environment.

A patient may not have the personal physical strength to abide the effects of a drug. Some patients are exquisitely sensitive to toxic effects. The major part of the problem of tardive dyskinesia appears to be that some patients are extraordinarily sensitive to the neurotoxic effects of dopamine-blocking drugs (see Chapter 10, this volume).

A patient who is profoundly suicidal may not tolerate the initial beneficial effects of drug treatment without activating some very deadly programs. Such patients are no more suicidal than when treatment first has its effect.

Severely demented patients and patients with severe Parkinson's disease reach a point where they are too far gone to respond favorably to pharmacotherapy. The same is true for schizophrenics, especially when the "deficit" symptoms have taken hold late in the course of the illness. When a patient reaches end state, he is not likely to respond to the specific effects of drug treatment.

This is also true for head injury patients, for whom recovery from coma may be enhanced with certain drugs, dopamine agonists for example; with severe head injuries, however, there may not be a neural matrix to sustain a drug effect.

This is also true of mentally retarded people, for whom drug treatment may reduce a negative behavior; if there is not a repertoire of positive behaviors to fill the void, however, what you will see is simply another kind of maladaptive behavior. The patient's repertoire of positive behaviors is an important clue to the success of pharmacotherapy. This is like the venerable idea of a physiological reserve, a concept that is used to describe events that develop around cardiac or hepatic decompensation. The idea of a patient's "internal economy" is really a kind of "psychological reserve."

There is a prejudice in neuropsychiatry against the use of more than one drug at a time. That has even been an issue is juridical proceedings against drug misuse in institutions and nursing homes. The prejudice against "polypharmacy" may be well taken in some instances at least, because it has often been an indication of misguided treatment. Like all prejudices, though, it is cogent only some of the time. There are plenty of occasions when more than one drug is necessary and beneficial.

The strongest argument against polypharmacy, however, is economic. If it is costly and time consuming to evaluate the effects of a single drug, it is four times as costly and time consuming to evaluate the effects of two.

And a Wider Economy

A wider economy, or an ecology. How much can the environment sustain, in the way of difficult behavior, as one experiments with drug-free baselines, slow titrations to optimal dose, as one eschews polypharmacy and tries to get a clear and unequivocal picture of one drug effect before introducing another? Is it possible to have one-to-one supervision, or two-to-one? Do the regulations tolerate physical restraint or time-out? Is the staff skilled in behavior management for times of crisis?

These issues first arose years ago, when we were beginning to withdraw large numbers of patients from neuroleptics, in some places, on a yearly basis. The practice quickly lost its appeal when it became clear that most units could not abide the behavioral instability that accompanied neuroleptic withdrawal, especially when a few bad actors were going down at the same time. The withdrawals were perfunctory and meaningless, because the economy of the unit could not sustain the additional programming that was necessary. Even today it is unwise to attempt a trial neuroleptic withdrawal unless there are resources available to cope with withdrawal-related difficulties. Issues like this, related to the economy of a residential unit, influence drug decisions by practitioners far more than anyone likes to admit.

We all are familiar with the admonition that drugs are no substitute for programming and should not be used as such. What is missing from this old saw is the fact that clinical decisions are not made on the basis of a one-time choice between "drugs" and "programming." They are made over and over again at team meetings and in periodic consultations, where the issue is not the drug as a substitute but this: the drug is a compensation for the programmatic deficiencies of the unit; or a means to raise the threshold of stimulation by a noisy disruptive environment; or an adjunct during a period of difficult transition; or something that allows a client to adjust to a community setting, whose behavior when drug free is really quite tolerable within an institution.

The third aspect of an ecology to drug treatment is the old belief that behaviors that are a reaction to an inappropriate or a toxic environment should not be handled pharmacologically. This, of course, is a Manichaean fallacy—etiology is biological or psychological, but never both, and never the product of an interaction. A "biochemical imbalance" should be treated with drugs, and a psychological problem should be treated behaviorally, or psychotherapeutically.

In fact, however, it is a matter of relative proportions not of absolute choices. The degree to which a behavior problem is an appropriate reaction to a disturbed environment, then to that degree will an attempt at drug intervention be antiphysiological. But that does not mean drug treatment will be unsuccessful in such cases. And it is known that even a normal physiological response—the stress response, for example, if it continues unabated—can lead to severe morbid development.

Structure

Structure, we have come to believe, is the essence of all behavioral and psychological treatments for neuropathic patients. Structure refers to an system of external controls and directions to behavior; a system that is understandable, gentle, and predictable. The events of the patient's day are "structured" when they are prearranged, guided, and given to little if any variation. The therapeutic focus is not on the patient or his disorder or his symptoms; it is, rather, on the environment of the patient and the direction and the contingencies that envelop his day.

Structure is necessary because it works. It is an idea that arose among people who actually treat patients, especially children with developmental disabilities and disorders of conduct. It has become an essential part of treatment, with very little attention to the theory or rationale behind it. It works, that is all. To the degree a patient's life is orderly and structured, to that degree he will do well. To the degree that his life is disordered and unstructured, to that degree he will do poorly.

The rationale behind our therapeutic preoccupation with structure is the handicap model. The social handicap that is most likely attendant on brain injury or developmental delay is a weakness in adaptation. This may be manifest as a low level of frustration in the face of difficult tasks; diminished flexibility in the face of changing sets or novel situations; and exaggerated response to stress. It may be manifest as panic in the face of change that one cannot integrate or understand, and this is what we see in autistic people; or as aggression when the unfamiliar is perceived as threatening, as we see in violent patients. The capacity to adapt is profoundly impaired, the ability to bend and be curious as the world unfolds, full of change and the unexpected.

If the handicap is a weakness of adaptation, the appropriate compensation is to give the patient less to adapt to. Structuring the patient's environment is the way to effect that result. The day is contrived to minimize the occurrence of unexpected things. Programming is a word we use to refer to the various elements of a structured environment, and how they are assembled in a therapeutic environment. It refers to the organization of therapies, training, social events, recreation, and periods of rest, all day, every day.

It is an administrative not a psychological term, because it refers to the design and administration of a structured environment. But it is more than simple administration, because the proper construction of a therapeutic program must be attentive to the psychological idiosyncrasies of the patients, or clients, as they are usually referred to in such circles. Structure and programming are the two key aspects of the ecology of the handicapped patient.

One cannot really understand the behavior of the handicapped patient, in neuropsychiatric terms, unless one first understands the environment of that patient. One cannot really appreciate behavior as a purely neuropathic event until one has established that the patient's ecology is properly structured.

Behavioral treatments are successful when they succeed in ordering and arranging the patient's environment. Structure and programming allow the patient to learn, from constant repetition, the "procedural learning" we have alluded to in our discussion of the Kluver–Bucy syndrome (see Chapter 9, this volume).

From the general to more specific principles of behavioral psychopharmacology.

Epilepsy Is First

The rule is that any psychiatric disorder may be a manifestation of epilepsy, or of a cerebral lesion that is epileptogenic, or the consequence of behavioral toxicity from an anticonvulsant drug. There are books written on this subject, so I will not expand further on the rule; it is the ramifications of the rule one should reiterate.

In some neuropathic patients, the threshold for diagnosis of epilepsy, or, if you will, "subclinical epilepsy," should be very low. This includes patients with lesions in areas that are known to be epileptogenic, like the frontal and temporal lobes; patients who have clinical problems like autism, that are probably related to deep frontotemporal injury; patients who have behavior disorders that are paroxysmal or episodic or even cyclic; patients who have nocturnal disorders; and patients with sensory and motor phenomena that are known to be associated with epilepsy.

Epilepsy is by definition the cooccurrence of a particular behavioral disturbance, a seizure, along with the demonstration of a defined electrical event in brain. The problem is that the first element is impossibly broad and the second is impossibly inaccurate. The neuropsychiatrist is all too likely to see patients whose behavioral disturbances are only vaguely suggestive of seizure, and whose EEG are suggestive of nothing at all. That kind of dilemma may be an obstacle to intelligent action, but it need not be a barrier.

The availability of the "psychotropic" anticonvulsants carbamazepine, valproate, and acetazolamide, and their favorable toxicity profiles when compared to the other psychotropes, should usually settle the issue in favor of a therapeutic trial. The usual scenario is a patient with paroxysmal outbursts of rage or self-injurious behavior who is referred to a neurologist who in turn decides that the patient does not have a seizure disorder. Then the patient sees a neuropsychiatrist who tries carbamazepine or valproate, and the problem is resolved.

The other scenario is a patient on phenobarbital or phenytoin or ethosuccimide with severe behavior problems, whose seizures are well controlled so that no change is necessary. In fact, the proper step is to try an alternative anticonvulsant, certainly before one would consider any psychotropic. If the patient is on carbamezepine, the proper step would be to evaluate the additional psychotropic effect of different blood levels; or the effect of concomitant treatment with valproate or acetazolamide or the effect of a change to valproate alone. Psychotropics should never be used until all the anticonvulsant alternatives are exhausted.

In Fever of Unknown Origin, Stop All Drugs

Even carbamezepine and valproate may have behavioral toxicity in some patients. In fact, any neuroactive drug may have behavioral toxicity. One never knows whether a new behavior problem is the consequence of drug toxicity until one has discontinued the drug.The general categories of behavior toxicity are stimulation, associated with the stimulants, antidepressants, carbamazepine, and valproate; disinhibition, associated with the barbiturates and benzodiazepines; and blunting, associated with the neuroleptics lithium and phenytoin. But these are only broad categories, and the rule, especially in neuropathic patients, is that treatment with any neuroactive drug can induce virtually any kind of reaction.

When in doubt, try a drug-free baseline. The longer the baseline, the likelier is the clinical picture to settle down or to clarify itself so an accurate diagnosis can be made and intelligent treatment started.

Overt Toxicity Is Not a Bad Thing

It is not a bad thing at all, especially when one considers the alternative. The really dangerous drugs are those which have subtle, long-term effects, toxic effects that sneak up on the patient over the years. The classic examples are neuroleptic neurotoxicity, tardive dyskinesia, and tardive akathisia. Not only do these effects arise slowly, after years of trouble-free prescription, but their early manifestations are usually masked by maintenance treatment. Phenytoin is the other classic: the slow progression of cognitive blunting, even to dementia, over years of treatment.

Nephrotoxicity with lithium could conceivably be the third example, although the significance of this effect is not really clear.

Better a drug that makes you sick after a few test doses—this can be monitored during the first few weeks of treatment; if a problem develops, the drug is stopped, an alternative is prescribed, and that is that. There are patients who simply cannot tolerate a dopamine agonist, or an antidepressant, or carbamazepine; their intolerance will be apparent within days. But if the initial dosing is well tolerated, there are hardly any long-term effects to worry about.

Drug teratogenicity is another example of covert toxicity. What is remarkable about the neuroactive drugs is how little they seem to have in the way of teratogenicity. Lithium, valproate, and phenytoin are probably the worst offenders in this category. The third category of general toxicity is sudden catastrophic toxicity that may arise at any point during the course of treatment. Once again, the paradigm is the unfortunate class of neuroleptic drugs, with agranulocytosis and malignant hyperthermia. These are major medical catastrophes that may arise out of the blue in patients who have had no previous record of drug sensitivity. They are impossible to predict even with the most careful monitoring, and the reactions may be fatal.

Sudden death in patients on maintenance neuroleptics may be a function of cardiac arrhythmia, although that point is not really settled. More commonly, it is the result of oropharyngeal dystonia with aspiration, or neuroleptic malignant syndrome. Sudden death from cardiac arrhythmia is more likely with the tricyclic antidepressants, and malignant hypertension may be the result of monoamine oxidase inhibitor treatment, especially after the ingestion of foods rich in tyramine or with cotreatment with sympathomimetic drugs.

Long-Term Drugs Require Long-Term Evaluation

Drugs are evaluated, for the most part, in short-term studies, and drug effects are usually defined in terms of the first weeks or months of treatment. This gives little solace to the physician who treats patients with medications that may be continued for years. One would prefer more guidance concerning long-term toxicity, especially after our unfortunate experience with the neuroleptics. Fenfluramine, a drug that was once proposed as "treatment" for autistic children, has now fallen into disfavor, largely because of unresolved fears concerning its long-term neurotoxicity. It is a healthy sign that fenfluramine fell into disfavor soon after theoretical concerns were raised about its long-term effects. We must be getting smarter. In 1968, George Crane issued stern warnings about the danger of neuroleptic overuse, but hardly anyone paid him attention until 10 years later.

The more practical issue over long-term treatment is not toxicity, because only a few of our drugs cause such problems. The more salient issue is long-term efficacy. A drug-free baseline is probably the only way to decide whether treatment is necessary after it has continued for several years. That is no problem for a hyperactive kid on a stimulant, or for a depressed patient who becomes euthymic.

But it can be a major issue for patients with severe psychiatric disorders, who may become floridly psychotic, violent, suicidal, or self-injurious; and for patients with severe forms of epilepsy. Or for patients with disorders like mania or schizophrenia, who may not relapse until months after drug withdrawal, long after they have been placed in a community setting or have moved away from regular follow-up visits.

Yet it is an important issue to address, because drug effects may change over the years, and a drug that is effective at one point in time, like a stimulant for a postconcussion patient, may grow ineffective or toxic as the months pass. Neuroleptics may control hyperactive disorganized behavior for some time, but after years of treatment, if the patient develops tardive akathisia, the drugs may actually be the *cause* of hyperactive disorganized behavior.

The long-term management of patients on neuroactive drugs is no small matter, because there are serious complications along the way; for example, if a patient's "lithium space" is suddenly expanded and a maintenance dose is no longer sufficient; if a temporal lobe psychotic, well controlled on anticonvulsants and neuroleptics, suddenly becomes depressed and suicidal; or if a head injury patient on dopamine agonists suddenly becomes irritable or agitated. Long-term drugs require long-term evaluation.

Doses are Empirical

Doses are decided empirically, when treatment begins and over the long term. It is appropriate to evaluate the full range of doses of psychoactive drugs, because they may behave quite differently at different doses. Stimulants at very low doses may be sedating and may cause lassitude or dysphoria, and higher doses may be required to correct problems with inattention or hyperactivity. Neuroleptics can cause tics at low doses, probably a presynaptic effect, while higher doses will suppress tics. At low doses, neurolyptics may improve attention and cognitive performance, while higher doses may lead to cognitive blunting. At low doses, carbamazepine may control seizures, but higher doses may cause seizures. The same appears to be true for amantadine. Some of the tricyclic antidepressants seem to have a therapeutic window. Low doses of the D1 dopamine receptor antagonist fluphenazine can control SIB while higher doses will cause akathisia and make the SIB even worse.

High blood levels of lithium seem to be required to control acute mania, while lower levels are usually sufficient for maintenance. The blood levels of carbamazepine or valproate that are required to control seizures may not be sufficient to control severe behavior problems.

Finding the optimal dose seems to be a function of endless "tinkering," going higher and lower in slow small increments, and repeating the process at intervals. This is even more important when a patient enters adolescence or senescence and his metabolic profile changes abruptly.

"Yes-No" Drugs

We experimented for years with different ways of evaluating hyperactive children on stimulant drugs, with rating scales, direct behavior observations, neuropsychological tests, educational tests, and even physiological measures like endocrine and cardiovascular responses. We learned, however, that no laboratory device was more reliable or more accurate than the consensus of opinion over the issues of behavior change and academic performance. That is because stimulants either work very well, or they do not work; the response is either dramatic, or the drug is not effective. No one needs convincing if the drug really works, and if it does not, no one needs to be convinced either. That was our introduction to a "yes–no" drug; it either works, or it doesn't.

The foil is a drug that "takes the edge off," that exercises a small degree of tranquilization, that does not really change the key target behaviors but only mitigates their severity to a degree. The classic example of such an effect is the use of neuroleptics in aggressive children.

When one is testing a specific hypothesis about a neuropsychiatric problem, with a clinical trial, it is preferable to begin with a "yes–no" drug. If you are looking for an answer, it is always better to try a drug that will give you one. The issue is also an economic issue, and it is appropriate to begin the hypothesis-testing process by choosing a drug that will give the answer within a short span of time and within a relatively narrow dose range. That, of course, is the supreme advantage of the dopamine agonists. Often a test dose or two of a stimulant in a hyperactive child, or of amantadine in an agitated coma-recovery patient, will yield as much information as a month on lithium or carbamazepine or a beta blocker.

In some clinical circumstances one is faced with a bewildering array of legitimate therapeutic choices. A patient with explosive rage attacks may respond to lithium, carbamazepine, valproate, a beta blocker, a dopamine agonist, or an antidepressant. An agitated coma-recovery patient may respond to any from *that* list, or to a calcium channel blocker, an opiate antagonist, buspirone, or a benzodiazepine. A self-injurious patient may respond to any from that list, or to a D1 antagonist or a serotonergic drug. The simple economy of practice should guide one's choice first to the simpler drugs, with clearer effects after only a few doses and with a limited range of possible doses.

You Do Not Know Until You Try

Surgical residents learn early that the only way to get an answer is to do a laparotomy. Psychopharmacology is, in a sense, a surgical specialty, because it too asks simple questions that can only be answered by undertaking a therapeutic intervention. One can never really tell if a cyclothymic patient is really bipolar, but one can decide if lithium will abate the problem. We will never settle the issue or "subclinical epilepsy," but we can measure the effects of carbamazepine for a paroxysmal behavior disorder. And you never can tell how well a drug will do until you try.

This is not to recommend a hair-trigger on the decision to prescribe psychopharmaceuticals. The converse rule, is to wait, and see how events transpire, or never make a decision until you have to. But it is not fair to deprive a patient the opportunity to experience the effects that a drug may confer. The decision is easier if it concerns whether to continue a drug than if concerns whether even to begin; it is easier because it is based on real information, not idle prediction.

Monitoring Is No Substitute for Intelligence

One is always impressed at the physician who lays his (or her) stethoscope on every patient's chest, at the neurologist who never fails to elicit a knee-jerk, or the psychopharmacologist who orders a blood level at every visit. There is a ritual to it that protects the image of the guild, and which redeems the fees we charge. But the examination of the patient is not a ritual. It is a scientific exploration; it is hypothesis testing, and the examination we do is rational, not ritual.

Monitoring the physical and psychological state of the patient on psychopharmaceutical agents should be organized around specific questions: What does one expect to see, as a consequence of treatment? What are the specific side effects one is worried about? What element of the exam should be documented, and how frequently should it be done?

Every drug requires its own exam, its own battery of tests and laboratory measures. This is discussed, of course, in Chapter 3. The examination may have a ritual, because that protects against errors of omission, but it also must have a rationale, because that guarantees that we will think and continue to think even after the work becomes routine.

Afterword

I began to write this book 3 years ago, after I had finished a monograph on mental retardation for the American Psychiatric Association. As I was working on that project, I realized that the behavioral problems of retarded people really ought to be considered in a wider context, in relation to the problems of patients with traumatic brain injuries and to some of the neurobehavioral disorders of childhood. The problems of "special populations" would make more sense, it occurred to me, if there were at least some attempt at a wider synthesis.

My intention was to have something that would supplement the lectures and consultations I was called on to give around the country; something that would place clinical recommendations in the wider context of neuroscientific investigation. After a talk, people would ask what could they read, and there was no single source to direct them to. Now there is, warts and all.

When I began, I was a research scientist at the University of North Carolina, working at the Biological Sciences Research Center under Morrie Lipton, and at the Division for Disorders of Development and Learning (DDDL) under Harrie Chamberlain. Their lives' work was a powerful influence upon my own, and their signature is always beneath my own, on everything I write.

By the time the book was finished, I had left the University, to expand my clinical work with head injury patients and mentally retarded patients around the country. Clinical practice actually released me to finish the book, and I had time and the freedom to think about what was to go into the book and also what it was, think about what was to go into the book and also what it was for. It was something to read, not to sit idly on a shelf as an occasional reference. It was for practitioners who needed to know not only what to do but why; not only the how of neuropsychiatric practice, but the rationale for it.

It would include only topics that I had handled in my practice and my research; when a contention is weak, by way of "scientific" justification, the reader may be assured that its strength and conviction come of extensive clinical experience—trial and error in the Neuropsychiatry Clinic, now on Rosemary Street in Chapel Hill, and at our rehabilitation centers, and at mental retardation facilities from Kinston, North Carolina, to Grand Junction, Colorado. It is a mean and shallow thought to consider such experience less "scientific" than the drivel that may be published in a peer-reviewed journal or passed with high marks by a granting agency. Clinical practice is the foundation of medical science. It is a dangerous thing to remove the "science" of medicine so far from the people who actually do it. In many places, in this book, one perceives the ill consequence of having done so.

If the selection of topics may seem idiosyncratic, that is because it is; it is based on the particular course of my own clinical career. The reader is invited to learn from my mistakes, no one else's.

Not to say, however, that all the work was done by one person. Most of the chapters are based on work I did with friends and colleagues: Steve Schroeder, George Breese, Randy Evans, Jay Fahs, John Ratey, Tom Clay, Mark Chandler, Bob Hicks, Pam Keenan, Dave Cox, Jarrett Barnhill, and Debra Patterson. Most the bright ideas that are contained herein are theirs; all the mistakes are mine. (Or is the other way around?)

Now, to acknowledge the real sources of this book, may I offer this list:

First, my sturdy Underwood, an IBM PS-2. It has the intellectual strength of a university; it is faster, and its rules make more sense. Its range is beyond my skill to discover, it is *perestroika* in a very small package.

Second, my patients, their families, and my professional colleagues. They, after all, are the only reason for the book, and they are the source of all its intelligence. They have contrived a series of remarkable experiments; they collected the data, collated it, and they ran a sophisticated statistical analysis. Then they laid it on my desk. All I did was write it up.

Finally, Frances, my wife, and Dieter and John, my sons. Not only did they support this thing, but, more important, they tolerated it. All the time the author had for this project was time that they, very graciously, lent to him. One can only wish for an appropriate way to return their grace.

Perhaps, by way of return, it is this:

When I started to write 3 years ago, I was sure that I would dedicate the book to my father, Tom Gualtieri, who died in 1976. He was, after all, my first teacher; he still is. He was a surgeon in Brooklyn, New York, where I grew up. He had gone to Columbia College in 1925, and to the College of Physicians and Surgeons in 1929, and I followed him 40 years later. My childhood was full of his stories from university, and from his practice. He used to say, "You have a moral responsibility to be intelligent."

When I was 5, my brother Leo was born, profoundly handicapped. In those days, when physicians were not at all wealthy and there was no Association for Retarded Citizens (ARC), a retarded child was an extraordinary burden. My mother carried the weight of the day to day, but it was Tom who carried the heavier weight of suffering. Nothing in his classical education had prepared him to understand the irrational, egregious suffering of a severely brain-damaged child.

And so it seemed natural, after I had been a physician for 20 years, working in the fields that had been so difficult for my father, to write this book and to dedicate it to his memory.

But that is old history. On January 4, 1990—10 days ago—Anthony Powell, our third son, was born. Perhaps it is better, then, to turn one's thoughts not to former unhappiness but to new work to do. To Tony, then, and to his brothers and sisters around the world born this year, I shall dedicate this book. May they live in peace, and may they share, equally, the fruits of our precious Earth. Would that they be free of the afflictions I have written to you about; and when afflictions come, as they must, may they treat them more kindly, and with better skill.

Appendices

APPENDIX 1
The Movement and Behavior Scale

The Movement and Behavior Scales (MABS) can be used by nurses to rate patients for symptoms of tardive akathisia. It can be used for surveys, to identify cases for medical examination, or for serial evaluation of tardive akathisia cases.

MOVEMENT AND BEHAVIOR
RATING SCALE

Patient's Name _____   Rater _____

Facility _____   Friday's Date ___/___/___

Please rate the individual's movements/behavior using the following scale. Rate the items based on behavior observed during the past week (Mon-Fri) in a number of settings, such as during school, meals, etc. Circle the number that indicates your global impression of the severity of each item listed. Circle NA (not applicable) when an item can not be rated due to physical handicaps or barriers.

Stereotypies: Rate the severity of persistent and stereotyped repetition of words, posture, or movements. Each item indicates the general location from which the behaviors originate. Do not rate self-injurious behavior.

Motor Activity: Rate voluntary movements. Do not rate involuntary or dyskinetic movements. Do not rate self-injurious behavior (SIB).

NA = Not Applicable 0 = absent 1 = minimal 2 = mild 3 = moderate 4 = severe
---

Stereotypies

1. Upper extremities	NA	0	1	2	3	4
2. Lower extremities	NA	0	1	2	3	4
3. Trunk	NA	0	1	2	3	4
4. Neck, shoulders, and head	NA	0	1	2	3	4
5. Oral (vocal)	NA	0	1	2	3	4

Motor Activity

6. Rocking from foot-to-foot	NA	0	1	2	3	4
7. Walking on the spot	NA	0	1	2	3	4
8. Pacing	NA	0	1	2	3	4
9. Fidgety movements (exclude stereotypies and SIB)	NA	0	1	2	3	4
10. Restlessness (exclude stereotypies and SIB)	NA	0	1	2	3	4

General Behavior

11. Dysphoria (unhappy, sad, fretful)	NA	0	1	2	3	4
12. Self-injurious behavior	NA	0	1	2	3	4
13. Sleep disturbances	NA	0	1	2	3	4
14. Aggression toward others	NA	0	1	2	3	4
15. Noncompliance	NA	0	1	2	3	4
16. Agitation	NA	0	1	2	3	4

COMMENTS: _____

APPENDIX 2
The Self-Injurious Behavior Questionnaire

The Self-Injurious Behavior Questionnaire (SIBQ) is a 25 item rating scale to rate SIB and other maladaptive behaviors in retarded people. It can be used for surveys, to identify index cases; it can also be used to evaluate individual patients over time. It is reliable, and very drug responsive. There are normative data on the SIBQ, so facilities can use the results of a SIBQ survey to compare their population (or staff perceptions of the population) to that of other facilities.

SIB-Q

Name: _____ Date: _____

Rater: _____ Position: _____

Current medications: _____

Please consider the individual's behavior in settings you are familiar with, over the past week. Circle the appropriate number for each item:

> 0 = Not a problem
> 1 = Minimal problem
> 2 = Mild problem
> 3 = Moderate problem
> 4 = Severe problem

Self-injurious behavior (SIB):

1. Frequency of SIB	0	1	2	3	4
2. Severity of SIB	0	1	2	3	4
3. Restraints used for SIB	0	1	2	3	4
4. Presence of self-inflicted bruises	0	1	2	3	4
5. Presence of self-inflicted wounds or tissue damage	0	1	2	3	4
6. Physical aggression toward others	0	1	2	3	4
7. Difficulty sleeping	0	1	2	3	4
8. Stereotypic, repetitive movements	0	1	2	3	4
9. Excessive yelling or screaming	0	1	2	3	4
10. Overly active	0	1	2	3	4
11. Destructive to property or objects	0	1	2	3	4
12. Eating non-food items (Pica)	0	1	2	3	4
13. Tantrums	0	1	2	3	4
14. Peculiar or bizarre behavior	0	1	2	3	4
15. Doesn't follow directions, noncompliant	0	1	2	3	4
16. Difficulty paying attention, easily distracted	0	1	2	3	4
17. Poor motor coordination	0	1	2	3	4
18. Poor performance in class/workshop	0	1	2	3	4
19. Withdrawn, isolated	0	1	2	3	4
20. Mood changes quickly, emotionally labile	0	1	2	3	4
21. Hostile, angry	0	1	2	3	4
22. Nervous, anxious	0	1	2	3	4
23. Irritable	0	1	2	3	4
24. Unhappy, sad, cries easily	0	1	2	3	4
25. Agitated	0	1	2	3	4

TOTAL _____

Comments:

12/87

APPENDIX 3
The TDAK

The TDAK (pronounced tee-dak) is a structured medical examination scale for tardive dyskinesia, since the first section includes the venerable AIMS exam. It also includes a number of elements that are consistent with tardive akathisia. It is the preferred instrument for TD monitorring in facilities for the mentally handicapped, where the problem of tardive akathisia is so prevalent.

TARDIVE DYSKINESIA AND TARDIVE AKATHISIA: EXAMINATION

Patient's Name _____   Rater _____

Location _____   Exam Date ___/___/___

AIMS Exam: Rate involuntary movements and rate the highest severity observed. Rate movements that occur upon activation one less than those observed spontaneously.

Stereotypies Exam: Rate severity of persistent and stereotyped repetition of words, posture, or movements based on your global impression. Each item indicates the general location from which the behaviors originate. Do not rate self-injurious behavior.

TDAK Exam: Rate voluntary movements and affective behavior. Rate severity of each item based on your global impression. Do not rate involuntary or dyskinetic movements.

Hyperactivity Exam: Rate severity of hyperactivity and motor actions based on your global impression. Do not rate dyskinetic movements or stereotypies.

```
NA = Not Applicable  0 = absent  1 = minimal  2 = mild  3 = moderate  4 = severe
```

AIMS Exam

1. Muscles of facial expression	NA	0	1	2	3	4	
2. Lips and perioral area	NA	0	1	2	3	4	
3. Jaw	NA	0	1	2	3	4	
4. Tongue	NA	0	1	2	3	4	
5. Upper extremities	NA	0	1	2	3	4	
6. Lower extremities	NA	0	1	2	3	4	
7. Neck, shoulders, and hips	NA	0	1	2	3	4	____

Stereotypies Exam

1. Upper extremities	NA	0	1	2	3	4	
2. Lower extremities	NA	0	1	2	3	4	
3. Trunk	NA	0	1	2	3	4	
4. Neck, shoulders, and head	NA	0	1	2	3	4	
5. Oral (verbal)	NA	0	1	2	3	4	____

TDAK Exam

1. Rocking from foot-to-foot	NA	0	1	2	3	4	
2. Walking on the spot	NA	0	1	2	3	4	
3. Pacing	NA	0	1	2	3	4	
4. Fidgety (exclude stereotypies)	NA	0	1	2	3	4	
5. Dysphoria	NA	0	1	2	3	4	____

Hyperactivity Exam

1. Restless	NA	0	1	2	3	4	
2. Self-injurious behavior	NA	0	1	2	3	4	____

COMMENTS: _____

_____

References

APA. APA Task Force on Vitamin Therapy in Psychiatry. Unpublished, 1973.

Abarbanel J, Herishanu Y, Frisher S. Encephalopathy associated with baclofen. Ann Neurol 1985;17(6):617-618.

Abe K. Lithium prophylaxis of periodic hypersomnia. Br J Psychiatry 1977;130:312-313.

Achte KA, Hillbom E, Aalberg V. Post traumatic psychoses following war brain injuries. Rehabilitation Institute for Brain Injured Veterans in Finland, 1967.

Adams DJ, Lueders H. Hyperventilation and 6-hour EEG recording in evaluation of absence seizures. Neurology 1981;31:1175-1177.

Adams JH, Mitchell DE, Graham DK,. Diffuse brain damage of immediate impact type. Brain 1977;100:489-502.

Adler LA, Angrist B, Reiter S, Rotrosen J. Neuroleptic-induced akathisia: a review. Psychopharmacology 1989;97(1):1-11.

Adler L, Angrist B, Peselow E, Corwin J, Rotrosen J. Noradrenergic mechanisms in akathisia: treatment with propranolol and clonidine. Psychopharmacol Bull 1987a;23(1):21-23.

Adler L, Angrist B, Peselow E, Reitano J, Rotrosen J. Clonidine in neuroleptic-induced akathisia. Am J Psychiatry 1987b;144:235-236.

Adler LE, Bell J, Kirch D, Friedrich E, Freedman R. Psychosis associated with clonidine withdrawal. Am J Psychiatry 1982;139(1):110.

Ahmad S. Phantom limb pain and propranolol. Br Med J 1979;1:415.

Ahsanuddin K. Side effects of clonidine. Am J Psychiatry 1982;139(8):1083.

Aicardi J. Epilepsy in children. New York: Raven Press, 1986.

Albibi R, McCallum RW. Metoclopramide: pharmacology and clinical application. Ann Intern Med 1983;98:86-95.

Albright PS, Burnham WM. Development of a new pharmacological seizure model: effects of anticonvulsants on cortical- and amygdala-kindled seizures in the rat. Epilepsia 1980;21:681-689.

Alhadeff L, Gualtieri CT, Lipton M. Toxic effects of water-soluble vitamins. Nutr Rev 1984;42:33-40.

Alldredge BK, Lowenstein DH, Simon RP. Seizures associated with recreational drug abuse. Neurology 1989;39:1037-1039.

Allen D, Lader M. Interactions of alcohol with amitryptiline, fluoxetine and placebo in normal subjects. Int Clin Psychopharmacol 1989;4 (suppl 1):7-14.

Allen D, Baylay A, Lader M. A comparative study of the interaction of alcohol with aldipem, lorazepam and placebo in normal subjects. Int Clin Psychopharmacol 1988;3:327-341.

Allen RM. Role of amantadine in the management of neuroleptic-induced extrapyramidal syndromes: overview and pharmacology. Clin Neuropharmacol 1983;6:S64-S73.

Altshuler LL, Conrad A, Kovelman JA, Scheibel A. Hippocampal pyramidal cell orientation in schizophrenia. Arch Gen Psychiatry 1987;44(12):1094.

Altura BT, Altura BM. Phencyclidine, lysergic acid diethylamide, and mescaline: cerebral artery spasms and hallucinogenic activity. Science 1981;212:1051-1052.

Alvarez N. Discontinuance of neuroleptic medications in patients with developmental disabilities and diagnosis of epilepsy. AJMR 1989;93:593-599.

Alves WA, Colohan ART, O'Leary TJ, Rimel RA, Jane JA. Understanding posttraumatic symptoms after minor head injury. J Head Trauma Rehabil 1986;1:1-12.

Amaducci L, Lippi A. Risk factors and genetic background for Alzheimer's disease. Acta Neurol Scand 1988;77(suppl 116):13-18.

Aman MG, Singh NN. Aberrant behavior checklist. 1983 (unpublished).

Amassian VE, Stewart M, Quirk GJ, Rosenthal JL. Physiological basis of motor effects of a transient stimulus to cerebral cortex. Neurosurgery 1987;20(1):74-93.

Ambrosini PJ, Fried J. Preliminary report: amantadine hydrochlorde in childhood enuresis. Clin Psychopharmacol 1984;4:223-235.

Ananth J. Current psychopathological theories of tardive dykinesia and their implications for future research. Neuropsychobiology 1982;8:210-222.

Ananth J, Sangani J, Noonan JPA. Amantadine therapy for drug-induced extrapyramidal signs and depression. Psychiatr J Univ Ottawa 1977;1:27-33.

Anderson LT, Campbell M, Grega DM, Perry R, Small AM, Green WH. Haloperidol in the treatment of infantile autism: effects on learning and behavioral symptoms. Am J Psychiatry 1984;141:1195-1202.

Anderson PH, Nielsen EB. The dopamine D1 receptor: biochemical and behavioral aspects. Adv Exp Med Biol 1976;204:73-92.

Andrasik F, Ollendick T, Turner SM, Hughes JR. Single case study: Pharmacological treatment of aggressive behavior and emesis in the Cornelia de Lange syndrome. J Nerv Ment Dis 1979;167(12):764-766.

Andy OJ, Jurko MF. Seizures and pain. Clin Electroencephalogr 1985;16 (4):195-201.

Angrist B, Rotrosen J, Gershon S. Differential effects of amphetamine and neuroleptics on negative vs. positive symptoms in schizophrenia. Psychopharmacology (Berlin) 1980;72:17-18.

Annegers JF, Grabow JD, Groover RD, Laws ER, Elverback LR, Kurland LT. Seizures after head trauma: a population study. Neurology 1980a;30:683-689.

Annegers JF, Grabow JD, Kurland LT, Laws ER. The incidence, causes and secular trends of head trauma in Olmsted County, Minnesota. Neurology 1980b;30:912-919.

Aoki FY, Sitar DS. Amantadine kinetics in healthy elderly men: implications for influenza prevention. Clin Pharmacol Ther 1985;37(2):137.

Aoki FY, Sitar DS. Clinical pharmacokinetics of amantadine hydrochloride. Clin Pharmacokinet 1988;14:35-51.

Aoki FY, Stiver HG, Sitar DS, Boudreault A, Ogilvie RI. Prophylactic amantadine dose and plasma concentration-effect relationships in healthy adults. Clin Pharmacol Ther 1979;37(2):128.

APA Task Force. Tardive dyskinesia. Washington, DC: American Psychiatric Association, 1979.

APA Task Force. Tardive dyskinesia. Washington, DC: American Psychiatric Association, 1991.

Appenzeller O. Post-traumatic headaches. In: Dalessio DJ, ed. Wolff's headache and other head pain. New York: Oxford University Press, 1987:289-303.

Aranko K, Seppala T, Pellinen J, Mattila MJ. Interaction of diazepam or lorazepam with alcohol. Psychomotor effects and bioassayed serum levels after single and repeated doses. Eur J Clin Pharmacol 1985;28:559-565.

Arieti S. Interpretation of schizophrenia. New York: Basic Books, 1974.

Arnsten AFT, Goldman-Rakic PA. Adrenergic mechanisms in prefrontal cortex. Science 1985;230:1273-1276.

Aronson TA, Shukla S, Hirschowitz J. Clonazepam treatment of five lithium-refractory patients with bipolar disorder. Am J Psychiatry 1989;146(1):77.

Arora RC, Meltzer HY. Serotonergic measures in the brains of suicide victims: 5-HT2 binding sites in the frontal cortex of suicide victims and control subjects. Am J Psychiatry 1989;146(6):730-736.

Asano T, Spector S. Identification of inosine and hypoxanthine as endogenous ligands for the brain benzodiazepine-binding sites. Proc Natl Acad Sci USA 1979;76:977-981.

Asher SW, Aminoff MJ. Tetrabenzamine and movement disorders. Neurology 1981;31:1051-1054.

Atkinson WL, Arden NH, Patriarca PA, Leslie N, Lui K-J, Gohd R. Amantadine prophylaxis during an institutional outbreak of type A (H1N1) influenza. Arch Intern Med 1986;146:1751-1756.

Atsmon A, Blum I, Steiner M, Latz A, Wijsenbeek H. Further studies with propranolol in psychotic patients. Psychopharmacologia 1972;27:249-254.

Atsom A, Blum I, Moaz B. The short-term effects of adrenergic blocking agents in a small group of psychotic patients: preliminary clinical observations. Psychiatr Neurol Neurochirurgia 1971;74:251-258.

Ayd FJ, Jr. Fluoxetine: An antidepressant with specific serotonin uptake inhibition. Int Drug Ther Newsl 1988;23(2):5-12.

Babington RG. The pharmacology of kindling. In: Hanin I, Usdin E, eds. Animal models in psychiatry and neurology. New York: Pergamon, 1967:141-149.

Bacher NM, Lewis HA. Low-dose propranolol in tardive dyskinesia. Am J Psychiatry 1980;137:495-597.

Bachmann KM, Modestin J. Neuroleptic-induced panic attacks in a patient with delusional depression. J Nerv Ment Dis 1987;175(6):373-375.

Bakchine S, Chain F, Lhermitte F. Syndrome de Kluver-Bucy humain complet apres une encephalite a herpes simplex type 2. Rev Neurol (Paris) 1986;142(2):126-132.

Bakchine S, Lacomblez L, Benoit N, Parisot D, Chain F, Lhermitte F. Manic-like state after bilateral orbitofrontal and right temporoparietal injury: efficacy of clonidine. Neurology 1989;39:777-781.

Baker SP, O'Neill B, Karpf RS. The injury fact book. Lexington, Mass: DC Heath & Co, 1984.

Baldessarini RJ. Chemotherapy in psychiatry. Cambridge: Harvard University Press, 1977.

Ballenger JC, Post RM. Therapeutic effects of carbamazepine in affective illness: a preliminary report. Commun Psychopharmacol 1978;2:159-175.

Ballenger JC, Post RM. Carbamezepine in manic-depressive illness: a new treatment. Am J Psychiatry 1980;137:782-790.

Ballenger JC, Reuss VI, Post RM. The atypical clinical picture of adolescent mania. Am J Psychiatry 1982;139:602-606.

Balon R. Buspirone for attention deficit hyperactivity disorder. J Clin Psychopharmacol 1990;10:77.

Balster RL. The behavioral pharmacology of phencyclidine. In: Meltzer HY, ed. Psychopharmacology, the third generation of progress. New York: Raven Press, 1987:1573-1580.

Bankier A, Haan E, Birrell R. Letter to the editor: familial occurrence of Brachmann-de Lange Syndrome. Am J Med Genet 1986;25:163-165.

Bareggi SR, Porta M, Selenati A, et al. Homovanillic acid and 5-hydroxyindole acetic acid in the CSF of patients after a severe head injury. I.Lumbar CSF concentration in chronic brain post-traumatic syndromes. Eur Neurol 1975;13:528-544.

Barltrop D. The prevalence of pica. Am J Dis Child 1966;112:116-123.

Barnes SE, Bower BD. Sodium valproate in the treatment of intractable childhood epilepsy. Dev Med Child Neurol 1975;17:175-182.

Barnes TRE, Braude WM. Akathisia variants and tardive dyskinesia. Arch Gen Psychiatry 1985;42:874-878.

Barnhill LJ, Gualtieri CT. Late-onset psychosis after closed head injury. Neuropsychiatry Neuropsychol Behav Neurol 1989;2:211-218.

Bartak L, Rutter M. Differences between mentally retarded and normally intelligent autistic children. J Autism Child Schizophr 1976;6:108-120.

Barth JT, Macciochi SN, Giordani B, Rimel R, Jane JA, Boll TJ. Neuropsychological sequelae of minor head injury. Neurosurgery 1983;13:529-533.

Bartus RT, Dean RL, Fisher SK. Cholinergic treatment for age-related memory disturbances: dead or barely coming of age?. In: Crook T, Bratus RT, Ferris S, Gershon S, eds. Treatment development strategies for Alzheimer's disease, Madison, Conn: Mark Powley, 1986:421-450.

Baskin DS, Hosobuchi Y. Naloxone reversal of ischaemic neurological deficits in man. Lancet 1981;2:272.

Bauman M, Kemper TL. Histoanatomic observations of the brain in early autism. Neurology 1985;35:866-874.

Baumeister AA, Forehand R. Effects of extinction of an instrumental response on stereotyped body rocking in severe retardates. Psychol Rec 1971;21:235-240.

Bear DM, Fedio P. Quantitative analysis of interictal behavior in temporal lobe epilepsy. Arch Neurol 1977;34:454-467.

Beaudry P, Fontaine R, Chouinard G, Annable L. Clonazepam in the treatment of patients with recurrent panic attacks. J Clin Psychiatry 1986;47:83-85.

Beck B. Epidemiology of Cornelia de Lange's syndrome. Acta Paediatr Scand 1976;65:631-638.

Becker RE, Dufresne RL. Perceptual changes with brupropion, a novel antidepressant. Am J Psychiatry 1982;139(9):1200.

Beckwith B, Courk D, Schumacher K. Failure of naloxone to reduce self-injurious behavior in two developmentally disabled females. Appl Res Ment Retard 1986;7:183-188.

Beckwith B, Courk D, Schumacher K. Effectiveness of naloxone in reducing self-injurious behavior in two developmentally disabled females. 1984 (Unpublished).

Behrman S. Mutism induced by phenothiazines. Br J Psychiatry 1972;121:599-604.

Belin C, Larmande P. Transitory spatial disorder with propranolol. N Engl J Med 1985;312(12):790-791.

Bender L, Cobrinik L, Faretra G, Sankar DVS. The treatment of childhood schizophrenia with LSD and UML. In: Rinkel M, ed. Biological treatment of mental illness. New York: L.C. Page, 1966.

Benson F, Miller BL, Signer SF. Dual personality associated with epilepsy, multiple personality and the illusion of possession. Arch Neurol 1986;43:471-474.

Berg L, Miller JP, Storandt M, et al. Mild senile dementia of the Alzheimer type: 2. Longitudinal assessment. Ann Neurol 1988;23:477-484.

Berg R. A case of Tourette's syndrome treated with nefedipine. Acta Psychiatr Scand 1985;72:400-401.

Berkson G. Abnormal stereotyped motor acts. In: Zubin J, Hunt HF, eds. Comparative Psychopathology. New York: Grune & Stratton, 1967:76-94.

Berkson G. Repetitive stereotyped behaviors. Am J Ment Defic 1983;88(3):239-246.

Berkson G, Manson WA. Stereotyped movements of mental defectives IV. The effects of toys and the character of the acts. Am J Ment Defic 1964;68:511-524.

Berkson G, Mason WA, Saxon SV. Situation and stimulus effects on stereotyped behaviors of chimpanzees. J Comp Physiol Psychol 1963;56:786-792.

Berridge MJ. Inositol trisphosphate, calcium, lithium, and cell signaling. JAMA 1989;262(13):1834-1841.

Berrios GE, Samuel C. Affective disorder in the neurological patient. J Nerv Ment Dis 1987;175:173-176.

Bertino J, Walker JW Jr. Reassessment of theophylline toxicity: serum concentrations, clinical course, and treatment. Arch Intern Med 1987;147:-19203.

Betts TA. Depression, anxiety, and epilepsy. Epilepsy Psychiatry 1981;60-71.

Bickerstaff ER. Basilar artery migraine. Lancet 1961;1:15-17.

Bieliauskas LA, Glantz RH. Depression type in Parkinson disease. J Clin Exp Neuropsychology 1989;11(5):597.

Biemond A. The conduction of pain above the level of thalamus opticus. Arch Neurol Psychiatry 1956;75:231-244.

Bier DM, Kaplan SL, Havel RJ. The Prader-Willi syndrome: regulation of fat transport. Diabetes 1977;26:874-881.

Binder LM. Persisting symptoms after mild head injury: a review of the postconcussive syndrome. J Clin Exp Neuropsychology 1986;8(4):323-346.

Bing R. Uber Einige bemerkenswerte Begleiterscheinungen der exrapyramidalen Rigiditat (Akathesie - Mikrographie - Kinesia paradoxica). Schweiz Med Wochenschr 1923;53:167-171.

Bisno AL, Shulman ST, Dajani AS. The rise and fall (and rise?) of rheumatic fever. JAMA 1988;259:728-729.

Black DW, Winokur G, Nasrallah A. Suicide in subtypes of major affective disorder. Arch Gen Psychiatry 1987;44:878-880.

Blass JP, Gleason P, Brush D, DePonte P, Thaler H. Thiamine and Alzheimer's disease. Arch Neurol 1988;45:833-836.

Blazer D, Swartz M, Woodbury M, Manton KG, Hughes D, George LK. Depressive syndromes and depressive diagnoses in a community population. Arch Gen Psychiatry 1988;45:1078-1084.

Blier P, de Montigny C, Chaput Y. Modifications of the serotonin systems by antidepressant treatments: implications for the therapeutic response in major depression. J Clin Psychopharmacol Baltimore 1987;7(6):24s.

Block RL, Berchou R. Alprazolam and lorazepam effects on memory acquisition and retrieval processes. Biol Biochem Behav 1984;20:233-241.

Bloom DM, Tourjman SV, Vasavan Nair NP. Verapamil in refractory schizophrenia: a case report. Prog Neuropsychopharmacol Biol Psychiatry (Oxford) 1987;11:185-188.

Blum A, Tempey FW, Lynch WJ. Somatic findings in patients with psychogenic polydipsia. J Clin Psychiatry 1983;44:55-56.

Blumbergs PC, Jones NR, North JB. Diffuse axonal injury in head trauma. J Neurol Neurosurg Psychiatry 1989;52:838-841.

Blumer D. Psychiatric aspects of epilepsy. Washington, DC: American Psychiatric Press, 1984.

Blumstein SE. Neurolinguistic disorders: language-brain relationships. In: Filskov SB, Boll TJ, eds. Handbook of clinical neuropsychology. New York: John Wiley & Sons, 1981:227-256.

Bobruff A, Gardos G, Tarsy D, Rapkin RM, Cole JO, Moore P. Clonazepam and phenobarbital in tardive dyskinesia. Am J Psychiatry 1981;138(2):189.

Bogerts B, Meertz E. Basal ganglia and limbic system pathology in schizophrenia. Arch Gen Psychiatry 1985;42:784-790.

Bondareff W, Mountjoy CQ, Roth M, Rossor MN, Iverson LL, Reynolds GP. Age and histopathologic heterogeneity in Alzheimer's disease. Arch Gen Psychiatry 1987;44(5):412-417.

Bonnici F. Antidiuretic effect of clofibrate and carbamazepine in diabetes insipidus: studies on free water clearance and response to a water load. Clin Endocrinol 1973;2:265-275.

Boone KB, Miller BL, Rosenbert L, Durazo A, McIntyre H, Weil M. Neuropsychological and behavioral abnormalities in an adolescent with frontal lobe seizures. Neurology 1988;38(4):583-586.

Borg J, Gershon S, Alpert M. Dose effects of smoked marijuana on human cognitive and motor functions. Psychopharmacologia 1975;42:211-218.

Borison RL, Diamond BI. Treatment of extra-pyramidal side effects: amantadine versus benzotropine. World J Psychosynthesis 1984;16:40-43.

Borison RL. Amantadine in the management of extrapyramidal side effects. Clin Neuropharmacol 1983;6(1):557-563.

Bouchard RH, Pourcher E, Vincent P. Fluoxetine and extyramidal side effects. Am J Psychiatry 1989;146:1352-1353.

Bougousslavsky J, Ferrazzini M, Regli F, Assal G, Tanabe H, Delaloye-Bischof A. Manic delirium and frontal-like syndrome with paramedian infarction of the right thalamus. J Neurol Neurosurg Psychiatry 1988;51:116-119.

Boulenger J-P, Uhde TW, Wolff EA, Post RM. Increased sensitivity to caffeine in patients with panic disorders. Arch Gen Psychiatry 1984;41:1067-1072.

Bowden CL, Sarabia F. Diagnosing manic-depressive illness in adolescence. Comp Psychiatry 1980;21:263-269.

Braff DL, Silverton L, Saccuzzo DP, Janowsky DS. Impaired speed of visual information processing in marijuana intoxication. Am J Psychiatry 1981;138:613-617.

Branconnier RJ, Cole JD, Dessain EC, et al. The therapeutic efficacy of pramiracetam in Alzheimer's disease: preliminary observations. Psychopharmacol Bull 1983;19:726-730.

Brandt J, Seidman LJ, Kohl D. Personality characteristics of epileptic patients: a controlled study of generalized and temporal lobe cases. J Clin Exp Neuropsychol 1985;7 (1):25-38.

Brase DA, Myer EC, Dewey WL. Minireveiw: possible hyperendorphinergic pathophysiology of the Rett syndrome. Life Sci 1989;45:359-366.

Braude WM, Barnes TRE. Late-onset akathisia — an indicant of covert dyskinesia: two case reports. Am J Psychiatry 1983;140:611-612.

Braunhofer J, Zicha L. Eroffnet Tegretal neue Therapiemoglichkeiten bei bestimmen neurologischen und endokrinen Krankheitsbildern. Med Welt 1989;36:1875-1880.

Bray GA, Dahms WT, Swerdloff RS, Fisher RH, Atkinson RL, Carrel RE. The Prader-Willi syndrome: a study of 40 patients and a reveiw of the literature. Medicine (Baltimore) 1983;62(2):59-80.

Breese GR, Baumeister AA, McCown T Jr, et al. Behavioral differences between neonatal and adult 6-hyroxydopamine-treated rats to dopamine agonists: relevance to neurological symptoms in clinical syndromes with reduced brain dopamine. J Pharmacol Exp Ther 1984;231(2):343-354.

Breese GR, Baumeister AA, Napier CT, Frye GD, Mueller RA. Evidence that D-1 dopamine receptors contribute to the supersensitive behavioral responses induced by L-dehydroxyphenylaline in rats treated neonatally with 6-hydroxydopamine J Pharmacol Exp Ther 1985;235(2):287-295.

Breese GR, Hulebak KL, Napier TC, Baumeister AA, Frye GD, Mueller RA. Enhanced muscimol-induced behavioral responses after 6-OHDA lesions: relevance to susceptibility for self-mutilation behavior in neonatally lesioned rats. Psychopharmacology 1987;91:356-362.

Breggin PR. Psychiatric drugs: hazards to the brain. New York: Springer, 1983.

Breier A, Charney DS, Nelson JC. Seizures induced by abrupt discontinuation of alprazolam. Am J Psychiatry 1984;141(12):1606-1607.

Brenner A, Wapnir RA. A pyridoxine-dependent behavioral disorder unmasked by isoniazid. J Dis Child 1978;132:773-776.

Brent DA, Crumrine PK, Varma RR, Allan M, Allman C. Phenobarbital treatment and major depressive disorder in children with epilepsy. Pediatrics 1987;80:909-917.

Brin M. Abnormal tryptophan metabolism in pregnancy and with the oral contraceptive pill. 1. Specific effects of an oral estrogenic contraceptive steroid on the tryptophan oxygenase and two aminotransferase activities in livers of ovariectomized-adrenalectomized rats. Am J Clin Nutr 1971;24:699-703.

Briones DR, Rosenthal SH. Changes in urinary free Catecholamines and 17-ketosteroids with cerebral electrotherapy (electrosleep). Dis Nerv Syst 1973;34:57.

Brod TM. Fluoxetine and extrapyramidal side effects. Am J Psychiatry 1989;146:1353.

Broekkamp CLE, van Dongen PAM, van Rossum JM. Neostriatal involvement in reinforcement and motivation. In: Cools AR, Lohman AHM, van den Berken JHL, eds. Psychobiology of the striatum. Amsterdam: Elsevier/North-Holland, 1977:61-72.

Brogden RN, Heel RC, Speight TM, Avery GS. Trazadone: A review of its pharmacological properties and therapeutic use in depression and anxiety. Drugs 1981;21(6):401-429.

Brogna CG, Lee SI, Dreifuss FE. Pilomotor seizures magnetic resonance imaging and electroencephalographic localization of originating focus. Arch Neurol 1986;43:1085-1086.

Brooks N, Symington C, Beattie A, Campsie L, Bryden J, McKinlay W. Alcohol and other predictors of cognitive recovery after severe head injury. Brain Injury 1989;3:235-246.

Brooks SC, Lessin BE. Treatment of lithium-induced nephrogenic diabetes insipidus and schizoaffective psychosis with carbamazepine. Am J Psychiatry 1983;140:1077-1078.

Brown CS, Wittkowsky AK, Bryant SG. Neuroleptic-induced catatonia after abrupt withdrawal of amantadine during neuroleptic therapy. Pharmacotherapy 1986;6(4):193-195.

Brown GL, Wilson WP. Parkinsonism and depression. South Med J 1972;65:540-545.

Brown RG, Marsden CD. How common is dementia in Parkinson's disease? Lancet 1984;2:1262-1264.

Brown S, Schafer EA. An investigation into the functions of the occipital and temporal lobes of the monkey's brain. Philos Trans R Soc London 1888;179b:303-327.

Brown SW, Reynolds EH. Cognitive impairment in epileptic patients. In: Reynolds EH, Trimble MR, eds. Epilepsy and psychiatry. Edinburgh: Churchill Livingstone, 1981:147-164.

Browne TR. Clonazepam. N Engl J Med 1978;299(15):812-816.

Bruetsch WL. Late cerebral sequelae of rheumatic fever. Arch Intern Med 1944;73:472-476.

Brumback RA, Weinberg WA, Herjanic BL. Epileptiform activity in the electroencephalogram induced by lithium carbonate. Pediatrics 1975;56:831-834.

Bruno F. Buspirone in the treatment of alcoholic patients. Psychopathology 1989;22(suppl 1):49-59.

Bruun RD. Clonidine treatment of Tourette Syndrome. In: Friedhoff AJ, eds. Gilles de la Tourette Syndrome. New York: Raven Press, 1982.

Bryson Y, Sakati N, Nyhan WL, Fish CH. Self-mutilative behavior in the Cornelia de Lange syndrome. Am J Ment Defic 1971;76(3):319-324.

Buchhalter JR, Dichter MA. Effects of valproic acid in cultured mammalian neurons. Neurology 1986;36(2):259-262.

Buchwald NA, Hull CD, Levine MS, Villablanca J. The basal ganglia and the regulation of response and cognitive sets. In: Brazier MAB, ed. Growth and development of the brain. New York :Raven Press, 1975:171-189.

Bucy PC, Kluver H. An anatomical investigation of the temporal lobe in the monkey. J Comp Neurol 1955;103:151-252.

Bullard DE. Diencephalic seizures: responsiveness to bromocriptine and morphine. Ann Neurol 1987;21:609-611.

Bunney B, DeReimer S. Effect of clonidine on dopaminergic neuron activity in the substantia nigra: possible indirect mediation by noradrenergic regulation of the serotonergic raphe system. In: Friedhoff AJ, Chase TN, eds. Gilles de la Tourette syndrome. New York: Raven Press, 1982:99-104.

Burke RE, Fahn S, Jankovic J, Marsden CD, Lang AE, Gollomp S, Ilson J. Tardive dystonia: Late-onset and persistent dystonia caused by antipsychotic drugs. Neurology 1982;32:1335-1346.

Burroughs Wellcome. Wellbutrin tablets (bupropion hydrochloride). 1989 (unpublished).

Butlin AT, Wolfendale L, Danta G. The effects of anticonvulsants on memory function in epileptic patients: preliminary findings. Clin Exp Neurol

Byerley WF, Reimherr FW, Wood DR, Grosser BI. Fluoxetine, a selective serotonin uptake inhibitor, for the treatment of outpatients with major depression. J Clin Psychopharmacol 1988;8(2):112.

Byrne J, Arie T. Tetrahydroaminoacridine (THA) in Alzheimer's disease. Br Med J 1989;298:845-846.

Cade JFJ. Lithium salts in the treatment of psychotic excitement. Med J Austr 1949;36:349-352.

Caers LI, De Beukelaar F, Amery WK. Flunarizine, calcium-entry blocker, in childhood migraine, epilepsy, and alternating hemiplegi. Clin Neuropharmacol 1987;10(2):162-168.

Caille EJ. Effects of treatment with dipropylacetamide on vigilance, perception, decision-making capabilities and sleep of young normal adults. Psychol Med 1989;6:791-796.

Caine ED, Margolin DI, Brown GL, Ebert MH. Gilles de la Tourette's syndrome, tardive dyskinesia and psychosis in an adolescent. Am J Psychiatry 1978;135:241-243.

Caine ED, Polinski RJ. Haloperidol-induced dysphoria in patients with Tourette syndrome. Am J Psychiatry 1979;136(9):1216-1217.

Callaghan N, Garrett A, Goggin T. Withdrawal of anticonvulsant drugs in patients free of seizures for two years; a prospective study. N Engl J Med 1988;946: 318(15).942-946.

Campbell M, Fish B, Shapiro T, Floyd A. Acute responses of schizophrenic children to a sedative and a "stimulating" neuroleptic: a pharmacologic yardstick. Curr Ther Res 1972;14:759-766.

Campbell M, Adams P, Small AM, Tesch LM, Curren EL. Naltrexone in infantile autism. Psychopharmacol Bull 1988;24:135-139.

Campbell M, Anderson LT, Meier M, Cohen IL, Small AM, Samit C, Sachar EJ. A comparison of haloperidol and behavior therapy and their interaction in autistic children. J Am Acad Child Psychiatry 1978;17:640-655.

Campbell M, Anderson LT, Small AM, Perry R, Green WH, Caplan R. The effects of haloperidol on learning and behavior in autistic children. J Autism Dev Disord 1982;12(2):167-175.

Campbell M, Small AM, Collins PJ, Friedman E, David R, Genieser NW. Levodopa and levoamphetamine: a crossover study in schizophrenic children. Curr Ther Res 1976;18:70-86.

Carlson GA, Strober M. Manic-depressive illness in early adolescence. J Am Acad Child Adol Psychiatry 1978;17:138-153.

Carney MWP, Williams DG, Sheffield BF. Thiamine and pyridoxine lack in newly-admitted psychiatric patients. Br J Psychiatry 1979;135:249-254.

Carpenter S, Yassa R, Och R. A pathologic basis for Kleine-Levin syndrome. Arch Neurol 1982;39:25-28.

Carr DB, Bullen BA, Skrinar GS, Arnold MA, Rosenblatt M, Bietins IZ, Martin JB, McArthur JW. Physical conditioning facilitates the exercise-induced secretion of beta-lipotropin and beta-lipotropin in women. N Engl J Med 1981;305:560-563.

Carter CO. The inheritance of common congenital malformations. Prog in Med Genet 1965;4:59-84.

Carter G. The abrupt withdrawal of antiparkinsonian drugs in mentally handicapped patients. Br J Psychiatry 1983;142:166-168.

Casey DE. Tardive dyskinesia: reversible and irreversible. In: Casey DE, Chase TN, Christensen AV, Gerlach J, eds. Dyskinesia — research and treatment. Berlin/Heidelberg: Springer-Verlag, 1985.

Casey DE, Denney D. Pharmacologic characterization of tardive dyskinesia. Psychopharm 1977;54:1-8.

Casey DE, Gerlach J. Is tardive dyskinesia due to dopamine hypersensitivity. Clin Neuropharmacol 1986;9(s4):134-136.

Casey DE, Povisen UJ, Meidahl B, Gerlach J. Neuroleptic-induced tardive dyskinesia and Parkinsonism: changes during several years of continuing treatment. Psychopharmacol Bull 1986;22:250-253.

Cashman NR, Maselli R, Wollman RL, Roos R, Simon R, Antel JP. Late denervation in patients with antecedent paralytic poliomyelitis. N Engl J Med 1987;317:7-12.

Cassidy JW. Fluoxetine: a new serotonergically active antidepressant. J Head Trauma Rehabil 1989;4:67-70.

Castells S, Chakrabarti C, Winsberg BG, Hurwic M, Perel JM, Nyhan WL. Effects of L-5-hydroxytryptophan on monoamine and amino acids turnover in the Lesch-Nyhan syndrome. J Autism Dev Disord 1979;9:95-103.

Catsman-Berrevoets CE, Van Harskamp F. Compulsive presleep behavior and apathy due to bilateral thalamic stroke: response to bromocriptine. Neurology 1988;38:647-649.

Catsman-Berrevoets EC, Van Harskamp F, Appelhof A. Beneficial effects of physostigmine on clinical amnesic behaviour and neropsychological test results in a patient with a pest-encephalitic amnesic syndrome. J Neurol neurosurg Psychiatry 1986;49:1088-1089.

Caveness WF, Meirowsky AM, Rish BL. The nature of post-traumatic epilepsy. J Neurosurg 1979;50:545-553.

CDC/MMWR. Eosinophilia-Myalgia Syndrome - New Mexico. MMWR 1989;38:765-767.

Chadwick D, Reynolds EH, Marsden CD. Anticonvulsant-induced dyskinesias: a comparison with dyskinesias induced by neuroleptics. J Neurol Neurosurg Psychiatry 1976;39:1210-1218.

Chaffin DS. Phenothiazine-induced acute psychotic reaction: the "psychotoxicity" of a drug. Am J Psychiatry 1964;121:26-32.

Chamoye AS. Long-term learning deficits of mentally retarded monkeys. Am J Ment Defic 1984;88(4):352-368.

Chandler M, Gualtieri CT, Fahs, J.J. New psychpharmacology for handicapped People: stimulants, antidepressants, lithium, and propranolol. 1988 (Unpublished).

Chandler MC, Gualtieri CT. Amantadine: a medical, neuropsychological and psychiatric profile. In: Ratey JJ, ed. Mental retardation: developing pharmacotherapies. Washington, DC: American Psychiatric Press, in press.

Chandler MC, Barnhill JB, Gualtieri CT. Amantadine for the agitated head-injury patient. Brain Injury 1988;2:309-311.

Chandler MC, Barnhill LJ, Gualtieri CT, Patterson DR. Tryptophan antagonism of stimulant-induced tics. J Clin Psychopharmacol 1989;9(1):69.

Chandler MC, Gualtieri CT, Barnhill LJ. The neuropsychiatric examination of the child. In: Burrows G, Tonge B, Werry J, eds. Handbook of studies in child psychiatry. (in Press).

Charney DS, Sternberg DE, Kleber HD, Henninger GR, Redmond DE Jr. The clinical use of clonidine in abrupt withdrawal from methadone: effects on blood pressure and specific signs and symptoms. Arch Gen Psychiatry 1981;38:1273.

Chaudry RP, Waters BGH. Lithium and carbamazepine interaction: possible neurotoxicity. J Clin Psychiatry 1983;44:30-31.

Chavany JA. Role des causes occasionelles dans le determinisime du ramolissement cerebral (Reflections therapeutiques a le propos). Prat Med Francaise 1928;7:285-295.

Childs A. Naltrexone in organic bulimia. 1986 (unpublished).

Childs A. Naltrexolone in organic bulimia. Brain Injury 1990;1:49-55.

Childs A, Crismon ML. The use of cranial electrotherapy stimulation in post-traumatic amnesia: a report of two cases. Brain Injury 1988;2(3):243-247.

Choo PB, Bianchi GN. Brachmann-de Lange syndrome: A report of four cases. Aust Paediatr J 1965;1:236.

Chouinard G. Antimanic effects of clonazepam. Psychosomatics 1985;26(12):7-12.

Chouinard G, Jones BD. Neuroleptic-induced supersensitivity psychosis: clinical and pharmacologic characteristics. Am J Psychiatry 1980;137(1):16-21.

Chouinard G, Annable L, Langlois R. Absence of orthostatic hypotension in depressed patients treated with bupropion. Prog Neuro-Psychopharmacol 1981;5:483-490.

Chouinard G, Young SN, Annable L. Antimanic effect of clonazepam. Psychopathology 1983;451-466.

Chouinard G, Annable L, Mercier P, Ross-Chouinard A. A five-year follow-up study of tardive dyskinesia. Psychopharmacol Bull 1986;22(1):259-263.

Christensen E, Miller JE, Faurbye A. Neuropathological investigation of 28 brains from patients with dyskinesia. Acta Psychiatr Scand 1970;46:14-23.

Christodoulo GN, Kokkevi A, Lykouras EP. Effects of lithium on memory. Am J Psychiatry 1981;138:847-848.

Ciraulo DA, Barnhill J. Pharmacokinetic mechanisms of ethanol-psychotropic drug interactions. National Institute on Drug Abuse Research Monograph Series 1986;68:142-153.

Ciraulo DA, Barnhill J, Boxenbaum H. Pharmacokinetic interaction of disulfuram and antidepressants. Am J Psychiatry 1985;142:1373-1374.

Cirignotta F, Zucconi M, Mondini S, Lugaresi E. Writing epilepsy. Clin Electroencephalogr 1986;17 1:21-23.

Clancy RR, Kaplan KM, Baumgart S, Rosenberry KR. Neonatal theophylline neurotoxicity. Clin Pediatr 1985;24(3):168-170.

Clark M, Post RM. Carbamazepine, but not caffeine, is highly selective for adenosine A1 binding sites. Eur J Pharmacol 1989;164:399-401.

Clay TH, Gualtieri TC, Gullion C. Evans R.W. Clinical and neuropsychological effects of the novel antidepressant, buproprion. Psychopharmacol Bull 1988;24:143-148.

Clifford DB, Rutherford JL, Hicks FG, Zorumski CF. Acute effects of antidepressants on hippocampal seizures. Ann Neurol 1985;18:692-697.

Cloninger CR, Christiansen KO, Reich T, Gottesman II. Implications of sex differences in the prevalence of antisocial personality, alcoholism and criminality for familial transmission. Arch Gen Psychiatry 1978;35:941-951.

Coccaro EF, Siever LJ. Second generation antidepressants: a comparative review. J Clin Pharmacol 1985;25(4):241-260.

Coffey CE, Alston S, Heinz ER, Burger PC. Brain iron in progressive supranuclear palsy: clinical, magnetic resonance imaging, and neuropathological findings. J Neuropsychiatry 1989;1(4):400.

Cohen BM, Harris PZ, Altesman RI, et al. Amoxapine: neuroleptic as well as antidepressant? Am J Psychiatry 1982;139(9):1165-1167.

Coleman M. Serotonin and central nervous system syndromes of childhood: a review. J Autism Child Schizophr 1973;1:27-35.

Coleman M, Steinberg G, Tippett J, Bhagavan HN, Coursin DB, Gross M, Lewis C, DeVeau L. A preliminary study of the effect of pyridoxine administration in a subgroup of Biological hyperkinetic children: a double-blind comparison with psychiatry methylphenidate. Biol Psychol 1979;14(5):741-751.

Colenda CC. Buspirone in treatment of agitated demented patient. Lancet 1988;1169.

Collerton D, Fairbairn A, Britton P. Cognitive performance of medicated schizophrenics with tardive dyskinesia. Psychol Med 1985;15:311-315.

Colohan ART, Dacey RG, Alves WM, Rimel RM, Jane JA. Neurologic and neurosurgical implications of mild head injury. J Head Trauma Rehab 1986;1:13-21.

Comfort A. Phenelzine therapy: the doctor, the patient, and the wine and cheese party. J Oper Psychiatry 1982;13(1):37-40.

Cools AR, van den Bercken JHL. Cerebral organization of behaviour and the neostriatal function. In: Cools AR, Lohman AHM, van den Bercken JHL, eds. Psychobiology of the striatum. Amsterdam: North-Holland Biomedical Press, 1977:119-140.

Coombs C. Cerebral rheumatism. Practitioner 1912;88:99-106.

Cooper AF, Fowlie HC. Control of gross self-mutilation with lithium carbonate. Br J Psychiatry 1973;22:370-371.

Cope DN. The pharmacology of attention and memory. J Head Trauma Rehab 1986;1(3):34-42.

Corbett JA. Psychiatric morbidity and mental retardation. In: James FE, Smith RP, eds. Psychiatric illness and mental handicap. London: Gaskell Press, 1979.

Cowdry RW. Pharmacotherapy of borderline personality disorder. Alprazolam, carbamazepine, trifluoperazine, and tranylcypramine. Arch Gen Psychiatry 1988;45(2):111-119.

Coyle JT, Price DL, DeLong MR. Alzheimer's disease: a disorder of cortical cholinergic innervation. Science 1983;219:1184-1190.

Craft M, Ismail IA, Krishnamurti D, et al. Lithium in the treatment of aggression in mentally handicapped patients. Br J Psychiatry 1987;150:685-689.

Craig TJ, Behar R. Trends in the prescription of psychotropic drugs (1970-1977) in a state hospital. Compr Psychiatry 1980;21:336-345.

Crane G. Clinical psychopharmacology in its 20th year. Science 1973;181:124-128.

Creese I, Burt DR. Dopamine receptor binding enhancement accompanies lesion-induced behavioral supersensitivity. Science 1977;197:596-598.

Criswell H, Breese GR, Mueller RA. Evidence for adenosine dopamine interactions in the LNS. Soc Neurosci Abstr 1986;12:1007.

Criswell H, Mueller RA, Breese GR. Assessment of purine-dopamine interactions in 6-hydroxydopamine-lesioned Rats: evidence for pre-and postsynaptic influences by adenosine. J Pharmacol Exp Ther 1988;244(2):493-500.

Critchley M. Periodic hypersomnia and megaphagia in adolescent males. Brain 1962;85(4):628-657.

Crnic KA, Sulzbacher S, Snow J, Holm VA. Preventing mental retardation associated with gross obesity in the Prader-Willi syndrome. Pediatrics 1980;66(5):787-789.

Croog SH, Levine S, Testa MA, et al. The effects of Antihypertensive therapy on the quality of life. N Engl J Med 1986;314:1657-1664.

Crow TJ, Ball J, Bloom SR, et al. Schizophrenia as an anomaly of development of cerebral asymmetry: a postmortem study and a proposal concerning the genetic basis of the disease. Arch Gen Psychiatry 1989;46(12):1145-1150.

Cuetter AC. Sleep apnea and the Kleine-Levin syndrome. Mil Med 1985;150(5):286-288.

Culebras A, Magnana R. Neurological disorders and sleep disturbances. Semin Neurol 1987;7(3):277-284.

Cummings JL. Organic delusions. Br J Psychiatry 1985;146:184-197.

Cummings JL. Organic psychoses: delusional disorders and secondary mania. Psychiatry Clin North Am 1986;9(2):293-308.

Cummings JL, Duchen LW. Kluver-Bucy syndrome in pick disease: clinical and pathologic correlations. Neurology 1981;31:1415-1422.

Cummings JL, Mendez MF. Secondary mania with focal cerebrovascular lesions. Am J Psychiatry 1984;141:1084-1087.

Cummings JL, Gosenfeld LF, Houlihan JP, McCaffey T. Neuropsychiatric disturbances associated with idiopathic calcification of the basal ganglia. Biol Psychol 1983;18:591-599.

D'Alessandro R, Tinuper P, Ferrara R, et al. CT scan prediction of late post-traumatic epilepsy. J Neurol Neurosurg Psychiatry 1982;45:1153-1155.

D'Mello DA, McNeil JA, Harris W. Buspirone suppression of neuroleptic-induced akathisia: multiple case reports. J Clin Psychopharmacol 1989;9:151-152.

Daker MG, Chidiac P, Fear CN, Berry AC. Fragile X in a normal male: a cautionary tale. Lancet 1981;1:780.

Dalby MA. Antiepileptic and psychotropic effect of carbamazepine in the treatment of psychomotor epilepsy. Epilepsia 1971;12:325-334.

Dalby MA. Behavioral effects of carbamazepine. In: Penry JK, Daly DD, eds. Complex partial seizures and their treatment. New York: Raven Press, 1975:331-344.

Dalton K, Dalton MJT. Characteristics of pyridoxine overdose neuropathy syndrome. Acta Neurol Scand 1987;76:8-11.

Daly DD. Ictal clinical manifestations of complex partial seizures. In: Advances in Neurology. New York: Raven Press, 1975:57-83.

Daly JW, Bruns RF, Snyder SM. Adenosine receptors in the central nervous system: Relationship to the central actions of methylxanthines. Life Sci 1981;28:2083-2097.

Damasio AR, Van Hoesen GW. The limbic system and the localisation of herpes simplex encephalitis. J Neurol Neurosurg Psychiatry 1985;48:297-301.

Damlouji NF, Ferguson JM. Trazadone-induced delirium in bulimic patients. Am J Psychtry 1984;141(3):434.

Danford DE, Huber AM. Pica among mentally retarded adults. Am J Ment Defic 1982;87:141-146.

Daniels LE. Narcolepsy. Medicine 1934;13:1-122.

Davidoff E, Reifenstein EC. Treatment of schizophrenia with sympathomimetic drugs: benzedrine sulfate. Psychiatr Q 1939;127-144.

Davidoff RA. Antispasticity drugs: mechanisms of action. Ann Neurol 1985;17:107-116.

Davidson J. Seizures and bupropion: a review. J Clin Psychiatry 1989;50:256-261.

Davidson PW, Kleene BM, Carroll M, Rockowitz RJ. Effects of naloxone on self-injurious behavior: a case study. Appl Res Ment Retard 1983;4:1-4.

Davis JM. Comparative doses and costs of antipsychotic medication. Arch Gen Psychiatry 1976;33:858-861.

Davis KL, Rosenberg GS. Is there a limbic system equivalent of tardive dyskinesia? Biolog Psych 1979;14:699-703.

Davis RJ, Cummings JL. Clinical Variants of tardive dyskinesia. Neuropsychiatr, Neuropsychol Behav Neurol 1988;1(1):31-38.

Day JO. Water intoxication in psychogenic water drinkers taking thiazide diuretics. South Med J 1977;70:572-575.

de Carolis P, Baldrati A, Agati R, de Capoa D, D'Alessandro R, Sacquegna T. Nimodipine in episodic cluster headache: results and methodological considerations. Headache 1987;27:397-399.

Deicken RF. Captopril treatment of depression. Biol Psychol 1986;21:1425-1428.

Dejerine J, Roussy G. La syndrome thalamique. Rev Neurol (Paris) 1906;14:521-532.

Delaney R, Rosen AT, Mattson RH, Novelly RA. Memory function in focal epilepsy: a comparison of non-surgical unilateral temporal lobe and frontal lobe samples. Cortex 1980;16:103-107.

De Keyser J, Ebinger G, Herregodts P. Pathophysiology of akathisia. Lancet 1987;336.

de Lange C. Nouvelle observation du "typus amstelodamensis" et examen anatomopathologique de ce type. Arch Med Enfants 1938;41:193-203.

De Weid D. Hormonal influences on motivation learning and memory process. Hosp Prac [off] 1976;Jan:123-131.

de Lange C. Sur un type nouveau de de-degeneration (Typus Amstelodamensis). Arch Med Enfants 1933;36:713.

Delgado-Escueta AV, Mattson RH, King L. The nature of aggression during epileptic seizures. N Engl J Med 1981;305:711-716.

Delgado-Escueta AV, Kunze V, Waddell G, Boxley J, Nadel A. Lapse of consciousness and automatisms in temporal lobe epilepsy: a videotape analysis. Neurology 1977;27:144-155.

Dement WC, Guilleminault C. Sleep disorders: the state of the art. Hosp Prac [off] 1973;Nov:57-71.

Devane CL. Monitoring cyclic antidepressants. Clin Lab Med 1987;7:551-566.

De Vogelaer J. Carbamazepine in the treatment of psychotic and behavior disorders. Acta Psychiatr Belg 1981;81:532-541.

Dews PB. Caffeine. Berlin: Springer-Verlag, 1984.

Deykin EY, Macmahon B. The incidence of seizures among children with autistic symptoms. Am J Psychiatry 1979;136:1310-1312.

Diaz PM. Interaction of pentylenetetrazol and trimethadione on the metabolism of serotonin in brain and its relation to the anticonvulsant action of trimethadione. Neuropharmacology 1974;13:615-621.

Dimond SJ, Brouwers EYM. Increase in power of human memory in normal man through use of drugs. Psychopharmacology 1976;49:307-309.

Divac I. Functions of the caudate nucleus. Acta Biol Exp (Warsaw) 1968;28(2):107-120.

Dongier S. Statistical study of clinical and electroencephalographic manifestations of 536 psychotic episodes occurring in 516 epileptics between clinical seizures. Epilepsia (amsterdam) 1959;1: pp. 117-142.

Dorian P, Sellers EM, Kaplan HL, Hamilton C, Greenblatt DJ, Abernathy D. Triazolam and ethanol interaction: kinetic and dynamic consequences. Clin Pharmacol Ther 1985;37:558-562.

Douyon R, Serby M, Klutchko B, Rotrosen J. ECT and Parkinson's disease revisited: a "naturalistic study." Am J Psychiatry 1989;146(11):1451.

Dubovsky SL. Calcium antagonists: a new class of psychiatric drugs. Psychiatr Ann 1986;16:724-728.

Dufresne RL, Weber SS, Becker RE. Bupropion hydrochloride. Drug Intell Clin Pharm 1984;18:957-964.

Dunwiddie TV, Worth T. Sedative and anticonvulsant effects of adenosine analogs in mouse and rat. J Pharmacol Exp Ther 1982;220:70-76.

Eaton LF, Menolascino FJ. Psychiatric disorders in the mentally retarded: types, problems, and challenges. Am J Psychiatry 1982;139:1297-1303.

Edwards H. The significance of brain damage in persistent oral dyskinesia. Br J Psychiatry 1970;116:271-275.

Eichelman B. Catecholamines and aggressive behavior. In: Usdin E, ed. Neuroregulators and psychiatric disorders. New York: Oxford University, 1977:146-150.

Eison AS, Temple DL. Buspirone: Review of its pharmacology and current perspectives on its mechanisms of action. Am J Med 1986;80:1-9.

Ekbom DA. Astehnia crurum paraesthetica ("irritable legs"). Acta Med Scand 1944;118:197-209.

El-Mallax H. Use of beta-blockers in neurology. Resid Staff Physician 1986;32(6):68-73.

Elian M, Bornstein B. The Klein-Levin syndrome with Intermittent electroencephalographic abnormalities. Electroencephalgr Clin Neurophysiol 1969;27:601-604.

Ellenberg JH, Hirtz DG, Nelson KB. Do seizures in children cause intellectual deterioration? N Engl J Med 1986;314:1085-1088.

Ellenberger HF. The discovery of the unconscious. New York: Basic Books, 1970.

Elliot FA. The neurology of explosive rage. Practitioner 1976;217:51-60.

Elliot FA. Propranolol for the control of the Belligerent behavior following acute brain damage. Ann Neurol 1977;489-491.

Elliot RL. Case report of a potential interaction between clonidine and electroconvulsive therapy. Am J Psychiatry 1983;140:1237-1238.

Ellis JM, Kishi T, Azuma J, Folkers K. Vitamin B6 deficiency in patients with a clinical syndrome including the carpal tunnel defect: biochemical and clinical response to therapy with pyridoxine Res Commun Chem Pathol Pharmacol 1976;13:743-757.

Elwes RDC, Johnson AL, Shorvon SD, Reynolds EH. The prognosis for seizure control in newly diagnosed epilepsy. N Engl J Med 1984;311:944-947.

Emerson R, D'Souza BJ, Vining EP, Holden KR, Mellitis ED, Freeman JM. Stopping medication in children with epilepsy; predictors of outcome. N Engl J Med 1981;304:1125-1129.

Emmrich H, von Zerssen D, Kissling W, et al. Therapeutic effects of sodium valproate in mania. Am J Psychiatry 1981;138:2.

Empson JAC. Does electrosleep induce natural sleep? Electroencephalogr Clin Neurophysiol 1973;35:663.

Emrich HM, v Zerssen D, Kissling W, Moller H-J, Windorfer A. Effect of sodium valproate on mania, the GABA-Hypothesis of affective disorders. Arch Psychiatr Nervenkr 1980;229:1-16.

Engelhardt DM, Polizos P, Waizer J, Hoffman SP. A double-blind comparison of fluphenazine and haloperidol on outpatient schizophrenic children. J Autism Child Schizophr 1973;3:128-137.

Epstein CM. Ranitidine and confusion. Lancet 1984;1(8385):1071.

Epstein FM, Ward JD, Becker DP. Medical complications of head injury. In: Head injury. Cooper PR, ed. Baltimore: Williams & Wilkins, 1987:390-421.

Erkulwater S, Pillai R. Amantadine and the end-stage dementia of Alzheimer's type. South Med J 1989;82(5):550-554.

Erwin CW, Linnoila M, Hartwell J, Erwin A, Guthrie S. Effects of buspirone and diazepam, alone and in combination with alcohol, on skilled performance and evoked potentials. J Clin Psychopharmacol 1986;6:199-209.

Escalante H, Grunspun H, Frotarpassoa O. Severe sex-linked mental retardation. J Gene Hum 1971;19:137.

Esiri MM. Herpes simplex encephalitis: an immunohistological study of the distribution of viral antigen within the brain. J Neurol Sci 1982;54:209-226.

Evans DA, Funkenstein H, Albert MS, et al. Prevalence of Alzheimer's disease in a community population of older persons. JAMA 1989;262:2551-2556.

Evans KR, Eikelboom R. Feeding induced by ventricular bromocriptine and amphetamine: a possible excitatory role for dopamine in eating behavior. Behav Neurosci 1987;101(4):591-593.

Evans RW, Amara I, Gualtieri CT. Methylphenidate and memory: dissociated Effects in hyperactive children. Psychopharmacol 1986a;90(2):211-216.

Evans RW, Clay TH, Gualtieri CT. Carbamazepine in pediatric psychiatry. J American Acad Child Adolesc Psychiatry 1987a;26:2-8.

Evans RW, Gualtieri CT. Carbamazepine: a neuropsychological and psychiatric profile. Clin Neuropharmacol 1985;8:221-241.

Evans RW, Gualtieri CT. Effects of piracetam on verbal memory in dyslexic children: a negative report. 1986 (unpublished).

Evans RW, Gualtieri CT. Motor performance in hyperactive children treated with imipramine. Percept Mot Skills 1988;66:763-769.

Evans RW, Gualtieri CT, Amara I. Methylphenidate and memory: dissociated effects in hyperactive children. Psychopharmacology 1986b;90:211-216.

Evans RW, Gualtieri CT, Patterson DR. Treatment of chronic closed head injury with psychostimulant drugs: a controlled case study and an appropriate evaluation procedure. J Nerv Ment Dis 1987b;175:106-110.

Fadda F, Gessa GL, Mosca E, Stefanini E. Different effects of the calcium antagonists nimodipine and flunarizine on dopamine metabolism in the rat brain. J Neural Transm 1989;75:195-200.

Faden AI. Opiate antagonists and thyrotropin-releasing hormone. II. Potential role in the treatment of central nervous system injury. JAMA 1984;252:1452-1454.

Faden AI. Neuropeptides and central nervous system injury: clincial implications. Arch Neurol 1986;43:501-503.

Faden AI. Pharmacotherapy in spinal cord injury: a critical review of recent

Faden AI, Jacobs TP. Effect of TRH analogs on neurologic recovery after experimental spinal trauma. Neurology 1985;35(9):1331-1334.

Fahn S. Treatment of tardive dyskinesia: use of dopamine-depleting agents. Clin Neuropharmacol 1983;6:151-158.

Fahn S. Therapeutic approach to tardive dyskinesia. J Clin Psychiatry 1985;46:19-24.

Fahn S. Drug Treatment of hyperkinetic movement disorders. J Clin Psychiatry 1987;7:192-207.

Fahs JJ. Anxiety disorders. In: American Psychiatric Association, ed. Treatments of psychiatric disorders. Washington, D.C.: American Psychiatric Association, 1989:14-19.

Famuyiwa OO, Eccleston D, Donaldson AA, Garside RF. Tardive dyskinesia and dementia. Br J Psychiatry 1979;135:500-504.

Farber JM. Psychopharmacology of self-injurious behavior in mentally retarded persons. National Center for the Study and Treatment of Head Injury 1986;296-302.

Faught E, Falgout J, Nidiffer FD, Dreifuss FE. Self-induced photosensitive absence seizures with ictal pleasure. Arch Neurol 1986;43:408-410.

Faught E, Peters D, Bartolucci A, Moore L, Miller PC. Seizures after primary intracerebral hemorrhage. Neurology 1989;39:1089-1093.

Favazza AR. Bodies under siege: self-mutilation in culture and psychiatry. Baltimore: Johns Hopkins University Press, 1987.

Feeney DM, Gonzalez A, Law WA. Amphetamine, haloperidol and experience interact to affect rate of recovery after motor cortex surgery. Science 1982;217:855-857.

Feeney DM, Bailey BY, Boyeson MG, Hovda DA, Sutton RL. The effect of seizures on recovery of function following cortical contusion in the rat. Brain Injury 1987;1(1):27-32.

Feeney DM, Walker AE. The prediction of posttraumatic epilepsy: a mathematical approach. Arch Neurol 1979;36:8-12.

Feldman H, Crumrine P, Handen BL, Alvin R, Teodori J. Methylphenidate in children with seizures and attention-deficit disorder. Am J Dis Child 1989;143:1081-1086.

Fenwick P. The nature and management of aggression in epilepsy. J Neuropsychiatry 1989;1(4):418.

Ferrier IN. Water intoxication in patients with psychiatric illness. Br Med J 1985;291:1594-1596.

Festinger L. A theory of social comparison processes. Hum Rel 1954;7:114-140.

Field JH. Epidemiology of head injury in England and Wales. Leicester: Willsons, 1976.

Filley CM, Jarvis PE. Delayed reduplicative paramnesia. Neurology 1987;37:701-703.

Finelli P, Pueschel SM, Padre-Mendoza T, O'Brien MM. Neurological findings in patients with the fragile-X syndrome. J Neurol Neurosurg Psychiatry 1985;48:150-153.

Fischman MW. Cocaine and the amphetamines. In: Meltzer HY, ed. Psychopharmacology: the third generation of progress. New York: Raven Press, 1987:1543-1553.

Fish B, Campbell M, Shapiro T, Floyd A. Comparison of trifluperidol, trifluperazine and chlorpromazine in preschool schizophrenic children: the value of less sedative antipsychotic agents. Curr Ther Res 1911;1969:589-595.

Fitten LJ, Perryman KM, Gross PL, Fine H, Cummins J, Marshall C. Treatment of Alzheimer's disease with short- and long-term oral THA and lecithin: a double-blind study. Am J Psychiatry 1990;147:239-242.

Fjalland B, Nielson IM. Enhancement of methylphenidate-induced stereotypies by repeated administration of neuroleptics. Psychopharmacologia1974;34:105-109.

Fleet WS, Valenstein E, Watson RT, Heilman KM. Dopamine agonist therapy for neglect in humans. Neurology 1987;37:1765-1770.

Flor-Henry P. Psychosis and temporal lobe epilepsy. Epilepsia 1969;10:363-395.

Flor-Henry P. On certain aspects of the localization of the cerebral systems regulating and determining emotions. Biol Psychiatry 1979;14:677-698.

Flor-Henry P, Koles ZJ. EEG studies in depression, mania and normals: evidence for partial shifts of laterality in the affective psychoses. Adv Biol Psychiatry 1980;4:21-43.

Folstein S, Rutter M. Infantile autism: a genetic study of 21 twin pairs. J Child Psychol Psychiatry 1977;18:297-321.

Fontaine R. Clonazepam for panic disorders and agitation. Psychosomatics 1985;26(2):13-18.

Forehand R, Baumeister AA. Body rocking and activity level as a function of prior motion restraint. Am J Ment Defic 1970a;74:608-610.

Forehand R, Baumeister AA. Effect of frustration on stereotyped body rocking: follow-up. Percept Motor Skills 1970b;31:894.

Fraser HS, Carr AC. Propranolol psychosis. Br J Psychiatry 1976;129:508-509.

Frederiksen S, D'Elia G, Holsten R. Influence of ACTH-4-10 and unilateral ECT on primary and secondary memory in depressive patients. Eur Arch Psychiatry Neurol Sci 1985;234:291-294.

Freinhar JP. Clonazepam treatment of a mentally retarded woman. Am J Psychiatry 1985;142(12):1536.

Freinhar JP, Alvarez WA. Clonazepam: A novel therapeutic adjunct. Int J Psychiatry Med 1985a;15(4):321-328.

Freinhar JP, Alvarez WH. Use of clonazepam in two cases of acute mania. J Clin Psychiatry 1985b;46(1):29-30.

French LR, Schuman LM, Mortimer JA, Hutton JT, Boatman RA, Christians B. A case-control study of dementia of the Alzheimer type. Am J Epidemiol 1985;121:414-421.

Frieden BD. Clinical issues on the physical restraint experience with self-injurious children. Res Retard 1977;4:1-6.

Frieden BD, Johnson HK. Treatment of a retarded child's feces smearing and coprophagic behavior. J Ment Defic Res 1979;23:55-61.

Friedman MJ, Culver CM, Ferrell RB. On the safety of long-term treatment with lithium. Am J Psychiatry 1977;134:1123-1126.

Friedmann M. Uber eine besonere schwere from von Folgezustanden nach Gehirnershutterung und uber den vasomotorischen Symtomenkomplex bei der selben in Allgemeinen. Arch Psychiatry 1892;23:230-267.

Frye GD, Baumeister AA, Crotty K, Newman KD, Kotria K. Evaluation of the role of antinociception in self-injurious behavior following intranignal injection of muscle. Neuropharmacology 1986;25:717-726.

Fryns JP. The fragile X syndrome: a study of 83 families. Clin Genet 1984;26:497-528.

Fryns JP. The female and the fragile X: a study of 144 obligate females carriers. Am J Med Genet 1986;23:157-169.

Fryns JP, Jacobs J, Kleczkowska A, van den Berghe H. The psychological profile of the fragile X syndrome. Clin Genet 1984;25:131-134a.

Fryns JP, Kleczkowska A, Kubien E, van den Berghe H. Cytogenetic findings in moderate and severe mental retardation. Acta Paediatr Scand Suppl 1984b;313:3-23.

Fukuda N, Yoshiaki S, Nagaway J. Behavioral and EEG alterations with brain stem compression and effect of TRH in chronic cats. Folia Pharmacol Jpn 1979;75:321-331.

Fuller RW, Wong DT. Fluoxetine: a serotonergic appetite suppressant drug. Drug Dev Res 1989;17:1-15.

Furgerson SM, Rayport M. Psychoses in epilepsy. In: Blumer D, ed. Psychiatric aspects of epilepsy. Washington,DC: American Psychiatric Press, 1984:229-270.

Furgeson BG. Kleine-Levin syndrome: a case report. J Child Psychol Psychiatry 1986;27(2):275-278.

Gadoth N, Lerman M, Garty B, Shuelewitz O. Normal intelligence in the Cornelia de Lange syndrome. Johns Hopkins Med J 1982;150:70-72.

Gallassi R, Morreale A, Lorusso S, Procaccianti G, Lugaresi E, Baruzzi A. Carbamazepine and phenytoin, comparison of cognitive effects in epileptic patients during monotherapy and withdrawal. Arch Neurol 1988;45:892-894.

Ganesh S, Rao JM, Cowie VA. Akathisia in neuroleptic medicated mentally handicapped subjects. J Ment Defic Res 1989;33:323-329.

Gardner DL, Cowdry RW. Development of melancholia during carbamezapine treatment in borderline personality disorder. J Clin Psychopharmacol 1986;6(4):236-239.

Gardos G, Casey DE. Clinical insights monograph: tardive dyskinesia and affective disorders. Washington, DC: American Psychiatric Press, 1984.

Gardos G, Cole JO, Schniebolk S, Salomon M. Comparison of severe and mild tardive dyskinesia: implications for etiology. J Clin Psychiatry 1987;48(9):359-362.

Garland H, Sumner D, Fourman P. Kleine-Levin syndrome: some further observations. Neurology 1965;15:1161-1167.

Garner SJ, Eldridge FL, Wagner PG, Dowell RT. Buspirone, an anxiolytic drug that stimulates respiration. Am Rev Respir Dis 1989;139:946-950.

Garside RF, Kay DWK. The genetics of stuttering. In: Andrews G, Harris MM, eds. The syndrome of stuttering. Heinemann, 1964.

Gartrell N. Increased libido in women receiving trazadone. Am J Psychiatry 1986;143(6):781-782.

Gastaut H, Zifkin BG, Mariani E, Puig JS. The long-term course of primary generalized epilepsy with persisting absences. Neurology 1986;36:1021-1028.

Gath A, Gumley D. Behaviour problems in retarded children with special reference to Down's syndrome. Br J Psychiatry 1986;149:156-161.

Gelenberg AJ, Mandel MR. Catatonic reactions to high-potency neuroleptic drugs. Arch Gen Psychiatry 1977;34:947-950.

Gelenberg AJ, Doller-Wojcik JC, Growden JH. Choline and lecithin in the treatment of tardive dyskinesia. Am J Psychiatry 1979;136:772-775.

Geller E, Ritvo ER, Freeman BJ, Yuwiler A. Preliminary observations on the effect of fenfluramine on blood serotonin and symptoms in three autistic children. N Engl J Med 1982;307:165-169.

Gelmers, HJ. Nimodipine in ischemic stroke. Clin Neuropharmacol 1987;10(5):412-422.

Gengo FM, Huntoon L, McHugh WB. Lipid-soluble and water-soluble b-Blockers: comparison of the central nervous system depressant effect. Arch Intern Med 1987;147:39-43.

George MS, Scott T, Kellner CH, Malcolm R. Abnormalities of the septum pellucidum in schizophrenia. J Neuropsychiatry 1989;1(4):385.

Gerbino L, Oleshansky M, Gershon SI. Clinical use and mode of action of lithium. In: Lipton MA, Dimascio A, Killiam KF, eds. Psychopharmacology: a generation of progress. New York: Raven Press, 1978:1261-1275.

Gerner R, Estabrook W, Steuer J, Jarvik L. Treatment of geriatric depression with trazadone, imipramine, and placebo: a double-blind study. J Clin Psychiatry 1980;41:216-220.

Gershon ES, Goldstein RE, Moss AJ, van Kammen DP. Psychosis with ordinary doses of propranolol. Ann Intern Med 1979;90:938-939.

Gershon S. Comparative side effect profiles of trazadone and imipramine; special reference to the geriatric population. Psychopathology 1984;17(2):39-50.

Gershon S, Newton R. Lack of anticholinergic side effects with a new antidepressant-Trazadone. J Clin Psychiatry 1980;41(3):100-104.

Gerstenbrand F, Poewe W. Aichner PF, Saltuari L. Kluver-Bucy syndrome in man: experiences with postraumatic cases. Neurosci Biobehav Rev 1983;7:413-417.

Giannini AJ, Houser WL, Louiselle RH, et al. Antimanic effects of verapamil. Am J Psychiatry 1984;141:1602-1603.

Gianutsos G, Moore KE. Differential behavioral and biochemical effects of four dopaminergic agonists. Psychopharmacology 1980;68:139-146.

Gianutsos G, Stewart C, Dunn JP. Pharmacological changes in dopaminergic systems induced by long-term administration of amantadine. Eur J Pharmacol 1985;110:357-361.

Gibson GE, Sheu KR, Blass JP, Baker A, Carlson KC, Perrino P. Reduced activities of thiamine-dependent enzymes in the brains and peripheral tissues of patients with Alzheimer's disease. Arch Neurol 1988;45:836-840.

Gilbert GJ. Periodic hypersomnia with bulimia: Kleine-Levin syndrome. Neurology 1964;14:844-850.

Gillberg C, Wahlstrom J, Hagberg B. A "new" chromosome marker common to the Rett syndrome and infantile autism? The frequency of fragile sites at X P22 in 81 children with infantile autism, childhood psychosis and the Rett syndrome. Brain Dev 1985;7(3):365-367.

Gillberg C, Wahlstrom J, Johansson R, Tornblom M, Albertsson-Wikland K. Folic acid as an adjunct in the treatment of children with the autism fragile-X syndrome (AFRAX). Dev Med Child Neurol 1986;28:624-627.

Gilleard CJ, Vaddad KS. Mood, memory, and performance and the severity of tardive dyskinesia. Percept Motor Skills 1986;63:1037-1038.

Giorguieff-Chesselet MF, Kernel ML, Wandscheer D, Glowinski J. Regulation of dopamine release by presynaptic nicotinic receptors on rat striatal slices: effect of nicotine in a low concentration. Life Sci 1979;25:1257-1262.

Giovannini M, Valsasina R, Longhi R. Serotonin and noradrenaline concentrations and serotonin uptake in platelets from hyperphenylalaninaemic patients. J Inherited Metab Dis 1988;11(3):285-290.

Gispen WH, Isaacson RL, Spruijt BM, et al. Melanocortins, neural plasticity and ageing. Prog Neuropsychol Biol Psychiatry 1986;10:416-426.

Gitlin MJ, Weiss J. Varapamil as maintenance treatment in bipolar illness: a case report. J Clin Psychopharmacol 1984;4(6):341-343.

Glass GV, Singer JE. Urban stress: experiments on noise and social stressors. New York: Academic Press, 1972:

Glazer W, Moore DC, Schooler NR, Brenner LM, Morgenston H. Tardive dyskinesia: a discontinuation study. Arch Gen Psychiatry 1984;41:623-627.

Gleiter CH, Nutt DJ. Chronic electroconvulsive shock and neurotransmitter receptors - an update. Life Sci 1989;44:985-1006.

Goa KL, Ward A. Buspirone: a preliminary review of its pharmacological properties and therapeutic efficacy as an anxiolytic. Drugs 1986;32:114-129.

Goddard GV, Douglas RM. Does the engram of kindling model the engram of normal long term memory?. Can J Neurol Sci 1975;2:385-394.

Goddard GV, McIntyre DC, Leech CK. A permanent change in brain function resulting from daily electrical stimulations. Exp Neurol 1969;25:295-330.

Godwin-Austen RB, Lee PN, Marnot MG, Stern GM. Smoking and Parkinson's disease. J Neurol Neurosurg Psychiatry 1982;45:577-581.

Goff DC, Garber J, Jenike MA. Partial resolution of ranitidine-associated delirium with physostigmine: case report. J Clin Psychiatry 1985;46:400-401.

Goh K, Herman MA, Campbell RG, Thompson D. Abnormal chromosome in Prader-Willi syndrome. Clin Gen 1984;26:597-601.

Golbe LI. Deprenyl as symptomatic therapy in Parkinson's disease. Clin Neuropharmacol 1988;11(5):387-400.

Gold MS, Pottash C, Sweeney DR, Kleber HD. Opiate withdrawal using clonidine: a safe, effective, and rapid nonopiate treatment. JAMA 1980;243(4):343-346.

Goldberg MA. The treatment of Kleine-Levin syndrome with lithium. Can J Psychiatry 1983;28:491-492.

Goldbloom DS, Kennedy SH, Kaplan AS, Woodside DB. Anorexia nervosa and bulimia nervosa. Can Med Assoc J 1989;140:1149-1153.

Golden RN, James SP, Sherer MA, Rudorfer MV, Sack DA, Potter WZ. Psychoses associated with bupropion treatment. Am J Psychiatry 1985;142(12):1459.

Goldman MB, Luchins DJ, Robertson GL. Mechanisms of altered water metabolism in psychotic patients with polydipsia and hyponatremia. N Engl J Med 1988;318:397-403.

Goldstein K. After-effects of brain injuries in war. New York: Grune & Stratton, 1948:

Goldstein M, Anderson LT, Reuben R, Dancis J. Self-mutilation in Lesch-Nyhan disease is caused by dopaminergic denervation. Lancet 1985a;1:338-339.

Goldstein M, Kuga S, Schimizu Y, Mueller E. The pathophysiological functions mediated by D1 dopamine receptors. 1985b; (unpublished).

Goldstein PC, Simpson G, Jubanyik K. Treatment effects of clonazepam upon neuropsychological and psychiatric concomitants of Meige's syndrome. 1986 (unpublished).

Golinko BE, Rennick PM, Lewis RF. Predicting stimulant effectiveness in hyperactive children with a repeatable neuropsychological battery. Prog neuropsychopharmacol 1981;5:65-68.

Gomez E, Mikhail AR. Treatment of methadone withdrawal with cerebral electrotherapy (electrosleep). Br J Psychiatry 1979;134:111.

Goutieres F, Aicardi J. Atypical presentations of pyridoxine-dependent seizures: a treatable cause of intractable epilepsy in infants. Ann Neurol 1985;17:117-120.

Grafman J, Jonas BS, Martin A, Intellectual function following penetrating head injury in Vietnam veterans. Brain 1988;111:169-184.

Graham DI, Adams JH, Gennarelli TA. Pathology of brain damage in head injury. In: Cooper PR, ed. Head injury. Baltimore: Williams & Wilkins, 1987:72-88.

Graham PJ, Rutter ML. Organic brain dysfunction and child psychiatric disorder. Br Med J 1968;3:695-700.

Grandin T, Scariano MM. Emergence labelled autistic. Novato, California: Arena Press, 1986.

Grant I, Alves W. Psychiatric and psychosocial disturbances in head injury. In: Levin HS, Grafman J, Eisenberg HM, eds. Neurobehavioral recovery from head injury. New York: Oxford University Press, 1987:232-261.

Granville-Grossman KL, Turner P. The effect of propranolol on anxiety. Lancet 1966;1:788-790.

Green LH. Kleine-Levin Syndrome: a case with EEG evidence of periodic brain dysfunction. Arch Neurol 1970;22:166-174.

Greenberg A, Coleman M. Depressed whole blood serotonin levels associated with behavioral abnormalities in the de Lange syndrome. Pediatrics 1973a;52(5):720-724.

Greenberg DA. Calcium channel antagonists and the treatment of migraine. Clin Neuropharmacol 1986;9(4):311-328.

Greenberg F, Robinson LK. Mild Brachmann-de Lange syndrome: changes of phenotype with age. Am J Med Genet 1989;32:90-92.

Greenblatt DJ, Shader RI. Drug Therapy: prazepam and lorazepam, two new benzodiazepines. N Engl J of Med 1978;299(24):1342-1344.

Greenblatt DJ, Shader RI, Abernethy DR. Drug therapy: current status of benzodiazepines. N Engl J of Med 1983;309(6):354-358.

Greenblatt DJ, Abernethy DR, Morse DS, Harmatz JS, Shader RI. Clinical importance of the interaction of diazepam and cimetidine. N Engl J Med 1984;310:1639-1643.

Greentree LB. Dangers of vitamin B6 in nursing mothers. N Engl J Med 1979;300:141-142.

Greenwald BS, Kramer-Ginsberg E, Marin DB, et al. Dementia with coexistent major depression. Am J Psychiatry 1989;146(11):1472.

Griffin JD, Carranza J, Griffith C, Miller LL. Bupropion: clinical assay for amphetamine-like abuse potential. J Clin Psychiatry 1983;44(5 Sec. 2):206-208.

Gronwall D, Wrightson P. Delayed recovery of intellectual function after minor head injury. Lancet 1974; 2:605-609.

Gronwall D, Wrightson P. Cumulative effect of concussion. Lancet 1975;2:995-997.

Gualtieri CT. Imipramine and children: a review and some speculations on the mechanism of drug action. Dis Nerv Syst 1977;38:368-375.

Gualtieri CT. The problem of tardive dyskinesia litigation. Psychiatr Aspects Ment Retard Rev 1985; 4(4):12-16.

Gualtieri CT. Pharmacotherapy and the neurobehavioral sequelae of closed head injury. Brain Injury 1988;2:101-129.

Gualtieri CT. The differential diagnosis of self-injurious behavior in mentally retarded people. Psychopharmacol Bull 1989b;25:358-363.

Gualtieri CT. The Kluver-Bucy syndrome. In: Gualtieri CT, ed. Neuropsychiatry and behavioral pharmacology. New York: Springer Verlag, 1990 (this volume).

Gualtieri CT. Mental retardation. In: APA Task Force, ed. Treatment of psychiatric disorders. Washington, DC: American Psychiatric Press, 1989a.

Gualtieri CT. The behavioral pharmacology of traumatic brain injury and the specific role of carbamazepine. Symposium Proceedings (in press).

Gualtieri CT. TMS: a system for prevention and control. In: Ratey JJ, ed. Mental Retardation: Developing Pharmacotherapies. Washington: American Psychiatric Press, 1990.

Gualtieri CT, Barnhill LJ. Tardive dyskinesia in special populations. In: Wolf ME, Mosnaim AD, eds. Tardive dyskinesia, biological mechanisms and clinical aspects. Washington, D.C.: American Psychiatric Press, 1988:137-154.

Gualtieri CT, Barnhill LJ, McGimsey J, Schell D. Tardive dyskinesia and other drug-induced movement disorders in children. J Am Acad Child Psychiatry 1980a;19:491-510.

Gualtieri CT, Chandler M, Coons T, Brown L. Amantadine: a new clinical profile for traumatic brain injury. Clin Neuropharmacol 1989;12:258-270.

Gualtieri CT, Cox DR. The delayed neurobehavioral sequelae of traumatic brain injury. Brain Injury 1990 (in press).

Gualtieri CT, Evans RW. Stimulant treatment for the neurobehavioral sequelae of traumatic brain injury. Brain Injury 1988;2:273-290.

Gualtieri CT, Evans RW, Patterson DR. The medical treatment of autistic people.

In: Schopler E, Mesibov GB, eds. Neurobiological Issues in Autism. New York: Plenum, 1987:373-388.

Gualtieri CT, Guimond M. Tardive dyskinesia and the behavioral consequences of chronic neuroleptic treatment. Dev Med Child Neurol 1981;23:255-259.

Gualtieri CT, Hawk B. Tardive dyskinesia and other drug-induced movement disorders among handicapped children and youth. J Appl Res Ment Retard 1980;1:55-69.

Gualtieri CT, Hicks RE. The neuropharmacology of methyphenidate and a neural substrate of childhood hyperactivity. Psychiatr Clin North Am 1985a;8(4):875-892.

Gualtieri CT, Hicks RE. Stimulants and neuroleptics in hyperactive children. J Am Acad Child Psychiatry 1985b;24(3):363-364.

Gualtieri CT, Hicks RE. An immunoreactive theory of selective male affliction. Behav Brain Sci 1985c;8:427-441.

Gualtieri CT, Hicks RE. Neuropharmacology of methylphenidate and a neural substrate for childhood hyperactivity. Psychiatr Clin North Am 1986;8(4):875-892.

Gualtieri CT, Hicks RE, Evans R, Patrick K. The clinical importance of methylphendate blood level determinations. In: Bloomingdale LM, ed. Attention deficit disorder. New York: Pergamon Press, 1983:81-100.

Gualtieri CT, Hicks RE, Levitt J, Conley R, Schroeder SR. Methylphenidate and Exercise: additive effects on motor performance, variable effects on the neuroendocrine response. Neuropsychobiology 1986a;15:84-88.

Gualtieri CT, Hicks RE, Patrick K, Schroeder SR, Breese G. Clinical correlates of methylphenidate blood levels. Ther Drug Monit 1984a;6:379-392.

Gualtieri CT, Keppel JM, Schroeder SR. Tardive dyskinesia: new facts and new recommendations. Psychiatr Aspects Ment Retard Rev 1986b; 5(1):1-6.

Gualtieri CT, Nygard NK. Rehabilitation for head injury, five years after the event. Rebound Q Res Rep 1988;1:16-26.

Gualtieri CT, Ondrusek MG, Finley C. Attention deficit disorder in adults. Clin Neuropharmacol 1985b; 8(4):343-356.

Gualtieri CT, Patterson DR. Neuroleptic-induced tics. Am J Psychiatry 1986;143(9):1176-1177.

Gualtieri CT, Quade D, Hicks RE, Schroeder SR. Tardive dyskinesia and the clinical consequences of neuroleptic treatment in children and adolescents. Am J Psychiatry 1984b; 141:21-23.

Gualtieri CT, Rojahn J, Staye J. The influence of neuroleptic drugs on prolactin secretion in children. Dev Med Child Neurol 1980b;22:515-524.

Gualtieri CT, Schroeder SR. Pharmacotherapy for self-injurious behavior: preliminary tests of the D1 hypothesis. Psychopharmacol Bull 1989;25:364-371.

Gualtieri CT, Schroeder SR. Pharmacotherapy for self-injurious behavior: preliminary tests of the D1 hypothesis. Prog Neuro-Psycholpharmacol (in press).

Gualtieri CT, Schroeder SR, Hicks RE, Quade D. Tardive dyskinesia in young mentally retarded individuals. Arch Gen Psychiatry 1986c;43:335-340.

Gualtieri CT, Sprague RL. Preventing tardive dyskinesia and preventing tardive dyskinesia litigation. Psychopharmacol Bull 1984;20(3):346-348.

Gualtieri CT, Sprague RL, Cole JO, Lipton MA. Tardive dyskinesia litigation and the dilemmas of neuroleptic treatment. J Psychiatry Law 1986d;14(1-2):187-216.

Gualtieri CT, van Bourgondien ME, Hartz C, Schopler E, Marcus L. A pilot study of pyridoxine treatment in autistic children. 1981 (unpublished).

Gualtieri CT, Wargin W, Kanoy R, et al. Clinical studies of methylphenidate serum levels in children and adults. J Am Acad Child Psychiatry 1982;21:19-26.

Guberman A, Cantu-Reyna G, Stuss D, Broughton R. Nonconvulsive generalized status epilepticus: clinical features, neuropsychological testing, and long-term follow-up. Neurology 1986;36:1284-1291.

Guess D, Rutherford G. Experimental attempts to reduce stereotyping among blind retardates. Am J Ment Defic 1967;71:984-986.

Guidice MA, Berchou RC. Post-traumatic epilepsy following brain injury. Brain Injury 1989;61:64-1987.

Gurd JM, Bessell NJ, Bladon RAW, Bamford JM. A case of foreign accent syndrome, with follow-up; clinical, neuropsychological and phonetic descriptions. Neuropsychologia 1988;26:237-251.

Guze BH, Baxter LR. Neuroleptic malignant syndrome. N Engl J Med 1985;313(3):163-166.

Haas JF, Cope DN. Neuropharmacologic management of behavior sequelae in head injury: a case report. Arch Phys Med Rehabil 1985;66:472-474.

Hagberg B, Aicardi J, Dias K, Ramos O. A progressive syndrome of autism, dementia, ataxia, and loss of purposeful hand use in girls: Rett's syndrome: report of 35 cases. Ann Neurol 1983;14:471-479.

Hagerman R, Kemper M, Hudson M. Learning disabilities and attentional problems in boys with the fragile X syndrome. Am J Dis Child 1985;136:674-677.

Hagerman RJ, Jackson AW, Levitas A, et al. Oral folic acid versus placebo in the treatment of males with the fragile X syndrome. Am J Med Genet 1986;23:241-262.

Haghes JD, Reed WD, Serjeant CS. Mental confusion associated with ranitidine. Med J Autism 1983;2(1):12-13.

Haigh D, Forsyth WI. The treatment of childhood epilepsy with sodium valproate. Dev Med Child Neurol 1975;17:743-748.

Hakola HPA, Laulumaa VA. Carbamazepine in treatment of violent schizophrenics. Lancet 1982;8285:1358.

Hale AS, Proctor AW, Bridges PK. Clomipramine, tryptophan and lithium in combination for resistant endogenous depression: seven case studies. Br J Psychiatry 1987;151:213-217.

Hale MS, Donaldson JO. Lithium carbonate in the treatment of organic brain syndrome. J Nerv Ment Dis 1982;170:362-365.

Hallett M, Cohen LG. Magnetism: a new method for stimulation of nerve and brain. JAMA 1989; 262(4):538-541.

Hambidge KM. zinc deficiency in man: Its origins and effects. Philos Trans Soc London (Biol) 1981;294(1071):129-144.

Hambidge KM, Silverman A. Pica with rapid improvement after dietary zinc supplementation. Arch Dis Child 1973;48:567-568.

Hamburg P, Weilburg JB, Cassem NH, Cohen L, Brown S. Relapse of neuroleptic malignant syndrome with early discontinuation of amantadine therapy. Comp Psychiatry 1986;27:272-275.

Hanesh S, Rao JM, Cowie VA. Akathisia in neuroleptic medicated mentally handicapped subjects. J Ment Defic Res 1989;33:323-329.

Hanley HG, Stahl SM, Freedman DX. Hyperserotonemia and amine metabolites in autistic and retarded children. Arch Gen Psychiatry 1977;34:521-531.

Harbaugh RE, Roverts DW, Coombs DW, et al. Preliminary report: intracranial cholinergic drug infusion in patients with Alzheimer's disease. Neurosurgery 1984;15(4):514-518.

Hariprasad MK, Eisinger RP, Nadler IM, Padmanabhan CS, Nidus BD. Hyponatremia in psychogenic polydipsia. Arch Intern Med 1980;140:1639-1642.

Harker LA, Kadatz RA. Mechanism of action of dipyridamole. Thrombosis Res 1983;(Suppl IV):39-46.

Harms HH, Wardeh G, Mulder AH. Adenosine modulates depolarization-induced release of 3H-noradrenaline from slices of rat brain mesocortex. Eur J Pharmacol 1978;49:305-309.

Harrell RF, Capp RH, Davis DR, Peerless J, Ravitz LR. Can nutritional supplements help mentally retarded children? An exploratory study. Proc Natl Acad Sci USA 1981;78(1):574-578.

Harrington RA, Hamilton CW, Brogden RN, et al. Drugs 1983;25:451-494.

Hardy PM. New insights into the physiology of aggression and self-injury: implications for behavioral and pharmacologic therapy. 1990 (Unpublished).

Harvey NS. Psychiatric disorders in parkinsonism: 2. Organic cerebral states and drug reactions. Psychosomatics 1986;27:177-184.

Haskovec L. Akathisie. Arch Bohemes Med Clin 1902;3:193-200.

Haskovec L. Nouvelles remarques sur l'akathisie. Nouv Iconograph Salpetriere 1903;16:287-296.

Hauser SL, DeLong, R Rosman NP. Pneumographic findings in the infantile autism syndrome. Brain 1975;98:667-688.

Hauser WA, Anderson VE, Loewenseon RB, McRoberts SM. Seizure recurrence after a first unprovoked seizure. N Engl J Med 1982; 307:522-528.

Hawkins DR, Taub JM, Van de Castle R. Extended sleep (hypersomnia) in young depressed patients. Am J Psychiatry 1985;142:905-910.

Hawley PP, Jackson LG, Kurnit DM. Sixty-four patients with Brachmann-de Lange syndrome: a survey. Am J Med Genet 1985;20:453-459.

Hayes PE, Kristoff CA. Adverse reactions to five new antidepressants. Clin Pharm 1986; 5:471-480.

Hayman MA, Abrams R. Capgras' syndrome and cerebral dysfunction. Br J Psychiatry 1977;130:68-71.

Hefti F, Weiner WJ. Nerve growth factor and Alzheimer's disease. Ann Neurol 1986;20(3):275-281.

Helfgott E, Rudel RG, Krieger J. Effect of piracetam on the single word and prose reading of dyslexic children. Psychopharmacol Bull 1984; 20:688-690.

Henderson AS. The epidemiology of Alzheimer's disease. Br Med Bull 1986;42:3-10.

Heninger GR, Charney DS, Sternberg DE. Lithium carbonate augmentation of antdepressant treatment: an effective prescription for treatment-refractory depression. Arch Gen Psychiatry 1983;40:1335-1342.

Henry DA, Lawson DH, Reavey P, Renfrew S. Hyponatremia during carbamazepine treatment. Br Med J 1977;1:83-84.

Henry GM, Weingartner H, Murphy DL. Influence of affective states and psychoactive drugs on verbal learning and memory. Am J Psychiatry 1973;130:966-971.

Herman BH, Hammock MK, Arthur-Smith A. Naltrexone decreases self-injurious behavior. Ann Neurol 1987;22:550-552.

Hermann BP, Riel P. Interictal personality and behavioral traits in temporal lobe and generalized epilepsy. Cortex 1981;17:125-128.

Hernandez-Peon R. Central action of G32883 upon transmission of trigeminal pain impulses. Pharmacol Exp 1965;12:73-80.

Herrman EC, Grabliks J, Engle C, Perlman PL. Antiviral activity of 1-adamantanamine (amantadine). Proc Soc Exp Biol Med 1960;103:625.

Herskowitz J, Rosman N. Pediatrics, Neurology and psychiatry — common ground. New York: MacMillian, 1982:377-378.

Herzog DB, Copeland PM. Eating disorders. N Engl J Med 1985;313(5):295-303.

Heston LL, White JA, Mastri AR. Pick's disease: clinical genetics and natural history. Arch Gen Psychiatry 1987;44(5):409-411.

Heyck H. Der Kopfschmerz. Stuttgart: Georg Thieme Verlag, 1975.

Heyman A, Wilkinson WE, Stafford JA, Helms MJ, Sigmon AH, Weinberg T. Alzheimer's disease: a study of epidemiologic aspects. Ann Neurol 1984;15:335-341.

Higgenbottam JA, Chow B. Sound-induced drive, prior motion restraint and reduced sensory stimulation effects on rocking behavior in retarded persons. Am J Ment Defic 1975;80:231-233.

Higgins ST, Bickel WK, O'Leary DK, Yingling J. Acute effects of ethanol and diazepam on the acquisition and performance of response sequences in humans. J Pharmacol Exp Ther 1987;243:1-8.

Hill BK, Balow EA, Bruinincks RH. A national study of prescribed drugs in institutions and community residential facilities for mentally retarded people. Minneapolis: University of Minnesota, 1983.

Hillbom M, Holm L. Contribution of traumatic head injury to neuropsychological deficits in alcoholics. J Neurol Neurosurg Psychiatry 1986;49:1348-1353.

Hillig U. On the genetics of the Rett syndrome. Brain Dev 1985;7(3):368-371.

Hiroshi I, Hidebumi H, Kaoru H, et al. Antipsychotic and prophylactic effects of acetazolamide (diamox) on Atypical Psychosis. Folia Psychiat Neurol Jpn 1984;38(4):425-436.

Hobson JA, English JT. Self-induced water intoxication. Ann Intern Med 1963;58:324-332.

Hoder EL, Cohen DJ. Repetitive behavior patterns of childhood. In: Levine M, Carey W, eds. Developmental and behavioral pediatrics. Philadelphia: W.B. Saunders, 1983:607-622.

Hoehn-Saric R, Merchant AF, Keyser ML, Smith VK. Effects of clonidine on anxiety disorders. Arch Gen Psychiatry 1981;38:1278-1282.

Hoeppner JB, Garron DC, Wilson RS, Koch-Weser MP. Epilepsy and verbosity. Epilepsia 1987;28(1):35-40.

Holdbourn AHS. Mechanics of head injuries. Lancet 1943;2:438-441.

Holliday W, Brasfield KH, Powers B. Grand mal seizures induced by maprotiline. Am J Psychiatry 1982;139(5):673-674.

Holm E, Kelleter R, Hamanon KF. Elektrophysiologische analyse der wirkungen von carbamazepin aug des behirn der katze. Pharmakopsychiatr Neuro-Psychopharmackol 1970;3:187-200.

Holm VA, Pipes PL. Food and children with Prader-Willi syndrome. Am J Dis Child 1976;130:1063-1067.

Holowach J, Thurston DL, O'Leary J. Prognosis in childhood epilepsy; follow-up study of 148 cases in which therapy had been suspended after prolonged anticonvulsant control. N Engl J Med 1972; 286:169-174.

Hooshmand H, Sepdham T, Vries JK. Kluver-Bucy syndrome, successful treatment with carbamazepine. JAMA 1974;229:1782.

Hoschl C. Verapamil for depression?. Am J Psychiatry 1983;140(8):1100.

Hosler DM, Craenen JM, Teske DW. Resurgence of Acute Rheumatic Fever. Am J Dis Child 1987;141:730-733.

Howard-Peebles PN, Friedman JM. Unaffected carrier males in families with fragile X syndrome. Am J Hum Genet 1985;37:956-964.

Hruska RE, Silbergeld EK. Increased dopamine receptor sensitivity after estrogen treatment using the rat rotation model. Science 1980;208:1466-1468.

Hsiao JK, Bartko JJ, Agren H, Rudorfer MV, Linnoila M, Potter WZ. Neuroendocrine response to 5-hydroxytryptophan in seasonal affective disorder. Arch Gen Psychiatry 1987;44(12):1086-1093.

Huber SJ, Paulson GW, Shuttleworth EC. Depression in parkinson's disease. Neuropsychiatry Neuropsychol Behav Neurol 1988;1:47-51.

Huf R, Schain RJ. Long-term experiences With carbamazepine in children with seizures. J Pediat 1981;97:310-312.

Hughes JD, Reed WD, Serjeant CS. Mental confusion associated with ranitidine. Med J Aust 1983;2(1):12-13.

Hunt RD, Minderaa RB, Ccohen DJ. Clonidine benefits children with attention deficit disorder and hyperactivity: report of a double-blind placebo-crossover therapeutic trial. J Am Acad Child Psychiatr 1985;24(5):617-629.

Hunter R, Blackwood W, Smith MC, Cummings JN. Neuropathological findings in three cases of persistent dyskinesia following phenothiazine medication. J Neurol Science 1968;7:263-273.

Hurwitz TA, Wada JA, Kosaka BD, Strauss EH. Cerebral organization of affect suggested by temporal lobe seizures. Neurol 1985;35(9):1335-1337.

Husby G, Van de Rijn I, Zabriskie JB, Abdin ZH, Williams RC. Antibodies reacting with cytoplasm of subthalamic and caudate nuclei neurons in chorea and acute rheumatic fever. J Exp Med 1976;144:1094-1110.

Illowsky BP, Kirch DG. Polydipsia and hyponatremia in psychiatric patients. Am J Psychiatry 1988;145:675-683.

Insel TR. Obsessive-compulsive disorder: new models. Psychopharmacol Bull 1988;24(3):365-369.

Insel TR, Murphy DL. The psychopharmacological treatment of obsessive-compulsive disorder: A review. J Clin Psychopharmacol 1981; 1:304-311.

International colloquium on temporal lobe epilepsy. Observations on the clinical symptomatology of bilateral partial or total removal of the temporal lobes in man. In: Baldwin, Bailey, eds. Temporal Lobe Epilepsy:, 1958:510-529.

Ioria LC, Barnett A, Leitz FH, Houser VP, Korduba CA. SCH 23390: A Potent Benzazepine Antipsychotic with Unique Interactions on Dopaminergic Systems. J Pharmacol Exp Ther 1983; 226:462-468.

Ishii N, Nishihara Y. Pellagra. Encephalopathy among tuberculous patients: its relation to isoniazid therapy. J Neurol Neurosurg Psychiat 1985; 48:628-634.

Itil TM, Soldatos C. Epileptogenic side effects of psychotropic drugs. JAMA 1980; 244:1460-1463.

Iversen S. Striatal function and stereotyped behaviour.In: Cools AR, Lohman AHM, van den Bercken JHL, eds. Psychobiology of the striatum. Amsterdam: North-Holland Biomedical Press, 1977:99-118.

Izquierdo I, Eias RD, Souza DO, et al. Review article: The role of opioid peptides in memory and learning. Behav Brain Res 1980;1:451-468.

Jack RA, Daniel DG. Possible interaction between phenelzine and amantadine. Arch Gen Psychiatry 1984; 41:726.

Jackson RD, Corrigan JD, Arnett JA. Amitriptyline for agitation in head injury. Arch Phys Med Rehab 1985; 66:180-181.

Jacobs B, Trulson M, Heym J, Steinfels G. On the role of CNS serotonin in the motor abnormalities of Tourette's syndrome: behavioral and single dose studies. In: Friedhoff AJ, Chase TN, eds. Gilles de la Tourette syndrome. New York: Raven Press, 1982:93-98.

Jacobs BL, Heym J, Rasmussen K. Action of hallucinogenic drugs at postsynaptic serotonergic receptors. Psychopharmacol Bull 1982; 18:168-172.

Jacome D. Carbamazepine-induced dystonia. JAMA 1979; 21:2262.

Jacome DE. Basilar artery migraine after uncomplicated whiplash injuries. Headache 1986; 26:515-516.

Jacome DE. EEG features in basilar artery migraine. Headache 1987; 27:80-83.

Jane JA, Rimel RW, Pobereskin LH, Tyson GW, Stewart O, Genarelli TA. Head Injury: basic and clinical aspects.In: Grossman RC, Gildenburg PL, eds. Outcome and pathology of head injury. New York: Raven Press, 1982:229-237.

Janowsky A, Sulser F. Alpha and beta adrenoceptors in brain. In: Meltzer HY, ed. Psychopharmacology: The third generation of progress. New York: Raven Press, 1987:249-256.

Jeavons PM, Clarke JE. Sodium Valproate in the Treatment of Epilepsy. Brit Med J 1974;2:584-586.

Jefferson JW. Beta-adrenergic receptor blocking drugs in psychiatry. Arch Gen Psychiatry 1974; 31:681-691.

Jefferson JW, Greist JH, Ackerman DL. Lithium Encyclopedia for clinical practice. Washington, DC: APA Press, 1983.

Jeffries JJ, LeFebvre A. Depression and mania associated with Kleine-Levin-Critchley syndrome. Can Psychiatr Assoc J 1973; 18:439-443.

Jennekens-Schinkel A, Eintzen AR, Lanser BK. A clinical trial with desglycinamide arginine vasopressin for the treatment of memory disorders in man. Prog Neuropsychopharmacol Biol Psychiat 1985; 9:273-284.

Jenner FA. Lithium and the question of kidney damage. Arch Gen Psychiatry 1979; 36:888-890.

Jennett B. Posttraumatic epilepsy. Adv Neurol 1979; 22:137-147.

Jennett B, Teasdale G. Management of head injuries. Philadelphia: F.A. Davis, 1981.

Jerussi TP, Glick SD. Apomorphine-induced rotation in normal rats and interaction with unilateral caudate lesions. Psychopharmacol 1975; 40:329-334.

Jeste D, Kerson CN, Wyatt RJ. Movement Disorders and Psychopathology. In: DV Jeste, Wyatt RJ, eds. Neuropsychiatric Movement Disorders. Washington, D.C.: APA Press, 1984.

Jeste DV, Lohr JB. Hippocampal pathologic findings in schizophrenia. Arch Gen Psychiatry 1989; 46(11):1019.

Joffe RT, Lippert GP, Grey TA, Sawa G, Horvath Z. Mood disorder and multiple schlerosis. Arch Neurol 1987;44:376-378.

Johnson AM, Lowe DM, Vigouret JM. Stimulant Properties of Bromocriptine on Central Dopamine Receptors in Comparison to Apomorphine, (+)-Amphetamine and L-dopa. Brit J Pharmacol 1976a; 56:59-68.

Johnson FN. Psychoactive Drugs and Stimulus Analysis: III. Adjustment of Behavioral Meaures for Drug-Induced Memory Effects and State Dependence: The Case of Chlorpromazine.Int J Neurosci 1983; 20:25-32.

Johnson HG, Ekman P, Friesen W, Nyhan WL, Shear C. A Behavioral Phenotype in th de Lange Syndrome. Pediatr Res 1976b; 10:843-850.

Jones RT. Tobacco Dependence. In: Meltzer HY, ed. Psychopharmacology The Third Generation of Progress. New York: Raven Press, 1987:1589-1595.

Jorm AF. Effects of cholinergic enhancement therapies on memory function in Alzheimer's disease: A meta-analysis of the literature. Austr J Psychiat 1986; 20:237-240.

Jose CJ, Mehta S, Perez-Cruet J. The syndrome of inappropriate secretion of antidiuretic hormone. Can J Psychiatry 1979; 24:225-231.

Joubin J, Pettrone CF, Pettrone FA. Cornelia de Lange's syndrome: A review article (with emphasis on orthopedic significance). Clin Orthop and Relat Res 1980; 171:180-185.

Jounela AJ, Lilja M.. Interactions between beta-blockers and clonidine. Ann Clin Res 1984; 16(4):181-182.

Judd LL, Hubbard B, Janowsky DS, et al. The effect of lithium carbonate on the cognitive functions of normal subjects. Arch Gen Psychiatry 1977; 34:335-357.

Judd LL, Squire LR, Butters N, Salmon DP, Paller KA. Effects of psychotropic drugs on cognition and memory in normal humans and animals. In: Meltzer HY, ed. Psychopharmacology: The third generation of progress. New York: Raven Press, 1987:1467-1475.

Julien RM, Hollister RP. Carbamazepine: mechanisms of action.In: Penry JK, Daly DD, eds. Complex partial seizures and their treatment. New York: Raven Press, 1975:263-277.

Jurko MF, Andy OJ, Webster CL. Disordered Sleep Following Thalamotomy. Clin ElectroEncephalogra 1971; 2:213-217.

Jus A, Villeneuve A, Gautier J, et al. Some remarks on the influence of lithium carbonate on patients with temporal epilepsy.Int J Clin Pharmacol 1973;7(1):67-74.

Kalachnik JE, Harder SR, Kidd-Nielsen P, Errickson E, Doebler M, Sprague RL. Persistent tardive dyskinesia in randomly assigned neuroleptic reduction, neuroleptic nonreduction, and no-neuroleptic-history groups: preliminary results. Psychopharmacol Bull 1984; 20:27-31.

Kalanie H, Niakan E, Harati Y, Rolak LA. Phenytoin-induced benign intracranial hypertension. Neurology 1986;36:443.

Kales A, Soldatos CR, Cadieux R, Bixler EO, Tan T, Scharf MB. Propranolol in the treatment of narcolepsy. Ann Intern Med 1979;91:741-743.

Kane J, Honigfeld G, Singer J, Meltzer H. Clozaril collaborative study group. Clozapine for the treatment-resistant schizophrenic. Arch Gen Psychiatry 1988; 45:789-796.

Kane JM, Smith JM. Tardive Dyskinesia, Prevalence and Risk Factors. Arch Gen Psych 1982; 39:473-481.

Kane JM, Woerner M, Weinhold P, Webner J, Kinon B.Incidence of Tardive Dyskinesia: Five Year Data from a Prospective Study. Psychopharm Bull 1984; 20(1):39-40.

Kang UJ, Burke RE, Fahn S. Natural History and Treatment of Tardive Dyskinesia. Movement Dis 1986; 1:193-208.

Kanner L. Child Psychiatry. Springfield: Charles C. Thomas, 1959.

Kapatos G, Kaufman S. Peripherally administered reduced pterins do enter the brain. Science 1981;212:955-956.

Kartsounis LD. Comprehension as the effective trigger in a case of primary reading epilepsy. J Neurol, Neurosurg, Psychiat 1988; 51:128-130.

Kastenholz KV, Crismon ML. Buspirone, A Novel Nonbenzodiazepine Anxiolytic. Clin Pharm 1984; 3:600-607.

Kasumatsu J, Pettigrew JD. Preservation of binocularity after monocular deprivation in the striata cortex of kittens treated with 6-hydroxydopamine. J Comp Neurol 1979;185:139-162.

Kasumatsu T, Pettigrew JD, Ary M. Cortical recovery from effects on monocular deprivation: acceleration with norepinephrine and suppression With 6-hydroxydopamine. J Neurophysiol 1981;45(2):139-162.

Kathol RG, Wilcox JA, Turner RD, Kronfol Z. Pharmacologic Approaches to Psychogenic Polydipsia. Prog Neuro-Psycho-Pharmacol and Biol Psychiat 1986; 10:95-100.

Katsuragi T, Ushijima I, Furukawa T. The clonidine-induced Sel B of mice involves purinergic mechanisms. Pharmacology & Biochemistry of Behavior 1984; 20:943-946.

Kaufman ME, Levitt H. A study of three stereotyped behaviors in institutionalized mental defective. Am J Ment Defic 1965;69:467-473.

Kawahata N, Nagata K. Case of Associative Visual Agnosia: Neuropsychological Findings and Theoretical Considerations. J of Clin Exp Neuropsyc 1989; 11(5):645.

Keaton W, Raskind M. Treatment of depression in the medically ill elderly with methylphenidate. Am J Psychiatry 1980;137:963-965.

Keck PE, Pope HG, Cohen BM, McElroy SL, Nierenberg AA. Risk factors for neuroleptic malignant syndrome. Arch Gen Psychiatry 1989;46(10):914-921.

Keck PE, Pope HG, McElroy SL. Frequency and Presentation of Neuroleptic Malignant Syndrome: A Prospective Study. Am J Psychiat 1987; 144(10):1344-1346.

Kellaway P. The William Osler Medal Essay. The Part Played by Electric Fish in the Early History of Bioelectricity and Electrotherapy. Montreal: McGill University, 1971:116.

Kelley JT, Abuzzahab FS. The antiparkinson properties of amantadine in drug-induced parkinsonism. J Clin Pharmacol 1971; 11(3):211-214.

Kendler KS, Heath AC, Martin NG, Eaves LJ. Symptoms of Anxiety and Symptoms of Depression: Same Genes, Different Environments? Arch Gen Psych 1987; 44(5):451-460.

Kerr TA, Kay DWK, Lassman LP. Characteristics of patients, type of accident, and mortality in a consecutive series of head injuries admitted to a neurosurgical unit. Br J Preventive Social Med 1971;25:179-185.

Kessler II, Diamond KL. Epidemiologic studies of Parkinson's Disease.I. Smoking and Parkinson's disease: a survey and explanatory hypothesis. Am J Epidemiology 1971; 94:16-25.

Khamnei AK. Psychosis, inappropriate antidiuretic hormone secretion, and water intoxication. Lancet 1984;1:963.

Killian GA, Holzman PS, Davis JM, et al. Effects of Psychotropic Medication on selected cognitive and perceptual Measures. J Abnorm Psychol 1984;93(1):58-70.

King JR, Hullin RP. Withdrawal symptoms from lithium: Four Case Reports and a Questionaire Study. Br J Psychiatry 1983; 143:30-35.

Kleber HD. Clinical Aspects of the Use of Narcotic Antagonists: The State of the Art.Internat'l J Addict 1977; 12:857-861.

Klein E, Bental E, Lerer B, Belmaker RH. Carbamazepine and haloperidol vs. placebo and haloperidol in excited psychoses. Arch Gen Psychiatry 1984; 41:165-170.

Klein E, Uhde TW. Controlled Study of Verapamil for Treatment of Panic Disorder. Am J Psych 1988; 145:431-434.

Klein RG. Pharmacotherapy of childhood hyperactivity: an update.In: Meltzer HY, ed. Psychopharmacology The Third Generation of Progress. New York:Raven Press, 1987:1215-1224.

Kleine W. Periodische Schlafsucht Mschr Psychaitr. Neurology 1925; 57:285.

Kline J, Reid KH. The acute periventricular injury syndrome: a possible animal model for psychotic disease. Psychopharm 1985; 87:292-297.

Klonoff DC, Andrews BT, Obana WG. Stroke associated with cocaine use. Arch Neurol 1989; 46:989-993.

Kluver H, Bucy KH. Preliminary analysis of functions of the temporal lobes in monkeys. Arch Neurol Psychiatr 1939; 42:979-1000.

Kluver H, Bucy PC. "Psychic blindness" and other symptoms following temporal lobectomy in Rhesus monkey. Am J Physiol 1937;119:352-353.

Kluver H, Bucy PC. An analysis of certain effects of bilateral temporal lobectomy in the rhesus monkey, with special reference to psychic blindness. J Psychol 1938;5:33-34.

Knesevich JW. Successful treatment of obsessive-compulsive disorder with clonidine hydrochloride. Am J Psychiatry 1982;139(3):364.

Knoll JH, Chudley AE, Gerrard JW. Fragile (X) X-Linked mental retardation.II. Frequency and replication pattern of fragile (X)(q28) in heterozygotes. Am J Hum Genet 1984;36:640-645.

Knott PJ, Hutson PH. Stress-induced stereotypy in the rat: neuropharmacological similarities to Tourette syndrome.In: Friedhoff AJ, Chase TN, eds. Gilles de la Tourette syndrome. New York: Raven Press, 1982:233-238.

Kogeorgos J, de Alwis C. Priapism and psychotropic medication. Br J Psychiatry 1986;149:241-243.

Kokmen E, Beard M, Offord KP, Kurland LT. Prevalence of medically diagnosed dementia in a defined United States population: Rochester, Minnesota, January 1, 1975. Neurology 1989;39:773-776.

Kopin I. Neurotransmitters and the Lesch-Nyhan syndrome. N Engl J Med 1981;305:1148-1150.

Kornetsky C. Hyporesponsivity of chronic schizophrenic patients to dextramphetamine. Arch Gen Psychiatry 1976;33:1425-1428.

Kotagal P, Rothner AD, Erenberg G, Cruse RP, Wyllie E. Complex partial seizures of childhood onset. Arch Neurol 1987;44:1177-1180.

Krahn DD, Mitchell JE. Case report of bulimia associated with increased intracranial pressure. Am J Psychiatry 1984;141(9):1099-1100.

Kraus JF. Epidemiology of head injury.In: Cooper PR, ed. Head injury. Baltimore: Williams & Wilkins, 1987:1-19.

Krauthammer C, Klerman GL. Secondary mania: manic syndromes associated with antecedent physical illness or drugs. Arch Gen Psychiatry 1978;35:1333-1338.

Kreek MJ. Multiple drug abuse patterns and medical consequences.In: Meltzer HY, ed. Psychopharmacology: the third generation of progress. New York: Raven Press, 1987:1597-1604.

Krener PG, Abramowitz SI. Prediction of videotelemetry productivity from clinical screening parameters. J Am Acad Child Psychiatry 1985;24(5):597-602.

Kroth H. Cornelia de Lange Syndrome I bei Zwillingen (Amsterdamer Degenerationstyp). Archiv Kinderheilk 1965;173:273-283.

Kruck S. Pica in the mentally retarded.In: Treatments of psychiatric disorders. Washington, DC: American Psychiatric Association, 1989:51-53.

Krupp P. The effect of tegretol on some elementary neuronal mechanisms. headache 1969;9:42-46.

Krystal H. Trauma and affects. Psychoanol Study Child 1978;33:81-116.

Kumar D, Blank CE, Griffiths BL. Cornelia de Lange syndrome in several members of the same family. J Med Genet 1985;22:296-300.

Kupfer DJ, Himmelnoch JM, Schwartburg M, Anderson C, Byck R, Detre TP. Hypersomnia in manic-depressive disease. Dis Nerv Syst 1972;33:720-724.

Kusumo KS, Vaugn M. Effect of lithium salts on memory. Br J Psychiatry 1977; 131:453-457.

Kutcher S, Williamson P, MacKenzie S, Marton P, Ehrlich M. Successful clonazepam treatment of neuroleptic-induced akathisia in older adolescents and young adults: a double-blind, placebo-controlled study. J Clin Psychopharmacol 1989; 9(6):403.

Kyriakides M, Silverstone T, Jeffcoate W, Laurance B. Effect of Naloxone on hyperphagia in Prader-Willi syndrome. Lancet 1980;1:876-877.

Lachiewicz AM, Gullion CM, Spiridigliozzi GA, Aylsworth AS. Declining IQs of young males with the fragile X syndromes. Am J Ment Retard 1987; 292(3):272-278.

Lachman R, Funamura J, Szalay G. Gastrointestinal Abnormalities in the Cornelia de Lange syndrome. Mt Sinai J Med (NY) 1981;48(3):236-240.

Lacourt GC, Arendt J, Cox J, Beguin F. Microcephalic dwarfism with associated low amniotic fluid 5-hydroxyindole-3-acetic acid (5-HIAA). Helv Paediatr Acta 1977;32:149-154.

Lader M. Psychological effects of buspirone. J Linguist Psychiatr 1982;43(12 Sec. 2):62-68.

Lader M. B-Adrenoceptor antagonists in neuropsychiatry: an update. J Clin Psychiatry 1988;49:6.

Lahey BB, Schaughency EA, Frame CL, Strauss CC. Teacher ratings of attention problems in children experimentally classified as exhibiting attention deficit disorder with and without hyperactivity. J Am Acad Child Psychiatry 1985;24(5):613-614.

Lai F, Williams RS. A prospective study of Alzheimer disease in Down syndrome. Arch Neurol 1989;46:849-853.

Lakoski JM, Aghajanian GK, Gallager DW.Interaction of histamine H2-receptor antagonists with gaba and benzodiazepine binding sites in the CNS. Eur J Pharmacol 1983;88:241-245.

Lal S, Merbtiz CP, Grip JC. Modification of function in head-injured patients with sinemet. Brain Injury 1988;2(3):225-233.

Lambert P-A, Carraz G, Borselli S, Carrel S. Action Neuro-psychotrope d'un nouvel anti-epileptique: le Diamide. Ann Med Psychol (Paris) 1966;1:707-710.

Landfield PW, Baskin RK, Pitler TA. Brain aging correlates: retardation by hormonal-pharmacological treatments. Sci 1981;214(30):581-584.

Lang AE. Anticholinergic therapy in adult dystonia. Can J Neurol Sci 1986;13:42-46.

Langer DH, Rapoport JL, Brown GL, et al. Behavioral effects of carbidopa-levodopa in hyperactive Boys. J Am Acad Child Psychiatry 1982; 21:10-18.

Langer EJ. Mindfulness. New York: Addison-Wesley, 1989.

Lasala JM, Coscia CJ. Accumulation of a tetrahydroisoquinoline in phenylketonuria. Science 1979;203:283-284.

Lautin A, Angrist B, Stanley M, et al. Sodium valproate in schizophrenia: some biochemical correlates. Br J Psychiatry 1980;137:240-244.

Lavie P, Gadoth N, Gordan CR, Goldhammer G, Bechar M. Sleep patterns in Kleine-Levin syndrome. Electroencephalogr Clin Neurophysial 1979; 4927:369-371.

Lawson WB, Williams B, Pasion R. Effects of captopril on psychosis and disturbed water regulation. Psychopharmacol Bull 1988;24:176-178.

Lazarus A. Treating neuroleptic malignant syndrome. Am J Psychiatry 1984;141(8):1014-1015.

Leavitt A, Nuhad D, Davis C. Cornelia de Lange syndrome in a mother and daughter. Clin Genet 1985;28:157-161.

Leeton J. Depression induced by oral contraception and the role of vitamin B6 in its management. Austr N Z J Psychiatry 1974;8:85.

Legros JJ, Gilot P, Seron X, et al.Influence of vasopressin on learning and memory. Lancet 1978;:41-42.

Leibowitz SF. Noradrenergic function in the medial hypothalamus: potential relation to anorexia nervosa and bulimia.In: Pirke KM, Ploog D, eds. The psychobiology of anorexia nervosa. Berlin: Springer-Verlag, 1984:35-45.

Leijon G, Boivie J. Central post-stroke pain — a controlled trial of amitryptiline and carbamazepine. Pain 1989;36:27-36.

Leijon G, Boivie J, Johansson I. Central post-stroke pain — neurological symptoms and pain characteristics. Pain 1989;36:13-25.

Lejeune J, Maunoury C, Rethore MO, Prieur M, Raoul O. Site fragile Xq 17 et metabolisme des monocarbones: diminution significative de la frequence de la lacune chromosomique par traitement in vitro it in vivo. C R Acad Sci Ser D (Paris) 1981;292:491-493.

Lemberger L, Fuller RW, Zerbe RL. Use of specific serotonin uptake inhibitors as antidepressants. Clin Neuropharmacol 1985;8(4):299-316.

Lena B. Lithium in child and adolescent psychiatry. Arch Gen Psychiatry 1979;36(8):854-855.

Lennox WG, Lennox MA. Epilepsy and related disorders. London: J & A Churchill, 1960.

Leonard HL, Swedo SE, Rapoport JL, Koby EV, Lenane MC, Cheslow DL, Hamburger SD. Treatment of obsessive-compulsive disorder with clomipramine and desepramine in children and adolescents: a double-blind crossover comparison. Arch Gen Psychio 1989;46(12):1088-1092.

Lesch M, Nyhan WL. A familial disorder of uric acid metabolism and central nervous system function. Am J Med 1964;36:561-570.

Levenson JL. Neuroleptic malignant syndrome. Am J Psychiatry 1985;142(10):1137-1145.

Levin AB, Ramirez LF, Katz J. The use of stereotactic chemical hypophysectomy in the treatment of thalamic pain syndrome. J Neurosurg 1983;59:1002-1006.

Levin HS, Gary HE, High WM, et al. Minor head injury and the postconcussional syndrome: methodological issues in outcome studies.In: Levin HS, Grafman J, Eisenberg HM, eds. Neurobehavioral recovery from head injury. New York: Oxford University Press, 1987:262-275.

Levin HS, Grossman RG. Behavioral sequelae of closed head injury: a quantitative study. Arch Neurol 1978;35:720-727.

Levin M. Periodic somnolence and morbid hunger: a new syndrome. Brain 1936;59:494.

Levine AM. Case report: buspirone and agitation in head injury. Brain Injury 1988;2(2):165-167.

Levine DN, Finkelstein S. Delayed psychosis after right temporoparietal stroke or trauma: relation to epilepsy. Neurology 1982;32:267-272.

Levine LS, Glen MB, Wroblewski B, et al. Use of lithium carbonate and comprehensive behavioral treatment in two severely brain-injured patients. 1986 (unpublished).

Levine MJ, Gueramy M, Friedrich D. Psychophysiological responses to closed head injury. Brain Injury 1987; 1:171-181.

Levine R, Hoffman JS, Knepple ED, Kenin M. Long-term fluoxetine treatment of a large number of obsessive-compulsive patients. J Clin Psychopharmacol 1989;9(5):281.

Levitt P. Monoclonal antibody to limbic system neurons. Science 1984;223:299-301.

Levy AB, Bucher P, Votolato N. Myoclonus, hyperreflexia and diaphoresis in patients on phenelzine-tryptophan combination treatment. Can J Psychiatry 1985; 30:434-436.

Levy RH, Pitlick WH, Troupin AS, Green JR, Neal JM. Pharmacokinetics of carbamazepine in normal man. Clin Pharmacol Ther 1975;17:657-668.

Lewin E, Bleck V. Cyclic AMP accumulation in cerebral cortical slices: effect of carbamazepine, phenobarbital, and phenytoin. Epilepsia 1977;18:237-242.

Lewis DO, Pincus JH. Epilepsy and violence: evidence for a neuropsychotic-aggressive syndrome. J Neuropsychiatry 1989;1(4):413.

Lewis DO, Moy E, Jackson LD. Biopsychosocial characteristics of children who later murder: a prospective study. Am J Psychiatry 1985;142:1161-1167.

Lewis DO, Feldman M, Greene M, Martinez-Mustardo Y. Psychomotor epileptic symptoms in six patients with bipolar mood disorders. Am J Psychiatry 1984;141:1583-1586.

Lewis DO, Pincus JH, Feldman M, Jackson LD, Bard B. Psychiatric, neurological and psychoeducational characteristics of 15 death row inmates in the United States. Am J Psychiatry 1986;143:838-845.

Lewis JR. Valproic acid (depakene): a new anticonvulsant agent. JAMA 1978;240:2190-2192.

Lewis MH, Baumeister AA. Stereotyped mannerisms in mentally retarded persons: animal models and theoretical analyses.In: Ellis NR, ed.International review of research on mental retardation. New York: Academic Press, 1982.

Lewis NDC. The psychanalytic approach to the problems of children under 12 years of age. Psychol Rev 1926;13:424-443.

Lewitter FI, DeFries JC, Elston RC. Genetic models of reading disability. Behav Genet 1980;10:9-30.

Leys D. Rheumatic encephalopathy. Edinb Med J 1946;53:444-450.

Lezak MD. Neuropsychological assessment. New York: Oxford University Press, 1983.

Lieberman JA, Alvir J, Mukherjee S, Kane JM. Treatment of tardive dyskinesia with bromocriptine: a test of the receptor. Arch Gen Psychiatry 1989;46(10):908-913.

Lilly R, Cummings JL, Benson F, Frankel M. The human Kluver-Bucy syndrome. Neurology 1983;33:1141-1145.

Lindenbaum J, Healton EB, Savage DG, et al. Neuropsychiatric disorders caused By cobalamin deficiency in the absence of anemia or macrocytosis. N Engl J Med 1988;318(26):1720-1728.

Lindsay J, Ounsted C, Richards P. Long-term outcome in children with temporal lobe seizures. III: Psychiatric aspects in childhood and adult life. Dev Med Child Neurol 1979;21:630-636.

Lindsay J, Ounsted C, Richards P. Long-term outcome in children with temporal lobe seizures. IV: Genetic factors, febrile convulsions and the remission of symptoms. Dev Med Child Neurol 1980;22:429-439.

Lindstrom LH, Persseon E. Propranolol in chronic schizophrenia: a controlled study in neuroleptic-treated patients. Br J Psychiatry 1980;137:126-130.

Linnoila M, Buitoni M, Hietal O. The effect of sodium valproate on tardive dyskinesia. Br J Psychiatry 1976;129:114-119.

Lipinski JF, Zubenko GS, Cohen BM, Barreira PJ. Propranolol in the treatment of neuroleptic-induced Akathisia. Am J Psychiatry 1984;141(3):412.

Lipman RS. The use of psychopharmacological agents in residential facilities for the retarded.In: Menolascino F, ed. Psychiatric approaches to mental retardation. New York: Basic Books, 1970:387.

Lishman WA. Brain damage in relation to psychiatric disability after head injury. Br J Psychiatry 1968;114:373-410.

Lishman WA. Organic psychiatry, the psychological consequences of cerebral disorder. Oxford: Blackwell, 1987.

Livingston JE, MacLeod PM, Applegarth DA. Vitamin B6 status in women with postpartum depression. Am J Clin Nutr 1978;31:886-891.

Livingston S. Drug therapy for epilepsy. Springfield, Il: Charles C. Thomas, 1966.

Ljungberg T, Ungerstedt U. Reinstatement of eating by dopamine agonists in aphagic dopamine denervated rats. Physiol Behav 1976;16(3):277-283.

Lloyd KG, Hornykiewicz O, Davidson L. Biochemical evidence of dysfunction of brain neurotransmitters in the Lesch-Nyhan syndrome. N Engl J Med 1981;305:1106-1111.

Lockman LA. Absence seizures and variants. Neurol Clin 1985;3(1):19-29.

Lockwood AH. Medical problems of musicians. N Engl J Med 1989;320:221-227.

Lofts R. The effect of zinc on pica in a mentally retarded female. 1976 (unpublished).

Lofts R. Effect of zinc on pica in a mentally retarded female. 1986 (unpublished).

Loiseau P, Strube E, Brouset D, Buttlellochi S, Gomeni C, Morselli PL. Learning impairment in epileptic patients. Epilepsia 1983;24:183-192.

Loney J, Langhorne JE, Paternite CE. An empirical basis for subgrouping the hyperkinetic. Minimal brain dysfunction syndrome. J Abnorm Psychol 1978;37:431-441.

Lorrin M, Koran M. Medical evaluation of psychiatric patients: 1. Results in a state mental health system. Arch Gen Psychiatry 1989;46:733-740.

Lott IT. Down's syndrome, aging, and Alzheimer's disease: a clinical review. Ann NY Acad Scis 1982;396:15-27.

Lott IT, Lai F. Dementia in Down's syndrome: observations from a neurology clinic. Appl Res Ment Retard 1982;3:233-239.

Lou HC, Henriksen L, Bruhn P. Focal cerebral hypoperfusion in children with dysphasia and/or attention deficit disorder. Arch Neurol 1984;41:825-829.

Lourie RS, Layman EM, Millican FK. Why children eat things that are not food. Children 1963;10:143-146.

Lubs H. A marker X chromosome. Am J Hum Genet 1969;21:231-244.

Luchins DJ. Carbamazepine for the violent psychiatric patient. Lancet 1983;1:766-766.

Luria A, Naydin V, Tsvetkova L, et al. Restoration of higher cortical function following local brain damage.In: Vinkin RJ, Bruyn GW, eds. Handbook of clinical neurology. North Holland: Amsterdam, 1968:368-433.

Luria AR. The frontal lobes and the regulation of behavior.In: Pribram KH, Luria AR, eds. Psychophysiology of the frontal lobes. New York: academic Press, 1973:3-28.

Lutz EG. Alternative drug treatments in Tilles de la Tourette's syndrome. Am J Psychiatry 1977;134:98-99.

Lydiard RB, Laraia MT, Ballenger JC, Howell EF. Emergence of depressive symptoms in patients receiving alprazolam for panic disorder. Am J Psychiatry 1987;144(5):664.

MacDonald GW, Roy DL. Williams syndrome: a neuropsychological profile. J Clin Exp Neuropsychiatry 1988;10(2):125-131.

Maher BA. Principles of psychopathology. New York: McGraw-Hill, 1966.

Maher BA. Anomalous experience and delusional thinking: the logic of explanations.In: Otmanns TF, Maher BA, eds. Delusional beliefs. New York: Wiley, 1988.

Mamelak M, Buck L, Csima A, Price V, Smiley A. Effects of flurazepam and zopiclone on the performance of chronic insomniac patients: a study of ethalnol-drug interaction. Sleep 1987;10(suppl 1):79-87.

Manaka S, Takahashi H, Sana K. The difference between children and adults in the onset of post-traumatic epilepsy. Folia Psychiatry Neurol Jpn 1981;35(3):301-304.

Mandell AJ. From molecular biological simplification to more realistic central nervous system dynamics: an opinion.In: Judd J, Grove P, eds. Psychiatry: psychobiological foundations of clinical psychiatry. New York: Basic Books, 1986:361-366.

Mander AJ. Is there a lithium withdrawal syndrome? Br J Psychiatry 1986; 149:498-501.

Manfredi RL, Brennan RW, Cadieux RJ. Disorders of excessive sleepiness: narcolepsy and hypersomnia. Semin Neurol 1987;7(3):250-256.

Mannuzza S, Klein RG, Konig PH, Giampino TL. Hyperactive boys almost grown up: IV. Criminality and its relationship to psychiatric status. Arch Gen Psychiatry 1989;46(12):1073-1079.

Mansheim P. Treatment with propranolol of the behavioral sequelae of b rain damage. J Clin Psychiatry 1981;42:132.

Marcell PD, Stabler SP, Pedell ER, Allen RH. Quantitation of methylmalonic acid and other dicarboxylic acids in normal serum and urine using capillary gas chromatography-mass spectrometry. Anal Biochem 1985;150:58-66.

Marien M, Brien J, Jhamandas K. Regional release of (3H) dopamine from rat brain in vitro: effects of opioids on release induced by potassium, nicotine and l-glutamic acid. Can J Physiol Pharmacol 1982;61:43-60.

Mark VH, Ervin FR. Violence and the brain. New York: Harper & Row, 1970.

Marotta RF, Potegal M, Glusman M, et al. Dopamine Agonists Induce Recovery From Surgically-Induced Septal Rage. Nature 1977; 269(6):513-515.

Marsden CD.Investigation of dystonia. Adv Neurol 1988;50:35-44.

Martineau J, Garreau B, Barthelemy C, Callaway E, Lelord G. Effects of vitamin B6 on averaged evoked potentials in infantile autism. Biol Psychol 1981;16(7):627-641.

Masur H, Elger CE, Ludolph AC, Galanski M. Cerebellar atrophy following acute intoxication with phenytoin. Neurology 1989;39:432-433.

Mattella MJ, Aranko K, Seppala T. Acute effects of buspirone and alcohol on psychomotor skills. J Clin Psychiatry 1982;43(12 Sec. 2):56-60.

Mattes J. A pilot trial of amantadine in hyperactive children. Psychol Bull 1980;16(3):67-67.

Mattes JA. Propranolol for adults with temper outbursts and residual attention deficit disorder. J Clin Psychopharmacol 1986;6:299-302.

Matteson MT, Ivancevich JM. An exploratory investigation of CES as an employee stress management procedure. 1985 (unpublished).

Matthews CG, Harley JP. Differential psychological test performances in toxic and nontoxic adult epileptics. Neurology 1975;25:184-188.

Mattila MJ, Liljequist R, Seppala T. Effects of amitryptiline and mianserin on psychomotor skills and memory in man. Br J Clin Pharmacol 1978;5:53S-55S.

Mayeux R, Stern Y, Rosen J, Leventhal J. Depression, intellectual impairment and Parkinson disease. Neurology 1981;31:645-650.

McElroy SL, Keck PE, Pope HG. Sodium valproate: its use in primary psychiatric disorders. J Clin Psychopharmacol 1987;7:16-24.

McElroy SL, Keck PE, Pope HG, Hudson JI. Valproate in the treatment of rapid-cycling bipolar disorder. J Clin Psychopharmacol 1989;8:275-279.

McEntee WJ, Mair RG. Memory enhancement in Korsakoff's psychosis by clonidine: further evidence for a noradrenergic deficit. Ann Neurol 1980;7:466-470.

McEvoy JP, McCue M, Spring B, Mohs RC, Lavori PW, Farr R. The effects of amantadine vs. trihexyphenidyl on memory in elderly normal volunteers. Psychopharmacol Bull 1987;23(1):30-32.

McKinlay WW, Brooks DN, Martinage DP, Marshall MM. The short-term outcome of severe blunt head injury as reported by relatives of the injured person. J Neurol Neurosurg Psychiatry 1981;44:527-533.

McLean A, Stanton KM, Cardenas DD, Bergerud DB. Memory training combined with the use of oral physostigmine. Brain Injury 1987; 1:145-159.

McLeod NA, White LE. Trazadone in essential tremor. JAMA 1986;256(19):2675-2676.

McNeil GN, Shaw PK, Dock DS. Substitution of atenolol for propranolol in a case of propranolol-related depression. Am J Psychiatry 1982;139:9.

McQueen JK, Blackwood DHR, Harris P, Kalbag RM, Johnson A. Low risk of late post-traumatic seizures following severe head injury: implications for clinical trials of prophylaxis. J Neurol Neurosurg Psychiatry 1983;46:899-904.

Meldrum BS, Brierley JB. Prolonged epileptic Seizures in primates. Arch Neurol 1973;28:10-17.

Meldrum BS, Turski L, Schwarz M, Czuczwar SJ, Sontag KH. Anticonvulsant action of 1,3-dimethyl-5-aminoadamantane. Pharmacological studies in rodents and baboon. Naunyn-Schmiedeberg's Arch Pharmacol 1986;332:93-97.

Mello NK. Alcohol abuse and alcoholism: 1978-1987.In: Meltzer HY, ed. Psychopharmacology: the third Generation of progress. New York: Raven Press, 1987:1515-1520.

Meltzer HY, Lowy MT. The serotonin hypothesis of depression.In: Meltzer HY, ed. Psychopharmacology: the third generation of progress. New York: Raven Press, 1987:513-526.

Mendels J, Amin MM, Chouinard G, et al. A comparative study of bupropion and amitriptyline in depressed outpatients. J Clin Psychiatry 1983;44(5)2:118-120.

Mendez MF, Cummings JL, Benson F. Depression in Epilepsy. Arch Neurol 1986;43:766-770.

Menini C, Meldrum BS, Riche D, Silva-Comte C, 1980 Stutzmann JM. Sustained limbic seizures induced by intraamygdaloid kainic acid in the baboon:

symptomatology and neuropathological consequences. Ann Neurol 1980;8:501-509.

Menkes MM, Rowe JS, Menkes JH. A twenty-five year follow-up study on the hyperkinetic child with minimal brain dysfunction. Pediatrics 1967;39:393-399.

Merriman AE. Kleine-Levin syndrome following acute viral encephalitis. Biol Psychol 1986;21:1301-1304.

Messing RO, Closson RG, Simon RP. Drug-induced seizures: a ten-year experience. Neurology 1984;34:1582-1586.

Mesulam MM. Dissociative states with abnormal temporal lobe EEG: multiple personality and the illusion of possession. Arch Neurol 1981;38:176-181.

Mesulam MM. Low-dose haloperidol for stereotypic self-injurious behavior in the mentally retarded. N Endl J Med 1986;315:398-399.

Meunier G, Carraz G, Meunier Y. Pharmacodynamic properties of N-dipropylacetic acid. Therapie 1963;18:435-438.

Michels VV. Fragile sites on human chromosomes: description and clinical significance. Mayo Clin Proc 1985;60:690-696.

Mikkelson EJ. Low dose haloperidol for stereotypic self-injurious behavior in the mentally retarded. N Engl J Med 1986;315:398-399.

Mikkelsen EJ, Detlor J, Cohen DJ. School avoidance and social phobia triggered by haloperidol in patients with Tourette's syndrome. Am J Psychiatry 1981;138(12):1572-1576.

Milberg W, Albert M. Cognitive differences between patients with progressive supranuclear palsy and Alzheimer's disease. J Clin Exp Neuropsychol 1989;11(5):605.

Miller JG. Information overload and psychopathology. Am J Psychiatry 1976;133:627-634.

Miller LL, Branconnier RJ. Cannabis: effects on memory and the cholinergic limbic system. Psychol Bull 1983;93:441-456.

Minana MD, Portoles M, Jorda A, Grisolia S. Lesch-Nyhan syndrome, caffeine Model: increase of purine and pyrimidine enzymes in rat brain. J Neurochem 1984;43(6):1556-1560.

Minderaa RB, Anderson GM, Volkmar FR. Whole blood serotonin and tryptophan in autism: temporal stability and the effects of medication. J Autism Dev Disord 1989;19(1):129-136.

Mishkin M. Memory in monkeys severely impaired by combined but not by separate removal of amygdala and hippocampus. Nature 1978;275:297-298.

Mitchell JE, Christenson G, Jennings J, et al. A placebo-controlled, double-blind crossover study of naltrexone hydrochloride in outpatients with normal weight bulimia. J Clin Psychopharmacol 1989;9(2):94-97.

Mitchell JE, Groat R. A placebo-controlled, double-blind study of amitriptyline in bulimia. J Clin Psychopharmacol 1984;4:186-191.

Miyamoto M, Fukuda N, Narumi S, et al. V-Butyrolactone-v-cabonyl-histidyl-prolinamide citrate (DN-1417): a novel TRH analog with potent effects on the central nervous system. Life Sci 1981;28:861-869.

Mizuno T, Yugari Y. Prophylactic Effect of L-5-Hydroxytryptophan on Self-Mutilation in the Lesch-Nyhan Syndrome. Neuropadiatrie 1975; 6:13-23.

MMWR. Antiviral agents for influenza A. JAMA 1987;258(5):599-600.

Modell JG, Mountz JM, Curtis GC, Greden JF. Neurophysiologic dysfunction in basal ganglia/limbic striatal and thalamocortical circuits as a pathogenetic mechanism of obsessive-compulsive disorder. J Neuropsychiatry 1989;1(1):27-36.

Mohs RC, Breitner JCS, Silverman JM, Davis KL. Alzheimer's disease: morbid risk among first-degree relatives. Arch Gen Psychiatry 1987;44(5):405.

Moller H, von Zerssen D. Depressive states Occurring during the neuroleptic treatment of schizophrenia. Schizophr Bull 1982;8(1):109-117.

Molliver ME. Serotonergic neuronal systems: what their anatomic organization tells us about function. J Clin Psychopharmacol 1987;7(6):3s.

Monroe RR. Limbic ictus and atypical psychosis. J Nerv Ment Dis 1982;170:711-716.

Montanari C, Ferrari P, Bavazzano A. Urinary excretion of amantadine by the elderly. Eur J Clin Pharmacol 1975;8:349-351.

Moore DC, Bowers MB. Identification of a subgroup of tardive dyskinesia by pharmacological probes. Am J Psychiatry 1980;137:1202-1205.

Moretti C, Fabbri A, Gnessi L, Bonifacio V, Fraioli F, Isidori A. Pyridoxine (B6) suppresses the rise in prolactin and increases the rise in growth hormone induced by exercise. N Engl J of Med 1982;307(7):444-444.

Morgan MY, Jakobovits A, Elithorn A, James IM, Sherlock S. Successful use of bromocriptine in the treatment of a patient with chronic portasysyemic encephalopathy. N Engl J Med 1977;296(14):793-794.

Morley JE. The neuroendocrine control of appetite: the role of the endogenous opiates, cholecystokinin, TRH, gamma-amino-butyric-acid and the diazepam receptor. Life Sci 1980;27:335-368.

Morley JE, Levine AS. Stress-induced eating is mediated through endogenous opiates. Science 1980; 209:1259-1261.

Morrell F. Secondary epileptogenesis in Man. Arch Neurol 1985;42:318-335.

Morris HH, Estes ML. Traveler's amnesia. Transient global amnesia secondary to triazolam. JAMA 1987;258:945-946.

Morselli PL, Bossi L. Carbamazepine: absorption, distribution, and excretion.In: Woodbury DM, Penry JK, Piippenger CE, eds. Antiepileptic drugs. New York: Raven Press, 1982:465-482.

Mortimer JA, Christensen KJ, Webster DD. Parkinsonian dementia.In: Frederiks JAM, ed. Handbook of clinical neurology. Amsterdam: Elsevier 1985a:371-384.

Mortimer JA, French LR, Hutton JT, Schuman LM. Head injury as a risk factor for Alzheimer's disease. Neurology 1985b; 35:264-267.

Moscovitch M.Information processing and the cerebral hemispheres.In: Gazzaniga MS, ed. Handbook of behavioral neurobiology: neuropsychology. New York: Plenum, 1979:379-446.

Moss GR, James CR. Carbamazepine and lithium carbonate synergism in mania. Arch Gen Psychiatry 1983;40:588-588.

Mudd SH. Pyridoxine-responsive genetic disease. 1971 (unpublished).

Mueller K, Hsiao S. Pemoline-induced self-biting in rats and self-mutilation in the deLange syndrome. Pharmacol Biochem Behav 1980;13:627-631.

Mueller K, Nyhan WL. Pharmacologic control of pemoline-induced self-injurious behavior in rats. Pharmacol Biochem Behav 1982;16:957-963.

Mueller K, Nyhan WL. Clonidine potentiates drug-induced self-injurious behavior in rats. Pharmacol Biochem Behav 1983;18:891-894.

Mueller K, Saboda S, Palmour R, Nyhan WL. Self-injurious behavior produced in rats by daily caffeine and continuous amphetamine. Pharmacol Biochem Behav 1982;17:613-617.

Muenter MD, Whisnant J. Basal ganglia calcification, hypoparathyroidism, and extrapyramidal motor manifestations. Neurology 1968;18:1075-1083.

Mulick JA, Schroeder SR, Rojahn J. Chronic ruminative vomiting: a comparison of four treatment procedures. J Autism Dev Disord 1980b;10:203-213.

Mulick JA, Barbour R, Schroeder SR, Rojahn J. Overcorrection of pica in two profoundly retarded adults: analysis of setting effects, stimulus, and response generalization. Appl Res Memt Retard 1980a;1:241-252.

Muller HF, Dastoor DP, Klingner A, Cole M, Boillat J. Amantadine in senile dementia: Electroencephalographic and clinical effects. J Am Geriatr Soc 1979; 27:9-16.

Munetz MR, Cornes CL. Distinguishing akathisia and tardive dyskinesia: a review of the literature. J Clin Psychopharmacol 1983;3:343-349.

Mungas D.Interictal behavior abnormality in temporal lobe epilepsy. Arch Gen Psychiatry 1982;39:108-111.

Munsat TL. Serotonin and myoclonic seizures. N Engl J Med 1977;296(2):101-102.

Munyon WH, Salo R, Briones DF. Cytotoxic effects of neuroleptic Drugs. Psychopharmacology 1987;91(2):182-188.

Murakami JW, Courchesne E, Press GA, Yeung-Courchesne R, Hesselink JR. Reduced cerebellar hemisphere size and its relationship to vermal hypoplasia in autism. Arch Neurol 1989;46:689-694.

Murphy JM, Monson RR, Olivier DC, Sobol AM, Leighton AH. Affective disorders and mortality. Arch Gen Psychiatry 1987;44:473-480.

Murray EA, Mishkin M. Amygdalectomy impairs crossmodal association in monkeys. Science 1985;228:604-605.

Murray TJ. Amantadine therapy for fatigue in multiple sclerosis. Can J Neurol Sci 1985;12:251-254.

Naftchi NE. Functional restoration of the traumatically injured spinal cord in cats by clonidine. Science 1982;217:1042-1044.

Nahas GG. Cannabis: toxicological properties and epidemiological aspects. Med J Aust 1986;145:82-87.

Nardella MT, Sulzbacher SI, Worthington-Roberts BS. Activity Levels of Persons with Prader-Willi syndrome. Am J Ment Defic 1983;87(5):498-505.

Nasrallah HA, Fowler RC, Judd LL. Schizophrenic-like illness following head injury. Psychosomatics 1983;22:359-361.

Neal J. .In: Encephalitis. A clinical study. New York: Grune & Stratton, 1942:363-383.

Nelson KB, Ellenberg JH. Predictors of epilepsy in children who have experienced febrile seizures. N Engl J Med 1976;295:1029-1033.

Neppe VM. Carbamazepine as adjunctive treatment in nonepileptic chronic in patients with EEG temporal lobe abnormalities. J Clin Psychiatry 1983;44(9):326-331.

Neppe VM. Management of catatonic stupor with L-dopa. Clin Neuropharm 1988;11:90-91.

Newbold HL. Vitamin B-12: placebo or neglected therapeutic tool? Med Hypotheses 1989;28:155-164.

Newton RE, Marunycz JD, Alderdice MT, Napoliello MJ. Review of the side-effect profile of buspirone. Am J Med 1986;80:17-21.

Nielson EB, Lyon M. Evidence for cell loss in corpus striatum after long-term treatment with a neuroleptic drug fluphenthixol in rats. Psychopharmacology 1978;59:85-90.

Nishikawa T, Tanaka M, Tsuda A, Koga I, Uchida Y. Clonidine therapy for tardive dyskinesia and related syndromes. Clin Neuropharmacol 1984;7(3):239-245.

Nixon RA, Rothman JS, Chin W. Demeclocycline in the prophylaxis of self-induced water intoxication. Am J Psychiatry 1982;139:828-829.

Noetzel MJ. Theophylline neurotoxicity resulting in significant unilateral brain damage. Dev Med Child Neurol 1985;27:242-248.

Nolen WA. Carbamazepine, a possible adjunct of alternative to lithium in bipolar disorder. Psychiatr Scand 1983;67:218-225.

Noveske FG, Hahn KR, Flymm RJ. Possible toxicity of combined fluoxetine and lithium. Am J Psychiatry 1989;146(11):1515.

Novick NM. Drug abuse and drugs in sports. NY J Med 1973;73:2597-2600.

Noyes R, Kathol R, Claney J. Antianxiety effects of propranolol: a review of clinical studies.In: Klein DF, Rabkin J, eds. Anxiety- new research and changing concepts. New York: Raven Press, 1981:81-93.

Noyes R, Clancy J, Coryell WH, Crowe RR, Chaudhry DR, Domingo DV. A withdrawal syndrome after abrupt discontinuation of alprazolam. Am J Psychiatry 1985;142(1):114.

Nuzzo JL, Warfield CA. Thalamic pain syndrome. Hosp Pract 1985;32:32c-32j.

Nyhan WL. The Lesch-Nyhan syndrome. Annu Rev Med 1973;24:41-60.

Nyhan WL, Johnson HG, Kaufman IA, Jones KL. Serotonergic approaches to the modification of behavior in the Lesch-Nynan syndrome. Appl Res Ment Retard 1980;1:25-40.

O'Brien F. Treating self-stimulatory behavior.In: Matson JL, McCartney JR, eds. Handbook of behavior modification with the mentally retarded. New York: Plenum Press, 1981.

Ogura C, Okuma T, Nakazawa K, Kishimoto A. A treatment of periodic somnolence with lithiun carbonate. Arch Neurol 1976;33:143.

Oke A, Keller R, Meeford I. Lateralization of norepinephrine in human thalamus. Science 1978;200:1411-1413.

Okuma T, Inanaga K, Otsuki S. Comparison of the antimanic efficacy of carbamazepine and chlorpromazine: a double-blind controlled study. Psychopharmacology 1979;66:211-217.

Okuma T, Kishimoto A, Inoue K. Anti-manic and prophylactic effects of car bamazepine on manic-depressive psychosis: a preliminary report. Folia Psychiatr Neurol Jpn 1973;27:283-297.

Okuma T, Kishimoto A, Inoue K. Anti-manic and prophylactic effects of carbamazepine on manic-depressive psychosis. Seishin Igaku 1975;17:617-630.

Oliver AP, Luchins DJ, Wyatt RJ. Neuroleptic-induced seizures: an in vitro technique for assessing relative risk. Arch Gen Psychiatry 1982;39:206-209.

Olney JW, Labruyere J, Price MT. Pathological changes induced in cerebrocortical neurons by phencyclidine and related drugs. Science 1989;244:1360-1362.

Olsen TS, Hogenhaven H, Thage O. Epilepsy after stroke. Neurology 1987;37:1209101.-1211.

Olsson I, Steffenburg S, Gillberg C. Epilepsy in autism and autisticlike conditions: a populationbased studyo. Arch Neurol 1988;45(6):666-668.

Ommaya AK, Gennarelli TA. A cerebral concussion and traumatic unconsciousness: correlation of experimental and clinical observations on blunt head injuries. Brain 1974;97:633-654.

O'Neal M, Page N, Adkins WN, Eichelmann B. Tryptophan-Trazadone treatment of aggressive behavior. Lancet 1986; 2:859-860.

Ontiveros A, Fontaine R, Breton G, Elie R, Fontaine S, Dery R. Correlation of severity of panic disorder and neuroanatomical changes on magnetic resonance imaging. J Neuropsychiatry 1989;1(4):404.

Opitz JM. Editorial comments on the Brachmann-de lange syndrome.In: Yearbook of Pediatrics. Chicago: Year Book, 1965:502-504.

Opitz JM. Editorial comment: Brachmann-de Lange syndrome. Am J Med Genet 1985;22:89-102.

Opitz JM, Sutherland GR. Conference report: International Workshop on the fragile X and X-linked mental retardation. Am J Med Genet 1984;17:5-94.

Orlosky MJ. The Kleine-Levin Syndrome: a review. Psychosomatics 1982;23(6):609-621.

Pagon RA, Bennett FC, LaVeck B, Stewart KB, Johnson J. Williams syndrome: features in late childhood and adolescence. Pediatrics 1987;80(1):85-91.

Pakkenberg B. What happens in the leucotomised brain? A post-mortem study of brains from schizophrenic patients. J Neurol Neurosurg Psychiatry 1989;52:156-161.

Pandurangi AK, Devi V, Channabasavanna SM. Caudate Atrophy in irreversible tardive dyskinesia. J Clin Psychiatry 1980;41:229-231.

Paniak CE, Shore DL, Rourke BP. Recovery of memory after severe closed-head injury: dissassociations in recovery of memory parameters and predictors of outcome. J Clin Exp Neuropsychol 1989;11(5):631.

Panskepp JA. A neurochemical theory of autism. Trends Neurosci 1979;July:174-177.

Parnas J, Korsgaard S, Krautwald O, Jensen PS. Chronic psychosis in epilepsy. Acta Psychiatr Scand 1982;66:282-293.

Pashayan H, Whelan D, Guttman S, Fraser FC. Variability of the de Lange syndrome: report of 3 cases and genetic analysis of 54 families. J Pediatr 1969;75(5):853.

Pattison EM, Kahan J. The deliberate self-harm syndrome. Am J Psychiatry 1983;140:867-872.

Pauling L. On the orthomolecular environment of the mind: orthomolecular theory. J Psychiatry 1974;131:1251-1257.

Paulson GW, Rizvi CA, Crane GE. Tardive dyskinesia as a possible sequela of long-term therapy with phenothiazines. Clin Pediatr 1975;14:953-955.

Pearlman CA. Neuroleptic malignant syndrome: a review of the literature. J Clin Psychopharmacol 1986; 6:257-273.

Peck AW, Stern WC, Watkinson C.Incidence of seizures during treatment with tricyclic antidepressant drugs and bupropion. J Clin Psychiatry 1983;44(5):197-201.

Pecknold JC, Fleury D. Alprazolam-induced manic episode in two patients with panic disorder. Am J Psychiatry 1986;143(5):652.

Peet M, Middlemiss DN, Yates RA. Pharmacokinetic interaction between propranolol and chlorpromazine in schizophrenic patients. Lancet 1980;2:8-9.

Peet M, Middlemiss DN, Yates RA. Propranolol in schizophrenia: II. Clinical and biochemical aspects of combining propranolol with chlorpromazine. Br J Psychiatry 1981b;139:112-117.

Peet M, Bethell MS, Coates A, et al. Propranolol in schizophrenia: I. comparison of propranolol, chlorpromazine, and placebo. Bri J Psychiatry 1981a;139:105-111.

Penfield W, Gage L. Cerebral localization of epileptic manifestations. Arch Neurol Psychiatry 1933;30:709-727.

Pentel P. Toxicity of over-the-counter stimulants. JAMA 1984;252(14):1898-1903.

Perry R, Campbell M, Green WH, et al. Neuroleptic-related dyskinesias in autistic children: a prospective study. Psychopharmacol Bull 1985;21:140-143.

Peters NL, Anderson KC, Reid PR, Taylor GJ. Acute mental status changes caused by propranolol. Johns Hopkins Med J 1978;143:163-164.

Petersen RC, Stillman RC. Phencyclidine: a review. Washington, D.C.: national Institute on Drug Abuse, 1978:

Petrie WM, Ban TA. Propranolol in organic agitation. Lancet 1981;1(8215):324.

Petrie WM, Maffucci RJ, Woosley RL. Propranolol and Depression. Am J Psychiaty 1982; 139:92-94.

Phillips J. Self-injurious behavior in the community: a prevalence study. 1988 (unpublished).

Phillis JW.Interactions of the anticonvulsants dipheonylhydatoin and carbamazepine with adenosine on cerebral cortical neurons. Epilepsia 1984;25:765-772.

Phillis JW. Chlorpromazine and trifluoperazine potentiate the action of adenosine on rat cerebral cortical Neurons. Gen Pharmacol 1985;16:19-24.

Pickard JD, Murray GD, Illingworth R, et al. Effect of oral nimodipine on cerebral infarction and outcome after subarachnoid haemorrhage: british aneurysm nimodipine trial. Br Med J 1989;298:636-642.

Pintor C, Cella SG, Corda R, et al. Clonidine growth in children with impaired growth hormone secretion. Lancet 1985;:1482.

Platt JE, Campbell M, Green MH. Effects of lithium carbonate and halperidol or cognition in aggressive hospitalized school-age children. J Clin Psychopharmacol 1981;1:8-13.

Plum F, Posner JB. The Diagnosis of stupor and coma. Philadelphia: F. A. Davis, 1980.

Pollack MH, Tesar GE, Rosenbaum JF, Spier SA. Clonazepam in the treatment of panic disorder and agoraphobia: a one-year follow-up. J Clin Psychopharmacol 1986;6:302-304.

Pope HG Jr., Keck PE Jr., McElroy SL, Hudson JI. A placebo-controlled study of trazodone in bulimia nervosa. J Clin Psychopharmacol 1988;9(4):254-259.

Popoviciu L, Corforice O. Etude clinique et polygraphique au cours du nyc-thermere d'un cas de syndrome de Kleine-Levin-Critchley. Rev Romaine Neurol 1972; 9:229-248.

Poschel BPH, Marriot JG, Gluckman MI. Pharmacology Underlying the cognition-activating properties of pramiracetam (C1-879). Psychopharmacol Bull 1983;19:720-721.

Post RM, Ballenger JC, Uhde TW, Smith C, Robniow DR, Bunney WE. Effect of carbamazepine on cyclic nucleotides in CSF of patients with affective illness. Biol Psychiatry 1982a;17:1037-1045.

Post RM, Uhde TW, Ballenger JC. Efficacy of carbamazepine in affective disorders: implications for underlying physiological and biochemical substrates.In: Emrich HM, Okuma T, Muller AA, eds. Anticonvulsants in affective disorders. Amsterdam: Elsevier, 1984:93-115.

Post RM, Ballenger JC, Uhde TW, et al. Kindling and drug sensation: implications for the progressive development of psychopathology and treatment with Car-bamazepine.In: Sanler M, ed. The Psychopharmacology of anticonvulsants. Oxford: Oxford University Press, 1981.

Post RM, Uhde TW, Putnam FW, Ballenger JC, Berretini WH. Kindling and carbamazepine in affective illness. J Nerv Ment Dis 1982b;170:717-729.

Power KG, Jerrom DWA, Simpson RJ, Mitchell M. Controlled study of withdrawal symptoms and rebound anxiety after six week course of diazepam for generalised anxiety. Br Med J 1985;290:1246.

Powers PS, Gunderman RB. Kleine-Levin syndrome associated with fire setting. Am J Dis Child 1978;132:786-789.

Prader A, Labhart A, Willi H. Ein Syndrom Von Adipsoitas, Kleinwuchs, Kryp-torchismus and Oligophrenie Nach Myatonicartigem Zustand im Neugeborenenalter. Schweiz Med Wochenschr 1956;86.

Prange AJ, Wilson IC, Morris CE. Preliminary experience with tryptophan and lithium in the treatment of tardive dyskinesia. Psychopharmacol Bull 1973;9:36-37.

Pribram KH. The primate frontal cortex - executive of the brain.In: Pribram KH, Luria AR, eds. Psychophysiology of the frontal lobes. New York: Academic Press, 1973:293-314.

Pritchard PB, Lombroso CT, McIntyre M. Psychological complications of temporal lobe epilepsy. Neurology 1980;30:227-232.

Prober CG. Transitory spatial disorder With proporanolol. N Engl J Med 1985;312(12):790-791.

Pugsley TA, Poschel BPH, Downs DA, et al. Some pharmacological and neurochemical properties of a new cognition activator agent, piracetam (C1-879). Psychopharmacol Bulle 1983;19:721-726.

Purdy RE, Julien RM, Fairhurst AS, Terry MD. Effect of carbamazepine on the in vitro uptake and release of norepinephrine in adrenergic nerves of rabbit aorta and in whole brain synaptosomes. Epilepsia 1977;18:251-257.

Quattrone A, Samanin R. Decreased anticonvulsant activity of carbamazepine in 6-hydroxydopamine-treated rats. Eur J Pharmacol 1977;41:333-336.

Quitkin F, Rifkin A, Gochfeld L, Klein DF. Tardive dyskinesia: are first signs reversible? Am J Psychiatry 1977;134:84-87.

Rall TW. Central Nervous System Stimulants.In: The pharmacological basis of therapeutics, Gilman AG, Goodman LS, Rall TW, Murad F, eds. New York: Macmillan, 1985:589-603.

Ranson SW. Somnolence Caused by hypothalamic lesions in the monkey. Arch Neurol Psychiatry 1939;41:1-23.

Rao SM, Leo GJ, St Aubin-Faubert P. On the nature of memory disturbance in multiple sclerosis. J Clin Exp Neuropsychiatry 1989;11(5):699.

Rapoport JL, Wise SP. Obsessive-compulsive disorder: evidence for basal ganglia dysfunction. Psychopharmacol Bull 1988;24(3):380.

Rapaport M. Attention to competing Voice Voice Messages by Nonacute Schizophrenic Patients: Effects of Message Load, Drugs, Dosage Levels and Patient Background. J Nerv Ment Dis 1968; 146:404-411.

Rasmussen SA. Lithium and tryptophan augmentation in clomipramine-resistant obsessive-compulsive disorder. Am J Psychiatry 1984;141:1283-1285.

Ratey J, Greenberg MS, Linden KJ. Combination of treatments for attention deficit hyperactivity disorder. 1990 (Unpublished).

Ratey J, Gualtieri CT. Introduction. In Ratey JJ, ed. Mental retardation: developing pharmacotherapies. American Psychiatric Press: Washington, DC, 1990.

Ratey J, Sovner R, Mikkelsen E, Chmielinski HE. Buspirone therapy for maladaptive behavior and anxiety in developmentally disabled persons. J Clin Psychopharmacol (in press).

Ratey JJ, Mikkelsen EJ, Smith GB, et al. Beta-blockers in the severely and profoundly mentally retarded. J Clin Psychopharmacol 1989;6(2):103-107.

Ratey JJ, Sorgi P, Polakoff S. Nadolol as a treatment for akathisia. Am J Psychiatry 1985;142(5):640.

Realmuto GM, August GJ, Garfinkel BD. Clinical effect of buspirone in autistic children. J Clin Psychopharmacol 1989;9:122-124.

Realmuto GM, Garfinkel BD, Tuchman M, et al. Psychiatric diagnosis and be havioral characteristics of phenylketonuric children. Nerv Ment Dis 1986;174(9):536-540.

Reeves AC, Blum D. Hyperphagia, rage, and dementia Accompanying a ventro-median hypothalamic neoplasm. Arch Neurol 1969;20:616-624.

Regier DA, Boyd JH, Burke JD, et al. One-month prevalence of mental disorders in the United States based on five epidemiologic catchment area sites. Arch Gen Psychiatry 1988;45:977-986.

Reid AH. Schizophrenia in mental retardation: clinical features. Res Dev Disabil 1989;10:241-250.

Reifler BV, Teri L, Raskind M, et al. Double-blind trial of imipramine in Alzheimer's disease patients with and without depression. Am J Psychiatry 1989;146:45-49.

Reisberg B, Gershon S. Side effects associated with lithium therapy. Arch Gen Psychiatry 1979;36:879-887.

Reisberg B, Ferris SH, Gershon S. An overview of pharmacologic treatment of cognitive decline in the aged. Am J Psychiatry 1981;138(5):593-600.

Reisberg B, London E, Ferris SH, et al. Novel pharmacologic approaches to the treatment of senile dementia of the Alzheimer's type. Psychopharmacol Bull 1983;19:220-225.

Reiser G, Binmoller FJ, Koch R. Memantine-induced depolarization response in a neuronal cell line. Brain Res 1988;443:338-344.

Reiss AL, Feinstein C, Rosenbaum KN. Autism associated with Williams syndrome. J Pediatr 1985;106:247-249.

Reiss AL, Feinstein KE, Goldsmith TB, Rosenbaum K, Caruso MA. Psychiatric disability associated with the fragile X chromosome. Am J Med Genet 1986;23:393-401.

Reiss S. Psychopathology and mental retardation: survey of a developmental disabilities mental health program. Ment Retard 1982;20(3):128-132.

Rett A. Uber ein zerebral-atrophisches Syndrome bei Hyperammonamie. Bruder Hollinek 1966:

Reynolds EH. Chronic anti-epileptic toxicity: A review. Epilepsia 1975;16:319-352.

Reynolds EH, Trimble MR. Epilepsy & Psychiatry. Edinburgh: Churchill Livingstone, 1981:

Riblet LA, Gatewood CF, Mayol RF. Comparative Effects of trazadone and tricyclic antidepressants on uptake of selected neurotransmitters by isolated rat brain synaptosomes. Psychopharmacology 1979;63:99-101.

Richardson JW, Zaleski WA. Naloxone and self-mutilation. Biol Psychol 1983;18(1):99-101.

Richardson MA, Haugland G, Pass R, Craig TJ. The prevalence of tardive dys-kinesia in a mentally retarded population. Psychopharmacol Bull 1986;22:243-246.

Richelson E. Tricyclic antidepressants and neurotransmitter receptors. Psychiatry Ann 1979;9(4):16-31.

Richmond J, Eddy E. Rumination: a psychosomatic syndrome. Psych Res Rep 1957;8:1-11.

Rickels K, Schweitzer EE. Current pharmacotherapy of anxiety disorders.In: Meltzer HY, ed. Psychopharmacology: the third generation of progress. New York: Raven Press, 1987:1193-1203.

Riddle MA, Hardin MT, King R, Scahill L, Woolston JL. Fluoxetine treatment of children and adolescents with Tourette's and obsessive compulsive disorders: preliminary clinical experience. J Am Acad Child Adol Psychiatry 1990;29(1):45-48.

Rifkin A, Quitkin F, Klein DF. Akinesia: a poorly recognized drug-induced extrapyramidal behavioral disorder. Arch Gen Psychiatry 1975;32:672-674.

Rigler J. Uber die Folgen der Verletzungen auf Eisenbahnen, insbesondere der Verletzungen des Ruckenmarks. Berlin: G. Reimer, 1879.

Rigter H, Van Riezen H. Hormones and Memory.In: Lipton MA, Dimascib A, Killiam KF, eds. Psychopharmacology: a generation of progress. New York: Raven Press, 1978:677-689.

Rimel RA, Giordani B, Barth JT, Boll TJ, Jane JA. Disability caused by minor head injury. Neurosurgery 1981; 9:221-228.

Rimel RW, Giordani B, Barth JT, Jane JA. Moderate head injury: completing the clinical spectrum of brain trauma. Neurosurgery 1982;11:344-351.

Rimland B, Callaway E, Dreyfus P. The effect of high doses of vitamin B6 on autistic children: a double-blind crossover study. Am J Psych 1978;135:472-475.

Roberts JKA, Lishman WA. The use of the CAT head scanner in clinical psychiatry. Br J Psychiatry 1984;145:152-158.

Roberts WC. Recent Studies on the effects of beta blockers on blood lipid levels. Am Heart J 1989;117(3):709-714.

Robinson DS, Nies A, Ravaris CL, et al. Clinical pharmacology of phenelzine. Arch Gen Psychiatry 1978;35:629-635.

Robinson K, Wolfsberg E, Jones KL. Brachmann-de Lange syndrome: evidence for autosomal dominant inheritance. Am J Med Genet 1985;22:109-115.

Robinson RG, Szetela B. Mood change following left hemispheric brain Injury. Ann Neurol 1981; 9:447-453.

Robinson RG, Starr LB, Price TR. A two year longitudinal study of mood disorders following stroke: prevalence and duration at six months follow-up. Br J Psychiatry 1984;144:256-262.

Robinson RG, Starr LB, Kubos KL, Price TR. A two-year longitudinal study of post-stroke mood disorders: findings during the intitial evaluation. Stroke 1983b;14:736-741.

Robinson RG, Kubos KL, Starr LB, Rao K, Price TR. Mood changes in stroke patients: relationship to lesion location. Compr Psychiatry 1983a;24:555-566.

Rodenheffer RJ, Rommer JA, Wigley F, et al. Controlled double-blind trial of

Nifedipine in the treatment of Raynaud's phenomenon. N Engl J Med 1983;308(15):880-884.

Rodin EA. Carbamazepine (tegretol).In: Brown TR, Feldman RG, eds. Epilepsy diagnosis and management. Boston: Little Brown, 1983:203-214.

Rogers MP, Gittes RF, Dawson M, Reich P. Giggle Incontinence. JAMA 1982;247:1446-1448.

Rogers RC, Simensen RJ. Fragile X syndrome: a common etiology of mental retardation. Am J Ment Defic 1987;91:445-449.

Romney DM, Angus WR. A brief review of the effects of diazepam on memory. Psychopharmacol Bull 1984;20(2):313-316.

Rosebush P, Stewart T. A prospective analysis of 24 episodes of neuroleptic malignant syndrome. Am J Psychiatry 1989;146(6):717-725.

Rosen GD, Finklestein S, Stroll AL. Neurochemical asymmetries in the albino rat's cortex, striatum, and nucleus accumbens. Life Sci 1984;34:1143-1148.

Rosenbaum AH, Barry MJ. Positive therapeutic response to lithium in hypomania secondary to organic brain syndrome. Am J Psychiatry 1975;132(10):1072-1073.

Rosenblatt DS, Duschenes EA, Hellstrom FV, et al. Folic acid blinded trial in identical twins with fragile X syndrome. Am J Hum Genet 1985;37:543-552.

Ross D. The aprosodias functional-anatomic organization of the affective components of language in the right hemisphere. Arch Neurol 1981;38:561-569.

Ross ED, Rush AJ. Diagnosis and neuroanatomical Correlates of Depression in Brain-Damaged Patients. Arch Gen Psychiatry 1981;38:1344-1354.

Ross ED, Stewart RM. Akinetic mutism from hypothalmic damage: successful treatment with dopamine agonists. Neurology 1981;31:1435-1439.

Ross ED, Stewart RS. Pathological display of affect in patients with depression and right frontal brain damage. J Nerv Mental Dis 1987;175(3):165-172.

Ross RT. Behavioral correlates of levels of intelligence. Am J Ment Defic 1972;76:545-549.

Roupas van Lancker D, Kreiman J, Cummings J. Voice Perception deficits neuroanatomical correlates of phonagnosia. J Clin Exp Neuropsychol 1989;11(5):665.

Roy-Byrne PP, Joffe RT, Uhde TW, Post RW. Approaches to the evaluation and treatment of rapid-cycling affective illness. Br J Psychiatry 1984;145:543-550.

Rubin RT. Prolactin and Schizophrenia.In: Meltzer HY, ed. Psychopharmacology the: third generation of progress. New York: Raven Press, 1987:803-808.

Rudman D, Williams PJ. Megadose vitamins: use and misuse. N Engl J Med 1983;309(8):488-490.

Rudzik AD, Mennear JH. The mechanism of action of anticonvulsants. I: Diphenyl-hydantoin. Life Sci 1965;4:2373-2382.

Rumbaugh CL, Fang HCH. The effects of drug abuse on the brain. Resid Staff Physician 1978;April:47-55.

Rutherford WH, Merrett JD, McDonald JR. Symptoms at one year following concussion from minor head injuries.Injury 1979;10:225-230.

Rutter M, Graham P, Yule W. A Neuropsychiatric Study in Childhood. London: Heinemann, 1970:

Ryan JJ, Souheaver GT. The Role of sleep in Electrosleep Therapy for Anxiety. Dis Nerv Syst 1977;38:515.

Sadjapour K, Levine MJ, Bertram KW. Effects of Sinemet following left occipital lobectomy in early childhood. 1984 (unpublished).

Salazar AM, Jabbari B, Vance SC, Grafman J, Amin D, Dillon JD. Epilepsy after penetrating head injury. I. Clinical correlates: a report of the Vietnam Head Injury Study. Neurology 1985;35:1406-1414.

Salazar-Grueso EF, Rosenberg RS, Roos RP. Sleep apnea in livopontocerebellar degeneration: treatment with trazadone. Ann Neurol 1988;23(4):399-401.

Sale I, Kristall H. Schizophrenia following withdrawal from chronic phenothiazine administration: a case report. Aust & N Z J Psychiatry 1978;12:73-75.

Sallustro F, Atwell C. Body rocking, head banging and head rolling in normal children. J Pediatr 1978;93:704-708.

Saltz BL, Kane JM, Woerner MG, et al. Prospective study of tardive dyskinesia in the elderly. Psychopharmacol Bull 1989;25(1):52-56.

Sandman CA, Datta PC, Barron J, Hochler FK, Williams C, Swanson JM. Naloxone attenuates self-abusive behavior in developmentally disabled clients. App Res Ment Res 1983;4:5-11.

Sands S, Ratey J. The concept of noise. Psychiatry 1986;49:290-297.

Sandson TA, Lilly RB, Sodkol M. Kluver-Bucy syndrome associated with delayed post-anoxic leucoencephalopathy following carbon monoxide poisoning. J Neurol Neurosurg Psychiatry 1988; 51:156-157.

Sandyk R. Naloxone abolishes self-injury in a mentally retarded Child. Ann Neurol 1985;17(5):520.

Santamaria J, Tolosa E, Valles A. Parkinson's disease with depression: a possible subgroup of idiopathic parkinsonism. Neurology 1986;36:1130-1133.

Saran AS. Depression after minor closed head injury: Role of dexamethasone suppression test and antidepressants. J Clin Psychiatry 1985;46(8):335-338.

Sartori M, Pratt CM, Young JB. Torsade de Pointe Malignant cardiac arrhythmia induced by amantadine poisoning. Am J Med 1984;77:388-391.

Sawynok J. Monoamines as mediators of the antinociceptive effect of bacloflen. Naunym-Schmiedebergs Arch Pharmacol 1983;323:54-57.

Schacter S. The psychology of affiliation. Stanford: Stanford University Press, 1959.

Schain RJ, Ward JW, Guthrie D. Carbamazepine as an anticonvulsant in children. Neurology 1977;63:476-480.

Schakow D. Segmental set: a theory of the formal psychological deficit in schizophrenia. Arch Gen Psychiatry 1962;6:1-17.

Schauf CL, Davis FA, Marder J. Effects of carbamazepine on the ionic conductance of myxicola giant axons. J Pharmacol Exp Ther 1974;189:538-543.

Schaumberg H, Kaplan J, Windebank A, et al. Sensory neuropathy from pyridoxine abuse. N Engl J Med 1983;309:445-448.

Schaut J, Schnoll SH. Four cases of clonidine abuse. Am J Psychiatry 1983;140(12):1625.

Schenk L, Bear D. Multiple personality and related dissociative phenomena in patients with temporal lobe epilepsy. Am J Psychiatry 1981;138:10:1311-1316.

Scher M, Krieger J, Juergens S. Trazadone and Priapism. Am J Psychiatry 1983;140:1362-1363.

Scheyer RD, Haas DC. Pyridoxine in carpal tunnel syndrome. Lancet 1985;2:42-42.

Schmidt D. Adverse effects of antiepileptic Drugs. New York: Raven Press, 1982:

Schmidt D. Prognosis of chronic epilepsy with complex partial seizures. J Neurol Neurosurg Psychiatry 1984;47:1274-1278.

Schmitt H. Action de l'imipramine, de l'amitriptyline et de leurs derives monodemethyles sur les post decharges provoquers par l'excitation de certaines structures rhimencephaliques chez la lapin. Therapie 1966;21:675-675.

Schmitt R, Capo T, Boyd E. Cranial electrotherapy stimulation as a treatment for anxiety in chemically dependent persons. Alcohol Clin Exp Res 1986;10(2):158-160.

Schneiden H, Cox B. A comparison betwen amantadine and bromocriptine using the stereotyped behavior response test (SBR) in the rat. Eur J Pharmacol 1976;39:133-141.

Schneider LH, Murphy RB, Coons EE. Lateralization of striatal dopamine (D2) receptors in normal rats. Neurosci Lett 1982;33:281-284.

Schniedev H, Cox B. A comparison between amantadine and bromocriptine using the stereotyped behavior response test (SBR) in the rat. Eur J Pharmacol 1976;39:133-141.

Schonecker M. Ein eigentomliches Syndrom in oralen Bereich bei Megaphenapplikation. Nervenarzt 1957;28(35):

Schou M. Lithium in the treatment of psychiatric and non-psychiatric disorders. Arch Gen Psychiatry 1979;36(8):856-859.

Schreier HA. Use of propranolol in the treatment of post-encephalitic psychosis. Am J Psychiatry 1979;136:840-841.

Schroeder SR. Rumination.In: Treatments of psychiatric disorders. Washington, DC: American Psychiatric Association, 1989c:53-55.

Schroeder SR. Rectal digging, feces smearing, and coprophagy.In: Treatments of psychiatric disorders. Washington, DC: American Psychiatric Association, 1989b:43-44.

Schroeder SR. Abnormal Stereotyped Behaviors.In: American Psychiatric Association, ed. Treatments Of psychiatric disorders. Washington, D.C.: American Psychiatric Association, 1989a:44-49.

Schroeder SR, Mulick JA, Rojahn J. The definition, taxonomy, epidemiology, and ecology of self-injurious Behavior. J Autism Devord Dis 1980;10(4):417-432.

Schuckit MA. Alcohol and drug interactions with antianxiety medications. Am J Med 1987;82:27-33.

Schuster CR, Lewis M, Seiden LS. Fenfluramine: Neurotoxicity. Psychopharmacol Bull 1985;22(1):148-151.

Schwab RS, England AC, Poskanzer DC, Young RR. Amantadine in the Treatment of Parkinson's disease. JAMA 1969;208:1168-1170.

Schwab RS, Poskanzer DC, England AC, Young RR. Amantadine in Parkinson's disease. Review of more than two years experience. JAMA 1972;222:792-795.

Schwartz L, Swaminathan S. Maprotiline hydrochloride and convulsions: a case report. Am J Psychiat 1982;139:244-243.

Schwartz RD, McGee R, Keller KJ. Nicotinic cholinergic receptors labelled by (3H) acetylcholine in rat brain. Mol Pharmacol 1982;22:56-62.

Scoville WB, Milner B. Loss of Recent Memory After Bilateral Hippocampal Lesions. J Neurol Neurosurg Psychiatry 1957;20:11-21.

Scriver CR, Clow CL. Phenylketonuria: epitome of human biochemical genetics. N Engl J Med 1980;303(23):1336-1342.

Seashore MR, Friedman E, Novelly RA, Bapat V. Loss of Intellectual function in children with phenylketonuria after relaxation of dietary phenylalanine restriction. Pediatrics 1985;75(2):226-232.

Seegmiller JE, Rosenbloom FM, Kelly WN. Enzyme defect associated with a sex-linked human neurological disorder and excessive purine synthesis. Science 1967;155:1682-1684.

Seeman P. Brain Dopamine Receptors. Psych Rev 1981; 32(3):229-313.

Seidel WF, Cohen SA, Bliwise NG, et al. Buspirone: an anxiolytic without sedative effect. Psychopharmacol 1985;87:371-373.

Serby M, Resnick R, Jordan B, et al. Naltrexone and Alzheimer's disease. Progress in Neuropsychology and Biol Psychiatry 1986;10:587-590.

Shalat SL, Seltzer B, Pidcock C, Baker EL. Risk factors for Alzheimer's disease: a case-control study. Neurology 1987;37:1630-1633.

Sharpe PC, Berland WL. Mental Confusion and H-Receptor Blockers. Lancet 1980;2:924.

Shear CS, Nyhan WL, Kirman BH, Stern J. Self-mutilative behavior as a feature of the de Lange syndrome. J Pediatr 1971;78(3):506-509.

Sheard MH. Behavioral Effects of p-chlorophenylalanine: inhibition By Lithium. Behav Biol 1970a;5:71-73.

Sheard MH. Effect of lithium on footshock aggression in rats. Nature 1970b;228(b):284-285.

Sheard MH. Effect in the treatment of aggression. J Nerv Ment Disord 1975;160(2):108-118.

Sheppard GP. High-dose propranolol in schizophrenia. Br J Psychiatry 1979;134:470-476.

Shevitz SA, Jameison RC, Petre WM. Compulsive water drinking treated with high dose propanalol. J Nerv Mental Dis 1980;168:246-248.

Shewnon DA, Erwin RJ. Transient impairment of visual perception induced by single interictal occipital Spikes. J Clin Exp Neuropsychol 1989; 11(5):675.

Shields WD, Lake JL, Chugani HT. Amantadine in the treatment of refractory epilepsy: an open trial in ten patients. Neurology 1985;35:579-581.

Shopsin B. Bupropion's prophylactic efficacy in bipolar affective illness. J Clin Psychiatry 1983;44(5): Sec 2:163-169.

Shopsin B, Hirsch J, Gershon S. Visual hallucinations and propranolol. Biol Psychol 1975;10:105-107.

Shukla S, Godwin CD, Long LEB, Miller MG. Lithium-carbamazepine neurotoxicity and risk factors. Am J Psychiatry 1984;141:1604-1606.

Siever LJ. The effect of amantadine on prolactin levels and galactorrhea on neuroleptic-treated patients. J Clin Psychopharmacol 1981;1:2-7.

Silberman EK, Post RM, Nurnberger J, Theodore W, Boulenger J-P. Transient sensory, cognitive and affective phenomena in affective illness: a comparison with complex partial epilepsy. Br J Psychiatry 1985;146:81-89.

Sillanpaa M. Carbamazepine. Pharmacology and clinical uses. Acta Neurol Scand 1981;64(88):1-202.

Silver JM, Yudofsky SC. Documentation of aggression in the assessment of the violent Patient. Psychiatr Ann 1987;176: 375-384.

Silverstein FS, Faye , Johnston MV, Hutchinson RJ, Edwards NL. Lesch-Nyhan Syndrome: CSF neurotransmitter abnormalities. Neurology 1985;6:907-911.

Silverstein FS, Parrish MA, Johnston MV. Adverse behavioral reactions in children treated with carbamazepine. J Pediatr 1982;101:785-787.

Silverstone PH. Ranitidine and confusion. Lancet 1984;1(8385):1071.

Simeon JG, Volauka J, Trites R, et al. Electroencephalographic correlates in children with learning disorders treated with piracetam. Psychopharmacol Bull 1983;19:716-720.

Simpson GM. Neurotoxicity of major tranquilizers.In: Roizin L, Shiroki H, Grcevic N, eds. Neurotoxicology. New York: Raven Press, 1977:3.

Singh I. Prolonged oculogyric Crisis on Addition of nifedipine to neuroleptic medication regime. Br J Psychiatry 1987;150:127-128.

Singh MM, Kay SR. Dysphoric response to neuroleptic treatment in schizophrenia: its relationship to autonomic arousal and prognosis. Biol Psychiatry 1979;14(2):277-294.

Singh NN. Current trends in the treatment of self-injurious behavior. Adv in Pediatr 1981;28:377-440.

Singh NN, Bakker LW. Suppression of pica By overcorrection and physical restraint: a comparative analysis. J Autism Dev Dis 1984;14:331-341.

Singh NN, Dawson MJ. The prevalence of rumination in institutionalized mentally retarded children. 1980 (unpublished).

Singh NN, Millichamp CJ. Pharmacological treatment of self-injurious behavior in mentally retarded persons. J Autism Dev Disord 1985;15(3):257-267.

Singh S, Padi MH, Bullard H, Freeman H. Water intoxication in psychiatric patients. Br J Psychiatry 1985;146:125-131.

Sitland-Marken PA, Rickman LA, Wells BG, Mabie WC. Pharmacologic management of acute mania in pregnancy. J Clin Psychopharmacol 1989;9(2):78-87.

Skolnick P, Paul SM, Weissman BA. Preclinical pharmacology of buspirone hydrochloride. Pharmacotherapy 1984;4(6):308-314.

Slater E, Beard AW, Glithero E. The schizophrenia-like psychoses in epilepsy. Br J Psychiatry 1963; 10:93-97.

Slevin JT, Ferrara LP. Chronic valproic acid therapy and synaptic markers of amino acid neurotransmission. Neurology 1985;35(5):728-731.

Smith DF. Lithium and animal behavior. Montreal: Eden Press, 1977:1-66.

Smith DW, Jones KL. Recognizable patterns of human Malformation. Philadelphia: Saunders, 1982.

Smith JM, Baldessarini RJ. Changes in prevalence, severity, and recovery in tardive dyskinesia with Age. Arch Gen Psychiary 1980; 37:1368-1373.

Smith NJ, Espir ML, Baylis PH. Raised plasma arginine vasopressin concentration in carbamazepine-induced water intoxication. Br Med J 1977;2:804.

Smith RB, Day E. The effects of cerebral electrotherapy on short-term impairment in alcoholic patients.Int J Addict 1977;12:575.

Smith RC, Vroutis G, Johnson R, et al. Comparison of therapeutic response to long-term treatment with lecithin versus piracetam plus lecithin in patients with Alzheimer's disease. Psychopharmacol Bull 1989;20:542-545.

Smith WL, The effects of diphenylhydantoin on cognitive functions in man.In: . :, 1972: Smith, WL-(ed) Drugs, Development, and Cerebral Function, Springfield, Thomas Books

Smith WO, Clark ML. Self-induced water intoxication in schizophrenic patients. Am J Psychiatry 1980;137:1055-1060.

Snead OC, Hosey LC. Exacerbation of seizures in children by carbamazepine. N Engl J Med 1985;313:916-921.

Snyder SH. Opiate receptors in the brain. N Engl J Med 1977;296:266-271.

Snyder SH, Reynolds IJ. Calcium-antagonist drugs: receptor interactions that clarify therapeutic effects. N Engl J Med 1985;313(16):995-1001.

Solomon S, Hotchkiss E, Saravay SM, et al. Impairment of memory function by antihypertensive medication. Arch Gen Psychiatry 1983;40:1109-1112.

Sommerbeck KW, Theilgaard A, Rasmussen KE, Lohren V, Gram L, Wulff K. Valproate sodium: evaluation of so-called psychotropic effect. A controlled study. Epilepsia 1977;18:159-167.

Somni RW, Crismon ML, Bowden CL. Fluoxetine: a serotonin-specific, second generation antidepressant. Pharmacotherapy 1987;7(1):1-15.

Sonsalla PK, Golbe LI. Deprenyl as prophylaxis against Parkinson's disease. Clin Neuropharmacol 1988;11(6):500-511.

Sorgi PJ, Ratey JJ, Polakoff S. B-Adrenergic blockers for the control of aggressive behaviors in patients with chronic schizophrenia. Am J Psychiatry 1986;143:775-776.

Sovner R. Linking factors in the use of DSM III criteria with mentally Ill Retarded Persons. Psychopharmacology 1986; 22:1055-1059.

Sovner R. The treatment of typical and atypical bipolar disorder in mentally retarded persons with a valproic acid derivative, divalproex sodium. J Clin Psychopharmacol 1989;(In Press)

Sovner R, Hurley A. The management of chronic behavior disorders in mentally retarded adults with lithium carbonate. J Nerv Mental Dis 1981;169:191-195.

Sovner R, Hurley, AD. Do the mentally retarded suffer from affective illness? Arch Gen Psychiatry 1983;40:61-67.

Sprague RL, Baxley GB. Drugs used in the management of behavior in mental retardation.In: Wortis J, ed. Mental retardation and developmental disabilities. New York: Brunner/Mazel, 1978.

Sprague R, Werry J. Methodology of sychopharmacological studies With the retarded. In: Ellis N, ed. International review of research in mental retardation. New York: Academic Press, 1971:148-219.

Stabler SP, Marcell PD, Podell ER, Allen RH. Quantitation of total homocysteine, total cysteine, and methionine in normal serum and urine using capillary gas chromatography-mass spectrometry. Anal Biochem 1987;162:185-196.

Stahl SM. Akathisia and tardive dyskinesia: changing concepts. Arch Gen Psychiatry 1985;42:915-917.

Stahl SM. Basal ganglia neuropharmacology and obsessive-compulsive disorder: the obsessive-compulsive disorder hypothesis of basal ganglia dysfunction. Psychopharmacol Bull 1988;24(3):370-374.

Stahl SM, Berger PA. Bromocriptine, physosstigmine and neurotransmitter mechanisms in the dystonias. Neurology 1982;32:889-892.

Stahl SM, Davis KL, Berger PA. The neuropharmacology of tardive dyskinesia, spontaneous dyskinesia, and other ystonias. J Clin Psychopharmacol 1982;2(9):321-328.

Stapleton JM, Lind MD, Merriman VJ, Reid LD. Naloxone inhibits diazepam-induced feeding in rats. Life Sci 1979;24:2421-2425.

Starkstein SE, Boston JD, Robinson RG. Mechanisms of mania after brain injury: 12 case reports and a review of the literature. J Nerv Mental Dis 1988a;176:87-100.

Starkstein SE, Robinson RG, Price TR. Comparison of patients with and without poststroke major depression matched for size and location of lesion. Arch Gen Psychiatry 1988c; 45:247-252.

Starkstein SE, Robinson RG, Berthier ML, Parikh RM, Price TR. Differential Mood Changes Following Basal Ganglia vs Thalamic Lesions. Arch Neurol 1988b; 45:725-730.

Starkstein SE, Berthier ML, Lylyk PL, Casasco A, Robinson RG, Leiguarda R. Emotional behavior after a Wada test in a patient with secondary mania. J Neuropsychiatry 1989;1(4):408.

Straughan JL, Conradie EA. Buspirone - Frontrunner of a New Genre of Anxiolytics. S Afr Med J 1988; 75:441-444.

Stenson RL, Donlon PT, Meyer JE. Comparison of benztropine mesylate and amantadine HC1 in neuroleptic-induced extrapyramidal symptoms. Compr Psychiatry 1976; 17:763-768.

Stern WC, Harto-Truax N, van Wyck Fleet J, Miller L. Clinical profile of the novel antidepressant bupropion. In: Typical and Atypical Antidepressants: Clinical Practice, Costa E, Racagni G, eds. New York: Raven Press, 1982.

Stevens J. Striatal function and schizophrenias. In: Cools AR, Lohman AHM, van den Bercken JHL, eds. Psychobiology and the striatum. Amsterdam:North-Holland, 1977:173-194.

Stevens JR. Interictal Clinical Manifestations of Complex Partial Seizures. Advances in Neurology 1975; 11:85-112.

Stevens JR, Livermore A. Kindling of the mesolimbic dopamine system: animal model of psychosis. Neurology 1978;28:36-46.

Stevko RM, Balsley M, Segar EW. Primary polydipsia, compulsive water drinking. J Pediatr 1968; 73:845.

Stewart DJ, Gelston A, Hakim A. Effect of Prophylactic Administration of Nimodipine in Patients with Migraine. Headache 1988; 28:260-262.

Stewart RM, Growdon JH, Cancian D. Myoclonus After 5-Hydroxytryptophan in Rats with Lesions of Indoleamine Neurons in the Central Nervous System. Neurology 1976; 26:690-692.

Stockmeier CA, Martino AM, Kellar KJ. A Strong Influence of Serotonin Axons on B-Adrenergic Receptors in Rat Brain. Science 1985; 230:323-326.

Stone TW. Evidence for a non-dopaminergic action of amantadine. Neuroscience Letter 1977; 4:343-346.

Stores G, Hart J, Piran N. Inattentiveness in school children with epilepsy. Epilepsia 1978;19:169-175.

Strahan A, Rosenthal J, Kaswan M, Winston A. Three case Reports of acute Paroxysmal Excitement Associated With Alprazolam Treatment. Am J Psychiatry 1985;142(7):859.

Strang RR. The symptom of restless legs. Med J Aust 1967;24:1211-1213.

Strawn SK, Pederson CA, Evans DL. Alcohol precipitation of maprotiline-associated seizures (letter). South Med J 1988;81:1205-1206.

Strober M, Carlson G. Bipolar illness in adolescents with major depression. Arch Gen Psychiatry 1982;39:549-555.

Stromberg C, Suokas A, Seppala T. Interaction of alcohol with maprotiline or nomifensine: echocardiographic and psychometric effects. Eur J Clin Pharmacol 1988;35:593-599.

Strub RL, Black FW. The mental status examination in neurology. Philadelphia: F.A. Davis, 1985.

Struve FA, Willner WA. Cognitive dysfunction and tardive dyskinesia. Br J Psychiatry 1983;143:597-600.

Stuppaeck C, Barnas C, Miller C, Schwitzer J, Fleishhacker WW. Carbamazepine in the prophylaxis of mood disorders. J Clin Psychopharmacol 1990;10:39-42.

Sturzenegger MH, Meienberg O. Basilar artery migraine: a follow-up study of 82 cases. Headache 1985;25:408-415.

Summers WK, Majovsky LV, Marsh GM, et al. Oral tetrahydroaminoacridine in long-term treatment of senile dementia, Alzheimer type. N Engl J Med 1986;315(20):1241-1287.

Svensson TH. Feedback inhibition of brain noradrenaline neurons By tricyclic antidepressants: L-receptor mediation. Science 1978;202(8):1089-1091.

Swedo SE, Rapoport JL, Cheslow DL, et al. High Prevalence of obsessive-compulsive symptoms in patients with sydenham's chorea. Am J Psychiatry 1989;146:246-249.

Symons IE, Emson PC, Farman JV. Endogenous opioid poisoning. Br Med J 1982;284(6113):469-470.

Szechtman H, Nahmias C, Garnett ES, et al. Effect of neuroleptics on altered cerebral glucose Metabolism in schizophrenia. Arch Gen Psychiatry 1988;45(6):523-532.

Takezakl H, Hanaoka M. The use of carbamazepine in the control of manic-depressive psychosis and other manic depressive states. Seishin Igaku 1971;13:173-183.

Takrani LB, Cronin O. Kleine-Levin syndrome in a female patient. Can Psychiatr Assoc J 1976;21:315.

Tariot PN, Cohen RM, Sunderland T, L-deprenyl in Alzheimer's disease. Arch Gen Psychiatry 1987;44:427-433.

Tariot PN, Sunderland T, Weingarner H, et al. Low- and high-dose naloxone in dementia of the Alzheimer's type. Psychopharmacol Bull 1985;21:680-682.

Tarsy D, Baldessarini RJ. The pathophysiologic basis of tardive dyskinesia. Biol Psychiatry 1977;12(3):431-450.

Tarter RE. Intellectual and adaptive functioning in Epilepsy. Dis Nerv Syst 1972; 33:763-770.

Task Force on Tardive Dyskinesia, American Psychiatric Association. Task Force Report: Tardive Dyskinesia. Washington, D.C.: American Psychiatric Press, 1990.

Tate JL. Extrapyramidal symptoms in a patient taking haloperidol and fluoxetine. Am J Psychiatry 1989;146:399-400.

Taylor AE, Saint-Cyr JA, Lang AE, Kenny FT. Parkinson's disease and depression: a critical re-evaluation. Brain 1986;109:279-292.

Taylor DC. Factors influencing the occurrence of schizophrenia-like psychosis in patients with temporal lobe epilepsy. Psychol Med 1975;5:249-254.

Taylor DP, Hyslop DK, Riblet LA. Trazdone, a new nontricyclic antidepressant without anticholinergic Activity. Biochem Pharmacol 1989;29(15):2149-2150.

Taylor LP, Posner JB. Phenobarbital rheumatism in patients with brain tumor. Ann Neurol 1989;25:92-94.

Taylor MA, Abrams R. Catatonia prevalence and importance in the manic phase of manic depressive illness. Arch Gen Psychiatry 1977;34:1223-1225.

Teicher MH, Glod C, Cole JO. Emergence of intense suicidal preoccupation during fluoxetine treatment. Am J Psychiatry 1990; 147:207-210.

Tennant FS, Wild J. Naltrexone treatment for postconcussional syndrome. Am J Psychiatry 1987;144:813-814.

Terzian H, Dalle Ore GD. Syndrome of Kluver and Bucy: reproduced in man by bilateral removal of the temporal lobes. Neurology 1955;5(6):373-380.

Tetrud JW, Langston JW. The effect of deprenyl (selegiline) on the natural history of parkinson's disease. Science 1989;245:519-522.

Thacore VR, Ahmed M, Oswald I. The electroencephalography in a case of periodic hypersomnia. Electroencephalogr Clin Neurophysiol 1969;27:605-606.

Thase ME. Reversible dementia in down's syndrome. J Ment Defic Res 1982; 26:111-113.

Thase ME, Tigner R, Smeltzer DJ, Liss L. Age-related neuropsychological deficits in Down's syndrome. Biol Psychol 1984;19(4):571-585.

Theobald W, Kunz HA. Zur pharmakologic des antiepileptieums 5-carbamul-5H-ditenzo(b,f)azepin. Arzneim Forsch 1963;13:122-125.

Thomas P, McGuire R. Orofacial dyskinesia, cognitive function and medication. Br J Psychiatry 1986;149:216-220.

Thomas TH, Ball SG, Wales JK, Lee MR. Effect of carbamazepine on plasma and urinary levels of 8-arginine vasopressin (AVP). Clin Sci Mol Med 1977;53:10.

Thompson C, Obrecht R, Arendt FJ, Checkley SA. Neuroendocrine rhythms in a patient with Kleine-Levin syndrome. Br J Psychiatry 1985;147:440-443.

Thompson PJ, Trimble MR. Sodium valproate and cognitive functioning in normal volunteers. Br J Clin Pharmacol 1981;12:819-824.

Thompson R, Huppert F, Trimble M. Anticonvulsant drugs, cognitive function and memory. Acta Neurol Scand 1980;80:75-81.

Thompson TT. Prevention and early intervention with mentally retarded children with emotional and behavioral problems. 1985; (unpublished)

Thomsen IV. Late outcome of very severe blunt head trauma: a 10-15 year second follow-up. J Neurol Neurosurg Psychiatry 1984;47:260-268.

Thomsen IV. Late psychosocial outcome in severe blunt head trauma. Brain Injury 1987;1:131-143.

Thurston JH, Thurston DL, Hixon BB, Keller AJ. Prognosis in childhood epilepsy; additional follow-up of 148 children 15 to 23 years after withdrawal of anticonvulsant therapy. N Engl J Med 1982;306:831-836.

Tinklenberg JR, Taylor JL. Assessments of drug effects on human memory functions. In: Squires LR, Butters N, eds. Neuropsychology of memory. New York: Guilford Press, 1984:213-223.

Tinklenberg JR, Pigache R, Berger PA, et al. Desglycinamide-9-arginine-8-vasopressin in cognitively impaired patients. Psychopharmacol Bull 1982;18:202-204.

Titeler M. In: Dekker M, ed. Multiple dopamine receptors. New York: Marcel Dekker, 1983:38-55.

Tizard B. Observations of overactive imbecile children in controlled and uncontrolled Environments. Am J Ment Defic 1968;72:548-553.

Tkacz C, Hawkins DR. A preventive measure for tardive dyskinesia. J Orthomol Psychiatry 1981;10(2):119-123.

Toone BK. The psychoses of epilepsy and the functional psychoses. Br J Psychiatry 1982;141:256-261.

Townsend JJ, Baringer JR, Wolinsky JS, Progressive rubella panencephalitis. N Engl J Med 1975;292(19):990.

Tramontana MG, Sherrets SD. Brain impairment in child psychiatric disorders: correspondencies between neuropsychological and CT scan results. J Am Acad Child Psychiatry 1985;24(5):590-596.

Treffert DA. Marijuana use in schizophrenia: a clear hazard. Am J Psychiatry 1978; 135:1213-1217.

Trevathan E, Cascino G. Partial epilepsy presenting as focal paroxysmal pain. Neurology 1988;38:329-330.

Trimble MR. Non-monoamine oxidase inhibitors and epilepsy. Epilepsia 1978; 19:241-250.

Trimble MR. Anticonvulsant drugs, behaviour and cognitive abilities. Curr Dev in Psychopharmacol 1981; 6:65-91.

Trimble MR. The psychopharmacology of epilepsy. Chichester: Wiley, 1985.

Trimble MR, Cummings JL. Neuropsychiatric disturbances following brainstem lesions. Br J Psychiatry 1981;138:56-59.

Trimble MR, Zarifian E. Psychopharmacology of the Limbic System. Oxford: Oxford University Press, 1985.

Tryer P, Rutherford D, Huggerr T. Benzodiazepine withdrawal symptoms and propranolol. Lancet 1989;1:520-522.

Trzepacz PT, Murko AC, Gillespie MP. Progressive supranuclear palsy misdiagnosed as schizophrenia. J Nerv Ment Dis 1985;173:377-378.

Tsai L, Beisler JM. The development of sex differences in infantile autism. Br J Psychiatry 1983;142:373-378.

Tsai L, Tsuang MT. How can we avoid unnecessary CT scanning for psychiatric patients? J Clin Psychiatry 1981;42:452-454.

Tucker DM, Novelly RA, Walker PJ. Hyperreligiosity in temporal lobe epilepsy: redefining the relationship. J Nerv Ment Dis 1987;175 (3):181-184.

Tucker GJ, Price TR, Johnson VB, McAllister T. Phenomenology of temporal lobe dysfunction: a link to atypical psychosis - a series of cases. J Nerv Ment Dis 1986;174(6):348-356.

Turnbull DM, Howel D, Rawlins MD, Chadwick DW. Which drug for the adult epileptic patient: phenytoin or Valproate? Br Med J 1985; :815-819.

Turner G, Robinson H, Laing S, Purvis-Smith S. Preventive screening for the fragile X syndrome. N Engl J Med 1986;315(10):607-610.

Tyrer P, Rutherford D, Huggett T. Benzodiazepine withdrawal symptoms and propranolol. Lancet 1981;1:520-522.

Tyrer PJ, Lader MH. Response to propranolol and diazepam in somatic and psychic anxiety. Br Med J 1974;2:14-16.

Uhrbrand L, Faurbye A. Reversible and irreversible dyskinesia after treatment with perphenazine, chlorpromazine, reserpine, and electroconvulsive Therapy. Psychopharmacologia 1960;1:408-418.

Ungerstedt U. Adipsia and aphagia after 6-hydroxydopamine-induced degeneration of the nigro-striatal dopamine system. Acta Physiol Scand 1971;(Suppl)367:95-122.

Valenstein ES. Great and desperate cures. The rise and decline of psychosurgery and other radical treatments for mental illness. New York: Basic Books, 1986.

van der Kolk BA, Greenberg MS. The psychobiology of the trauma response: Hyperarousal, constriction and addiction to traumatic response, in psychological trauma. Washington, D.C.: American Psychiatric Press, 1987.

Van Gorp WG, Miller EN, Satz P, Visscher B. Neuropsychological performance in HIV-1 immunocompromised patients: a preliminary report. J Clin Exp Neuropsychiatry 1989;11(5):763.

Vanholder R, Lamieire N, Ringoir S. Long-term experience with the combination of clonidine and beta-adrenoceptor blocking agents in hypertension. Eur J Clin Pharmacol 1985;28:125-130.

Van Praag HM. Biogenic amines: new evidence of serotonin-deficient depressions, in depressive disorders. Stuttgart: JK Schattauer, 1978.

Van Putten T, Gelenberg AJ, Lavori PW, et al. Anticholinergic effects on memory: benztropine vs. amantadine. Psychopharmacol Bull 1987;23(1):26-29.

Van Wimersam Griedanus TJB, Jooles J, De Weid D. Hypothalamic neuropeptides and memory. Acta Neurochir 1985;75:99-105.

van Woerkom TCAM, Teelken AW, Mindenhoud JM. Difference in neurotransmitter metabolism in frontotemporal-lobe contusion and diffuse cerebral contusion. Lancet 1977;19:812-813.

Van Woert MH, Rosenbaum D, Howieson J, Bowers MB, Jr. Long-term therapy of myoclonus and other neurologic disorders with L-5-hydroxytryptophan and carbidopa. N Engl J Med 1977;296(2):70-75.

van Wyck Fleet J, Manberg PJ, Miller LL, et al. Overview of clinically significant adverse reactions to bupropion. J Clin Psychiatry 1983;44(5):191-195.

Vauhkonen K. Suicide among the male disabled with war injuries to the brain. Acta Psychiatr Neurol Scand 1959;137(Suppl):90-91.

Vecht CJ, van Woerkom TCAM, Teelken AW, Mindenhoud JM. Homovanillic acid and 5-hydroxyindoleacetic acid cerebrospinal fluid levels. Arch Neurol 1975;32:792-797.

Victor BS, Link NA, Binder RL, Bell IR. Use of clonazepam in Mania and Schizoaffective Disorders. Am J Psychiatry 1984;141:1111-1112.

Violon A, Demol J. Psychological sequelae after head trauma in adults. Acta Neurochirugica 1987;85:96-102.

Virkkunen M, De Jong J, Bartko J, Linnoila M. Psychobiological concomitants of history of suicide attempts among violent offenders and impulsive fire setters. Arch Gen Psychiatry 1989;46(7):604-606.

Volkmar FR, Nelson DS. Seizure disorders in autism. J Am Acad Child Adol Psychiatry 1990;29(1):127-129.

Voltolina EJ, Thompson SI, Tisue J. Acute organic brain syndrome with propranolol. Clin Toxicol 1971;4:357-359.

Volzke E, Doose H. Dipropylacetate in the treatment of epilepsy. Epilepsia 1973;14:185-193.

Waal HJ. Propranolol-induced depression. Br Med J 1967;2:50.

Wada JA. Pharmacologic prophylaxis in the kindling model of epilepsy. Arch Neurol 1977;34:389-395.

Wada JA, Sato M, Wake A, Green JR, Troupin AS. Prophylactic effects of phenytoin, phenobarbital and carbamazepine examined in kindled cat preparation. Arch Neurol 1976;33:426-434.

Waddington JI, Youssef HA. Late onset involuntary movements in chronic schizophrenia: age-related vulnerability to "tardive" dyskinesia independent of extent of neuroleptic medication. Ir Med J 1850;78(5):143-146.

Waddington JL. Tardive dyskinesia: a critical re-evaluation of the causal role of neuroleptics and of the dopamine receptor supersensitivity hypothesis. In: Callaghan N, Galvin R, eds. Recent research in neurology. London: Pitman, 1984.

Waddington JL, Youssef HA, Molloy AG, O'Boyle KM. Association of Intellectual Impairment, Negative Symptoms, and Aging with Tardive Dyskinesia: Clinical and Animal Studies. J Clin Psychiat 1985; 46(4):29-33.

Waid LR, Roberts J, Schneider SK. Naltrexone treatment for postconcussional syndrome. 1989; (UnPub)

Walker AE, Blumer D. The fate of World War II veterans with posttraumatic seizures. Arch Neurol 1989;46:23-26.

Walsh TL, Lavenstein B, Licamele WL, et al. Calcium Antagonists in the Treatment of Tourette's disorder. Am J Psych 1986; 143(1):1467-1468.

Walters A, Hening W, Chokroverty S, Fahn S. Opioid responsiveness in patients with neuroleptic-induced akathisia. Movement Disorders 1986; 1:119-127.

Ward AA, Kennard MA. Effect of Cholinergic Drugs on Recovery of Function Following Lesions of the Central Nervous System in Monkeys. Yale J Biol Med 1942; 15:189-228.

Warren M, Bick PA. Two case reports of trazodone-induced mania. Am J Psychiary 1984;141(9):1103.

Warren SA, Burns NR. Crib confinement as a factor in repetitive and stereotyped behavior in retardates. Ment Retard 1970;8:25-28.

Warrington SJ, Ankier SI, Turner P. Evaluation of possible interactions between ethanol and trazadone or amitryptiline. Neuropsychobiology 1986; 15 Suppl 1:31-37.

Wasterlain CG. Effects of epileptic seizures on brain ribosomes: Mechanism and relationship to cerebral energy metabolism. J Neurochem 1977; 29:707-716.

Waterman K, Purves SJ, Kosaka B, Strauss E, Wada JA. An epileptic syndrome caused by mesial frontal lobe seizure foci. Neurol 1987; 37:577-582.

Watson ST, Berger PA, Akil H, Mills MJ, Barchas JD. Effects of Naloxone on Schizophrenia: Reduction in Hallucinations in a Subpopulations of Subjects. Science 1978; 201:73-76.

Waxman SG, Geschwind N. The interictal behavioral syndrome of temporal lobe epilepsy. Arch Gen Psychiatry 1975; 32:1580-1586.

Weber MA, Drayer JIM, Laragh JH. The Effects of Clonidine and Propranolol, Separately and in Combination, on blood pressure and plasma renin activity in essential hypertension. J Clin Pharmacol 1978;233-240.

Wegner JT, Catalano F, Gibralter J, Kane JM. Schizophrenics with tardive dyskinesia. Arch Gen Psych iatry1985;42:860-865.

Weilburg JB, Mesulam MM, Weintraub S, Buonanno F, Jenike M, Stakes JW. Focal striatal abnormalities in a patient with Obsessive-Compulsive Disorder. Arch Neurol 1989;46:233-235.

Weintraub M, Evans P. Progabide: an experimental GABA-mimetic medication for epilepsy, spasticity, and movement disorders. Hosp formul 1985;20:1220.

Weischer ML. Uber die Antigressive Wirkung von Lithium. Psychopharmacologia 1969;15:245-254.

Weiss B, Santelli S. Dyskinesias evoked in monkeys by weekly administration of haloperidol. Science 1978;200:799-801.

Weiss G, Hechtman LT. Hyperactive children grown up. New York: Guilford, 1986.

Weiss GH, Salazar AM, Vance SC, Grafman JH, Jabbari B. Predicting posttraumatic epilepsy in penetrating head injury. Arch Neurol 1986;43:771-773.

Weiss MF. The treatment of insomnia through the use of electrosleep: an EEG study. J Nerv Ment Dis 1973;157:108.

Wertheimer N. The differential diagnosis of rheumatic fever in the histories of paranoid and non-paranoid schizophrenics. J Nerv Ment Dis 1957;125:637-641.

Wetzel CD, Squire LR, Janowsky DS. Methylphenidate impairs learning and memory in normal adults. Behav Neural Biol 1981; 31:413-424.

Wheatley D. Comparative effects of propanolol and chlordiazepoxide in anxiety states. Br J Psychiatry 1969;115:1411-1412.

White AJ. Cognitive impairment of acute mountain sickness and acetazolamide. Aviat Space Environ Medi 1984;July:598-602.

Whitehouse PJ, Martino AM, Wagster MV, et al. Reductions in (3H)nicotinic acetylcholine binding in Alzheimer's disease and Parkinson's disease. Neurology 1988;38:720-723.

Whyte J, Robinson KM. Pharmacological management of spasticity. In: Glenn MB, Whyte J, eds. Practical management of spasticity in children and adults. Philadelphia: Lea & Febiger (in press)

Wilcken B, Turner B. Homocystinuria: reduced folate levels during pyridoxine treatment. Arch Dis Child 1973;48:58-62.

Wilcox JA. perinatal distress and infectious disease as risk factors for catatonia. Psychopathology 1986;19:196-199.

Wilkinson DA. Examination of alcoholics by computed tomographic (CT) scans: a critical review. Alcohol Clin Exp Res 1982;6:31-45.

Williams M. Purinergic receptors and central nervous system function. In: Meltzer HY, ed. Psychopharmacology: the third generation of progress. New York: Raven Press, 1987:289-301.

Williams DT, Mehl R, Yudofsky S, Adams D, Roseman D. The effect of propranolol on uncontrolled rage outbursts in children and adolescents with organic brain dysfunction. J Am Acad Child Psychiatry 1982; 21:129-135.

Williams MJ, Harris RI, Dean BC. Controlled trial of pyridoxine in the premenstrual syndrome. J Int Med Res 1985;13(3):174-179.

Williamson PD, Spencer DD, Spencer SS, Novelly RA, Mattson RH. Complex partial seizures of frontal lobe origin. Ann Neurol 1985;18,(4):497-504.

Wilsher C, Melewski J. Effect of piracetam on dyslexics's verbal conceptualizing ability. Psychopharmacol Bull 1983;19:3-4.

Wilson GN, Dasouki M, Barr M. Further delineation of the dup(3q) Syndrome. Am J Med Gen 1985;22:117-123.

Wilson IC, Garbutt JC, Lanier CF, Moylan J, Nelson W, Prange AJ. Is there a tardive dysmentia? Schizophr Bull 1983;9(2):187-192.

Wilson JM, Young AB, Kelly WN. Hypoxanthine-guanine phosphoribosyl transferase deficiency: the molecular basis of the clinical syndromes. N Engl J Med 1983;309:900-910.

Wilson SAK. Morphinism. In: Bruce AN, ed. Neurology. Vol I, Part III. Baltimore: Williams & Wilkins, 1940:711.

Wilson WH. Reassessment of state hospital patients wiagnosed with schizophrenia. J Neuropsychiatry 1989;1(4):394.

Wing L. The handicaps of autistic children—a comparative study. J Child Psychol Psychiattry Allred Discip 1969;10:1-40.

Wing L, Gould J. Severe impairments of social interaction and associated abnormalities in children: epidemiology and classification. J Autism Dev Disord 1979;9:11-30.

Winkelman NW, Eckel JL. Brain in acute rheumatic fever; nonsupurative meningo-encephalitis rheumatica. Arch Neurol Psychiatey 1932;28:844-870.

Wise RA. Neuroleptics and operant behavior: the anhedonia hypothesis. Behav Brain Sci 1982;5:39-87.

Wolf ME, Ryan JJ, Mosnaim AD. Cognitive Functions in Tardive Dyskinesia. Psycho Med 1983;13:671-674.

Wolkowitz OM, Doran AR, Cohen MR, Cohen RM, Wise TN, Pickar D. Effect of naloxone on food consumption in obesity. N Engl J Med 1985;313(5):327.

Wolpert A, Quintos A, White L, Merlis S. Thiothixene and chlorprothixene in behavior disorders. Curr Ther Res 1968;10:566-569.

Wood PL, Nair NPV, Lal S, et al. Buspirone: a potential atypical neuroleptic. Life Sci 1983;33:269-273.

Woolf CM. Congenital cleft lip: a genetic study of 496 propositi. J Med Gene 1971;8:65-84.

Worrall EP, Moody JP, Naylor GJ. Lithium in nonmanic depressives: antiaggressive effect and red blood cell lithium values. Br J Psychiatry 1975;126:464-468.

Wright G, Galloway L, Kim J, Dalton M, Miller L, Stern W. Bupropion in the long-term treatment of cyclic mood disorders: mood-stabilizing effects. J Clin Psychiatry 1985;46(1):22-24.

Wu MJ, Ing TS, Soung LS, Daugirdas JT, Hano JE, Gandhi VC. Amantadine hydrochloride pharmacokinetics in patients with impaired renal function. Clin Nephrology 1982;17:19-23.

Wurtman RJ. Nutritional control of brain tryptophan and serotonin. In: Hayaishi O, Ishimura Y, Kido R, eds. Biochemical and medical aspects of tryptophan metabolism. Amsterdam: Elsevier North-Holland Biomedical Press, 1988:31-48.

Wurtman RJ, Fernstrom. Control of brain neuro-transmitters synthesis by precursor availability and nutritional State. Biochem Pharmacol 1976;25:1691-1696.

Wysowski DK, Baum C. Antipsychotic drug use in the United States, 1976-1985. Arch Gen Psychtry 1989;46(10):929-934.

Yagi G, Itoh H. Follow-up study of 11 patients with potentially reversible tardive dyskinesia. Am J Psychiatry 1987;144:1496-1498.

Yassa R, Iskandar H, Nastase C. Propranolol in the treatment of tardive akathisia: a report of two cases. J Clin Psychopharmacol 1988a;8:283-285.

Yassa R, Nair V, Schwartz G. Tardive dyskinesia: a two-year follow-up study. Psychosomatics 1984;25(11).

Yassa R, Iskander H, Nastase C, Camille Y. Carbamazepine and hyponatremia in patients with affective disorder. Am J Psychiatry 1988b;145:339-342.

Yassa R, Lal S, Korpassy A, Ally J. Nicotine exposure and tardive dyskinesia. Bio Psychol 1987;22:67-72.

Yeragani VK, Aleem A, Pohl R, Gershon S. Hypothesis: neuropharmacological basis of priapism. Clin Neuropharmacol 1987;10(2):93-95.

Yesavage JA, Leirer VO, Denari M, Hollister LE. Carry-over effects of marijuana intoxication on aircraft pilot performance: a preliminary report. Am J Psychiatry 1985;142:1325-1329.

Young B, Rapp RP, Norton JA, Haack D, Walsh JW. Failure of prophylactically administered phenytoin to prevent post-traumatic seizures in children. Child's Brain 1983;10:185-192.

Young RR, Delwaide PJ. Spasticity (first of two parts). N Engl J Med 1981; 304:28-29.

Yufofsky S, Williams D, Gorman J. Propranolol in the Treatment of Patients With Chronic Brain Syndrome. Am J Psych 1981; 138:218-330.

Zahn TP, Nurnberger Jr JI, Berrettini WH. Vilson's disease: psychiatric symptoms in 195 cases. Arch Gen Psychiatry 1989;46(12):1126-1136.

Zamektin A, Rapoport JL, Murphy DL, et al. Treatment of hyperactive children with monoamine oxdase inhibitors. Arch Gen Psychiatry 1985;42:962-976.

Zoghbi HY, Milstien S, Butler IJ, Cerebrospinal fluid biogenic amines and biopterin in Rett syndrome. Ann Neurol 1989;25(1):56-60.

Zohar J, Mueller EA, Insel TR, Zohar-Kadouch RC, Murphy DL. Serotonergic responsivity in obsessive-compulsive disorder. Arch Gen Psychiatry 1987;44:946.

Zola-Morgan S, Squire LR, Mishkin M. The neuroanatomy of amnesia: amygdala-hippocampus versus temporal stem. Science 1982;218:1337-1339.

Zubenko GS, Cohen BM, Lipinski JF, Jonas JM. Use of clonidine in the treatment of akathisia. Psychiatr Res 1984a; 13:253-259.

Zubenko GS, Cohen BM, Lipinski JF, Jonas JM. Clonidine in the treatment of mania and mixed bipolar disorder. Am J Psychiatry 1984b; 141(12):1617.

Index

Neuropsychiatry and Behavioral Pharmacology is concerned with the neuropsychiatric and behavioral consequences of brain injury, congenital and acquired. The clinical syndromes are described in practical terms, with special emphasis on pharmacologic management. The syndromes and their appropriate treatment are also dealt with in terms of their theoretical basis, that is, their brain-map, their anatomic and neurochemical underpinnings.

The book deals with the neuropsychiatric syndromes that may accompany traumatic brain injury, epilepsy, and mental retardation. Its range is from the common, childhood hyperactivity, for example, to the obscure, like Rheumatic Psychosis and the Kleine-Levin Syndrome. There are discussions of new treatments, like deprenyl, amantadine, buspirone, and the "serotonin cascade"; and new problems with old drugs, like tardive akathisia and the neuropathic effects of fenfluramine and "megavitamins."

Dr. Gualtieri is a consultant in neuropsychiatry to centers for brain injury patients and for developmentally handicapped individuals across the United States. A graduate of Columbia, he was for many years Research Scientist at the University of North Carolina. His clinical practice is now devoted to the patients who are described in this book.

ISBN 0-387-97314-1
ISBN 3-540-97314-1